Pediatric Emergency Medicine

Editor

PRASHANT MAHAJAN

PEDIATRIC CLINICS
OF NORTH AMERICA

www.pediatric.theclinics.com

Consulting Editor
BONITA F. STANTON

December 2018 • Volume 65 • Number 6

ELSEVIER

1600 John F. Kennedy Boulevard • Suite 1800 • Philadelphia, Pennsylvania, 19103-2899

http://www.theclinics.com

THE PEDIATRIC CLINICS OF NORTH AMERICA Volume 65, Number 6
December 2018 ISSN 0031-3955, ISBN-13: 978-0-323-64312-2

Editor: Kerry Holland
Developmental Editor: Casey Potter

The Pediatric Clinics of North America (ISSN 0031-3955) is published bimonthly by Elsevier Inc., 360 Park Avenue South, New York, NY 10010-1710. Months of issue are February, April, June, August, October, and December. Periodicals postage paid at New York, NY and additional mailing offices. Subscription prices are $216.00 per year (US individuals), $613.00 per year (US institutions), $292.00 per year (Canadian individuals), $816.00 per year (Canadian institutions), $338.00 per year (international individuals), $816.00 per year (international institutions), $100.00 per year (US students and residents), and $165.00 per year (international and Canadian residents and students). To receive students/resident rare, orders must be accompanied by name of affiliated institution, date of term, and the signature of program/residency coordinator on institution letterhead. Orders will be billed at individual rate until proof of status is received. Foreign air speed delivery is included in all *Clinics* subscription prices. All prices are subject to change without notice. **POSTMASTER:** Send address changes to *The Pediatric Clinics of North America*, Elsevier Health Sciences Division, Subscription Customer Service, 3251 Riverport Lane, Maryland Heights, MO 63043. **Customer Service: 1-800-654-2452 (US and Canada). From outside of the US and Canada: 1-314-447-8871. Fax: 1-314-447-8029. For print support, E-mail: JournalsCustomerService-usa@elsevier.com. For online support, E-mail: JournalsOnlineSupport-usa@elsevier.com.**

Reprints. For copies of 100 or more, of articles in this publication, please contact the Commercial Reprints Department, Elsevier Inc., 360 Park Avenue South, New York, NY 10010-1710. Tel.: 212-633-3874; Fax: 212-633-3820; E-mail: reprints@elsevier.com.

The Pediatric Clinics of North America is also published in Spanish by McGraw-Hill Inter-americana Editores S.A., Mexico City, Mexico; in Portuguese by Riechmann and Affonso Editores, Rua Comandante Coelho 1085, CEP 21250, Rio de Janeiro, Brazil; and in Greek by Althayia SA, Athens, Greece.

The Pediatric Clinics of North America is covered in *MEDLINE/PubMed (Index Medicus), Excerpta Medica, Current Contents, Current Contents/Clinical Medicine, Science Citation Index, ASCA, ISI/BIOMED,* and *BIOSIS.*

PROGRAM OBJECTIVE
The goal of the *Pediatric Clinics of North America* is to keep practicing physicians and residents up to date with current clinical practice in pediatrics by providing timely articles reviewing the state-of-the-art in patient care.

TARGET AUDIENCE
All practicing pediatricians, physicians and healthcare professionals who provide patient care to pediatric patients.

LEARNING OBJECTIVES
Upon completion of this activity, participants will be able to:
1. Review the application of quality improvement methodologies in the pediatric emergency department.
2. Discuss diagnostic decision making in the pediatric emergency department
3. Recognize new and evolving paradigms of acute care

ACCREDITATION
The Elsevier Office of Continuing Medical Education (EOCME) is accredited by the Accreditation Council for Continuing Medical Education (ACCME) to provide continuing medical education for physicians.

The EOCME designates this enduring material for a maximum of 15 *AMA PRA Category 1 Credit*(s)™. Physicians should claim only the credit commensurate with the extent of their participation in the activity.

All other healthcare professionals requesting continuing education credit for this enduring material will be issued a certificate of participation.

DISCLOSURE OF CONFLICTS OF INTEREST
The EOCME assesses conflict of interest with its instructors, faculty, planners, and other individuals who are in a position to control the content of CME activities. All relevant conflicts of interest that are identified are thoroughly vetted by EOCME for fair balance, scientific objectivity, and patient care recommendations. EOCME is committed to providing its learners with CME activities that promote improvements or quality in healthcare and not a specific proprietary business or a commercial interest.

The planning committee, staff, authors and editors listed below have identified no financial relationships or relationships to products or devices they or their spouse/life partner have with commercial interest related to the content of this CME activity:
Andrea Ana Almeida, MD; Lalit Bajaj, MD, MPH; Stuart Bradin, DO; Michele M. Carney, MD; James M. Chamberlain, MD; Todd P. Chang, MD, MAcM; Andrea T. Cruz, MD, MPH; Joy Ekezie, MB, BCH; Heidi R. Flori, MD; Chad Garthe, MD; Robert W. Grundmeier, MD; Andrew Nobuhide Hashikawa, MD, MS; Kerry Holland; Alison Kemp; Brandon C. Ku, MD; Matthew Thomas Lorincz, MD, PhD; Marisa C. Louie, MD; Marie M. Lozon, MD; Prashant Mahajan, MD, MPH, MBA; Rajkumar Mayakrishnan; Laura N. Medford-Davis, MD, MS; Russell Migita, MD; Raina Paul, MD; Elaine S. Pomeranz, MD; Lori Rutman, MD, MPH; Usha Sankrithi, MBBS, MPH, MD; Kathy N. Shaw, MD, MSCE; Hardeep Singh, MD, MPH; Kristen A. Smith, MD, MS; Rachel Stanley, MD, MHSA; Sarah Tomlinson, MD; Margaret Wolff, MD; George A. Woodward, MD, MBA; Hiromi Yoshida, MD, MBA.

The planning committee, staff, authors and editors listed below have identified financial relationships or relationships to products or devices they or their spouse/life partner have with commercial interest related to the content of this CME activity:
Jeffrey Schor, MD, MPH, MBA: has an employment affiliation with PM Pediatrics

UNAPPROVED/OFF-LABEL USE DISCLOSURE
The EOCME requires CME faculty to disclose to the participants:
1. When products or procedures being discussed are off-label, unlabelled, experimental, and/or investigational (not US Food and Drug Administration [FDA] approved); and
2. Any limitations on the information presented, such as data that are preliminary or that represent ongoing research, interim analyses, and/or unsupported opinions. Faculty may discuss information about pharmaceutical agents that is outside of FDA-approved labelling. This information is intended solely for CME and is not intended to promote off-label use of these medications. If you have any questions, contact the medical affairs department of the manufacturer for the most recent prescribing information.

TO ENROLL

To enroll in the *Pediatric Clinics of North America* Continuing Medical Education program, call customer service at 1-800-654-2452 or sign up online at http://www.theclinics.com/home/cme. The CME program is available to subscribers for an additional annual fee of USD 301.60.

METHOD OF PARTICIPATION

In order to claim credit, participants must complete the following:

1. Complete enrolment as indicated above.
2. Read the activity.
3. Complete the CME Test and Evaluation. Participants must achieve a score of 70% on the test. All CME Tests and Evaluations must be completed online.

CME INQUIRIES/SPECIAL NEEDS

For all CME inquiries or special needs, please contact elsevierCME@elsevier.com.

Contributors

CONSULTING EDITOR

BONITA F. STANTON, MD
Founding Dean, Hackensack Meridian School of Medicine at Seton Hall University, President, Academic Enterprise, Hackensack Meridian Health Robert C. and Laura C. Garrett Endowed Chair for the School of Medicine, Dean Professor of Pediatrics, Nutley, New Jersey, USA

EDITOR

PRASHANT MAHAJAN, MD, MPH, MBA
Professor of Emergency Medicine and Pediatrics, Vice-Chair, Department of Emergency Medicine, University of Michigan Medical School, Section Chief, Pediatric Emergency Medicine, CS Mott Children's Hospital of Michigan, Ann Arbor, Michigan, USA

AUTHORS

ANDREA ANA ALMEIDA, MD
Assistant Professor, Department of Neurology, Michigan Medicine, Co-Director of Sports Neurology, Michigan NeuroSport, Ann Arbor, Michigan, USA

LALIT BAJAJ, MD, MPH
Medical Director, Clinical Effectiveness, Children's Hospital Colorado, Professor of Pediatrics and Emergency Medicine, University of Colorado School of Medicine, Aurora, Colorado, USA

STUART BRADIN, DO
Associate Professor of Emergency Medicine and Pediatrics, Department of Emergency Medicine, University of Michigan Health System, Ann Arbor, Michigan, USA

MICHELE M. CARNEY, MD
Clinical Associate Professor, Departments of Emergency Medicine and Pediatrics, University of Michigan, Ann Arbor, Michigan, USA

JAMES M. CHAMBERLAIN, MD
Professor, Department of Pediatrics, Division of Emergency Medicine, Children's National Medical Center, George Washington University School of Medicine, Washington, DC, USA

TODD P. CHANG, MD, MAcM
Division Director for Research & Scholarship, Associate Fellowship Director, Pediatric Emergency Medicine, Associate Professor of Pediatrics (Educational Scholar), Keck School of Medicine of USC, Children's Hospital Los Angeles, Los Angeles, California, USA

ANDREA T. CRUZ, MD, MPH
Associate Professor, Department of Pediatrics, Sections of Emergency Medicine and Infectious Diseases, Baylor College of Medicine, Houston, Texas, USA

JOY EKEZIE, MB,BCh
Department of Pediatrics, Lagos University Teaching Hospital, Lagos, Nigeria

HEIDI R. FLORI, MD
Associate Professor, Pediatric Critical Care Medicine, University of Michigan School of Medicine, Ann Arbor, Michigan, USA

CHAD GARTHE, MD
Department of Emergency Medicine, The Ohio State University Medical Center, The Ohio State University, Columbus, Ohio, USA

ROBERT W. GRUNDMEIER, MD
Director of Clinical Informatics, Department of Biomedical and Health Informatics, Associate Professor of Pediatrics, Perelman School of Medicine, University of Pennsylvania, Children's Hospital of Philadelphia, Roberts Center, Philadelphia, Pennsylvania, USA

ANDREW NOBUHIDE HASHIKAWA, MD, MS
Associate Professor, Department of Emergency Medicine, Children's Emergency Services, Michigan Medicine, North Campus Research Complex, University of Michigan Injury Center, Ann Arbor, Michigan, USA

BRANDON C. KU, MD
Assistant Professor of Clinical Pediatrics, Department of Pediatrics, Perelman School of Medicine, University of Pennsylvania, Children's Hospital of Philadelphia, Philadelphia, Pennsylvania, USA

MATTHEW THOMAS LORINCZ, MD, PhD
Associate Professor, Department of Neurology, Michigan Medicine, Co-Director of Sports Neurology, Michigan NeuroSport, Ann Arbor, Michigan, USA

MARISA C. LOUIE, MD
Departments of Emergency Medicine and Pediatrics, Clinical Lecturer, University of Michigan Medical School, C.S. Mott Children's Hospital, Ann Arbor, Michigan, USA

MARIE M. LOZON, MD
Professor of Emergency Medicine and Pediatrics and Chief of Staff, Department of Emergency Medicine, University of Michigan Health System, Ann Arbor, Michigan, USA

PRASHANT MAHAJAN, MD, MPH, MBA
Professor of Emergency Medicine and Pediatrics, Vice-Chair, Department of Emergency Medicine, University of Michigan Medical School, Section Chief, Pediatric Emergency Medicine, CS Mott Children's Hospital of Michigan, Ann Arbor, Michigan, USA

LAURA N. MEDFORD-DAVIS, MD, MS
Assistant Professor, Department of Emergency Medicine, Baylor College of Medicine, Ben Taub General Hospital, Houston, Texas, USA

RUSSELL MIGITA, MD
Department of Pediatrics, Division of Emergency Medicine, Emergency Department, Seattle Children's Hospital, University of Washington School of Medicine, UW Medicine Center for Scholarship in Patient Care Quality and Safety, UWMC Health Sciences, Seattle, Washington, USA

RAINA PAUL, MD
Director of Quality Improvement, Pediatric Emergency Department, Division of Emergency Medicine, Advocate Children's Hospital, Park Ridge, Illinois, USA

ELAINE S. POMERANZ, MD
Assistant Professor, Departments of Pediatrics and Communicable Diseases, and Emergency Medicine, University of Michigan, Ann Arbor, Michigan, USA

LORI RUTMAN, MD, MPH
Department of Pediatrics, Division of Emergency Medicine, Emergency Department, Seattle Children's Hospital, University of Washington School of Medicine, Seattle, Washington, USA

USHA SANKRITHI, MBBS, MPH, MD
Medical Director, Urgent Care Services, Division of Emergency Medicine, Seattle Children's Hospital, Seattle, Washington, USA

JEFFREY SCHOR, MD, MPH, MBA
Founder and Managing Member, PM Pediatrics Management Group, Lake Success, New York, USA

KATHY N. SHAW, MD, MSCE
Professor, Department of Pediatrics, Perelman School of Medicine, University of Pennsylvania, Children's Hospital of Philadelphia, Philadelphia, Pennsylvania, USA

HARDEEP SINGH, MD, MPH
Professor, Center for Innovations in Quality, Effectiveness and Safety, Michael E. Debakey VA Medical Center, Department of Medicine, Section of Health Services Research, Baylor College of Medicine, Houston, Texas, USA

KRISTEN A. SMITH, MD, MS
Assistant Professor, Pediatric Critical Care Medicine, University of Michigan School of Medicine, Ann Arbor, Michigan, USA

RACHEL STANLEY, MD, MHSA
Division of Emergency Medicine, Associate Professor of Pediatrics, The Ohio State University, Nationwide Children's Hospital, Columbus, Ohio, USA

SARAH TOMLINSON, MD
Clinical Assistant Professor, Departments of Emergency Medicine and Pediatrics, University of Michigan, Ann Arbor, Michigan, USA

MARGARET WOLFF, MD
Clinical Associate Professor, Departments of Emergency Medicine and Pediatrics, University of Michigan, Ann Arbor, Michigan, USA

GEORGE A. WOODWARD, MD, MBA
Department of Pediatrics, Division of Emergency Medicine, Emergency Department, Seattle Children's Hospital, University of Washington School of Medicine, Seattle, Washington, USA

HIROMI YOSHIDA, MD, MBA
Department of Pediatrics, Division of Emergency Medicine, Emergency Department, Seattle Children's Hospital, University of Washington School of Medicine, Seattle, Washington, USA

Contents

Emergency medicine requires diagnosing unfamiliar patients with undifferentiated acute presentations. This requires hypothesis generation and questioning, examination, and testing. Balancing patient load, care across the severity spectrum, and frequent interruptions create time pressures that predispose humans to fast thinking or cognitive shortcuts, including cognitive biases. Diagnostic error is the failure to establish an accurate and timely explanation of the problem or communicate that to the patient, often contributing to physical, emotional, or financial harm. Methods for monitoring diagnostic error in the emergency department are needed to establish frequency and serve as a foundation for future interventions.

Several new studies have emerged in recent years that have attempted to aid emergency department providers in recognizing and treating pediatric patients with severe sepsis and septic shock. National guidelines and supporting literature are unanimous in recommendations that early recognition and timely therapeutics are necessary for improved survival and decreased morbidity. The literature is less concrete in defining how emerging advances in the field can aid in time-sensitive care of these patients. This article summarizes the recent literature as it pertains to the initial presentation of severe sepsis and septic shock in the pediatric patient within the emergency department.

In caring for critically ill children, recognition and management often begins in the pediatric emergency department. A seamless transition in care is needed to ensure appropriate care to the sickest of children. This review covers the management of critically ill children in the pediatric emergency department beyond the initial stabilization for conditions such as acute respiratory failure and pediatric acute respiratory distress syndrome, traumatic brain injury, status epilepticus, congenital heart disease, and metabolic emergencies.

use. There will be a discussion of the development of pediatric account-able care organizations and how payment mechanisms are evolving, and the challenges the pediatric ED may face in these new payment strategies.

Parents of pediatric patients seek appropriate high-quality care in a timely, cost-effective, and convenient manner. Pediatric urgent care offers a new and evolving delivery model that serves a growing demand by comple-menting services provided by the medical home and by pediatric emer-gency departments. Pediatric urgent care services are used by both nonprofit and for-profit sectors and include hospital and satellite clinics, free-standing clinics, retail-based clinics, and telemedicine services. The clinical scope is variable and there are distinct and unique operational con-siderations. Training models are evolving and further research is warranted.

Pediatric emergency medicine quality work continues to focus on the Na-tional Academies of Sciences, Engineering, and Medicine's 6 domains of quality, with a need for specific emphasis on equity and patient centered-ness. Adopting the principles of high-reliability organizations, pediatric emergency departments should become increasing transparent with benchmarking and collaboration across institutions in order to develop an infrastructure for quality and safety to improve the care of pediatric pa-tients in the emergency department.

The origins of quality improvement in health care trace back to industry. Lessons learned from the "flow production" system of the Ford Model-T assembly line in Michigan and the Toyota Production System led to direct applications of Lean and Six Sigma to improve health care systems. Emer-gency medicine is well suited as a testing and proving ground for quality improvement methodologies because of high patient volume and rapid turnover. This article reviews the history of quality improvement in health care, describes Lean principles in detail, and provides illustrative exam-ples of applications of Lean and quality improvement methodologies in the pediatric emergency department.

PEDIATRIC CLINICS OF NORTH AMERICA

THE CLINICS ARE AVAILABLE ONLINE!
Access your subscription at:
www.theclinics.com

Foreword

The Changing Role of Emergency Medicine

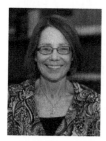

Bonita F. Stanton, MD
Consulting Editor

The role of the Emergency Department (ED) for both children and adults has changed considerably over the last several decades, with visits to the ED increasing by one-third in the decade between 1997 and 2007.[1] Beyond the critically important role of tending to children perceived to be in urgent need of health care, the pediatric ED is now used as an extension of the "safety net" for individuals without a primary care provider, including but not limited to low-income persons, an after-hours extension of private pediatricians' offices, a rapid diagnostic center, and a streamlined entryway for admissions. This substantial growth in the numbers of patients using EDs and the ever-widening scope of responsibility for the physicians serving the EDs includes all regions of the country.[1–3] Interestingly, despite this nationwide phenomenon, there is great variation by hospital in terms of the percent of patients admitted from the ED to the hospital.[4] Finally, the practice of emergency telemedicine is also rapidly expanding, along with a rapidly expanding set of telemedicine technologies to be mastered by the ED physician.[5]

This expansion of the role of the ED, for both children and adults, certainly complicates the role of the ED pediatrician and makes navigating the terrain of the ED more difficult for non-ED child health providers. In this artfully created issue, Dr Prashant Mahajan and the group of authors he has assembled address pediatric ED issues from a range of perspectives. Several articles address clinical issues of great importance for which there have been exciting advances (including true medical emergencies, such as sepsis and traumatic brain injury), diagnostic dilemmas, including child abuse and problems associated with adults presenting to a pediatric ED either because it is the closest ED or because the patient is suffering from a "pediatric" chronic disease. Other articles address broader issues, such as the need for rapid assessment and clinical decision making and what studies are needed to make such decisions in a timely fashion. There are several articles devoted to new technologies and to new health care systems

Pediatr Clin N Am 65 (2018) xv–xvi
https://doi.org/10.1016/j.pcl.2018.09.010
0031-3955/18/© 2018 Published by Elsevier Inc.

and algorithms designed to minimize the time from presentation to critical decision making (such as whether to admit or not admit the patient). Larger societal issues that pediatricians in the ED must be prepared to address are also discussed, including disaster preparedness.

In short, this is a fascinating and well-written collection of highly relevant and exciting developments in understanding how the modern pediatric ED functions. Every practicing child health provider will find the issue interesting and relevant to his or her practice. As well, child health providers working in emergency settings will find many useful updates and reviews in this issue.

Bonita F. Stanton, MD
Hackensack Meridian School of Medicine at Seton Hall University
340 Kingsland Street, Building 123
Nutley, NJ 07110, USA

E-mail address:
bonita.stanton@shu.edu

REFERENCES

1. Schur JD, Venkatesh AK. The growing role of emergency departments in hospital admissions. N Engl J Med 2012;367:391–3.
2. Tang N, Stein J, Hsia RY, et al. Trends and characteristics of US emergency department visits, 1997-2007. JAMA 2010;304:664–70.
3. Sood A, Penna FJ, Eleswarapu S, et al. Incidence, admission rates and economic burden of pediatric emergency department visits for urinary tract infection: data from the nationwide emergency department sample, 2006-2011. J Pediatr Urol 2015;11(5):246.e1-8.
4. Bourgeois FT, Monuteaux MC, Stack AM, et al. Variations in emergency department admissions rates in US children's hospitals. Pediatrics 2014;134(3):539–45.
5. Sharma R, Fleischut P, Barchi D. Telemedicine and its transformation of emergency care: a case study of one of the largest US integrated healthcare delivery systems. Int J Emerg Med 2017;10:21.

Preface

Pediatric Emergency Medicine

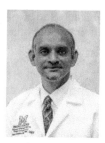

Prashant Mahajan, MD, MPH, MBA
Editor

It is an honor to be invited to guest edit this issue of the *Pediatric Clinics of North America* on *Pediatric Emergency Medicine*. Emergency medical services is an integral part of the US health care system. The Emergency Department (ED) is often the first point of contact to the health care system, and there are ~137 million annual ED visits, with ~25% of them by children. Although ~10% of all ED visits result in hospital admissions, ~50% of all hospitalizations come via the ED. The ED is the safety net for the US health care system, and as the only resource available 24/7, it is the point of contact for natural and man-made disaster management. Pediatric emergency care is constantly evolving due to macroeconomic forces, such as health care reform, opioid crisis, gun violence, and mental health emergencies. In addition, quality of care in pediatric emergencies is impacted by varying demand due to season or even time of the day and the need for rapid assessment and management of children with evolving illness all within a time-, information-, and resource-constrained setting.

Given the above background, it is easy to understand and justify the need for an entire issue of the *Pediatric Clinics of North America* dedicated to pediatric emergency care. However, it was challenging to limit the number of articles to a few topics. I have chosen to invite experts in pediatric emergency care and collaborators who are internationally recognized for their work and have created this issue of the *Pediatric Clinics of North America* of very pertinent, timely, readily applicable, and immediately useful topics that will appeal to providers across the spectrum of training and certification who manage ill and injured children.

The first article is focused on diagnostic errors. Assigning a diagnosis is an integral part of the provider-patient interaction. Diagnostic decision making is a highly cognitive and complex process that has not been studied in a robust manner. How clinicians make decisions, especially in children in the context of a chaotic ED environment where the illness is often evolving and details of the history are lacking and often the examination is performed in a hurried manner, predisposes to medical error. This

Pediatr Clin N Am 65 (2018) xvii–xix
https://doi.org/10.1016/j.pcl.2018.09.009
0031-3955/18/© 2018 Published by Elsevier Inc.

article discusses the recent National Academies of Medicine report (September 2015: Improving Diagnosis in Healthcare) and focuses on the current state-of-the-art knowledge on the pediatric ED aspect of diagnostic decision making.

The subsequent article deals with recent advances in the recognition, evaluation, management of pediatric sepsis, and the controversies surrounding recent evidence (or lack thereof) in sepsis management.

The evaluation and management of the adult patient presenting to a pediatric ED remain a challenge, and most pediatric emergency providers are not adequately trained to manage an adult who shows up at a pediatric ED. This article focuses on common conditions, differences in pathophysiology, as well as management of the "adult" who presents to the ED. In addition, the authors highlight the "adult" pediatric patient with chronic illnesses who has not yet been transitioned to an adult subspecialist.

There have been recent advances in the provision of critical care, especially the interventions in the "golden" hour in the ED before a critically ill or injured patient gets transported to the intensive care unit or a tertiary care facility. This article highlights the advances in management techniques, such as noninvasive ventilation, newer medications for resuscitation, and so forth.

Child abuse is extremely common (physical as well as sexual abuse). It is often underrecognized and in many instances completely missed. In the article on child abuse, the author focuses on the current state-of-the-art evaluation and management of a child with suspected child abuse and its medicolegal implications and discusses conditions that mimic child abuse.

Indications and interpretation of common investigations/tests in the ED is a very timely topic because a lot of investigations are added either without reason or without understanding the rationale. Indeed, many of us do need a handy reference on how to interpret the common tests that we order, when to order them, when not to order them, and the downstream implications of wrongly ordered or false positive/false negative tests in the ED. This practical article focuses on common blood and urine tests along with tips for interpretation of common radiographs and the electrocardiograph.

The article on recent advances in pediatric concussion and mild traumatic brain injury is very timely given the importance of sports as well as non-sports-related injuries that present to the ED, the need for reduction of radiation exposure, as well as diagnosing concussion in the ED setting.

The article on pediatric emergency care and impact on health care and implications for policy is pertinent because not much has been written on the policy implications as well as impact of recent changes in health care policy (Obamacare) on the pediatric ED. There is no comprehensive resource that is available for practicing providers that describes the rudiments of payment reform, explains the Emergency Medical Services for Children (EMSC) and how the EMSC Act has changed pediatric emergency care for the better over the last two decades.

There has been a recent surge in free-standing pediatric urgent care, adult urgent care, or minute clinics that manage pediatric patients, fast-tracks in the ED, and so forth; however, the impact on quality of care has not been very well documented. The article on pediatric urgent care focuses on its history, the current status of urgent care in the United States, the epidemiology of such visits, as well as impact on health care reimbursement and delivery in the United States.

The article on advances in medical education and implications for the pediatric ED workforce focuses on influence of the framework for adult learning as well as use of technologies, such as simulation and augmented reality. How has this impacted pediatric emergency medicine training, what are the applications and implications of such technologies in training the provider who manages pediatric emergencies, and what is the latest research on adult learning are some of the questions that are discussed in this article.

Safety and quality are always of interest to pediatric ED providers. The article on safety and quality focuses on current epidemiology and research on pediatric ED-based quality and safety, current benchmarks that are either developed in the pediatric ED or, more often than not, "handed down" from the adult ED settings as well as the policy implications on reimbursement, public disclosure, and transparency by institutions.

The article on optimizing resources and the impact of lean processes on ED operations focuses on the recent advances in the use of integrated facilities design process for building pediatric EDs that are optimized to patient care experience and flow, use of lean methods, as well as Six Sigma on ED throughput improvement.

The article on pediatric readiness and disaster management is a comprehensive article on the state of pediatric emergency readiness, the ability to manage pediatric aspects of disasters, the resources needed, as well as the implications on training, research, and policy to enhance outcomes.

Finally, recent advances in sensors, remote monitoring, use of newer monitors, newer instruments (such as C-Mac for airway management), use of newer EMRs that allow for predictive analytics, use of natural language processing and large data registries for ED care, ultrasound and its applications in the ED, and others are addressed in the article focusing on recent advances in technology and its applications to pediatric emergency care.

In summary, I have thoroughly enjoyed the opportunity to collate, edit, and interact with some of the brightest individuals, who have spared their time and shared their expertise that culminated in this issue of *Pediatric Clinics of North America* focused on pediatric emergency care. I sincerely hope that readers will reach out to this version, and individual articles will act as a valuable resource as we continue in our efforts to take care of the most vulnerable among us, our children.

Prashant Mahajan, MD, MPH, MBA
Department of Emergency Medicine
Pediatric Emergency Medicine
CS Mott Children's Hospital of Michigan
1540 East Hospital Drive
Room 2-737, SPC 4260
Ann Arbor, MI 48109-4260, USA

E-mail address:
pmahajan@med.umich.edu

Diagnostic Decision-Making in the Emergency Department

Laura N. Medford-Davis, MD, MS[a],*, Hardeep Singh, MD, MPH[b],
Prashant Mahajan, MD, MPH, MBA[c]

KEYWORDS

- Diagnostic error • Pediatric emergency medicine • Diagnosis • Cognition
- Reasoning • Patient safety

KEY POINTS

- Diagnostic errors have been defined by the National Academies of Sciences Engineering and Medicine as failures to establish an accurate and timely explanation of the patient's health problems or to communicate that explanation to the patient.
- Diagnosis requires hypothesis generation; questioning, examination, and testing to refine potential hypotheses; and verification of a final diagnosis.
- Competing priorities in the emergency department create time pressure that predisposes to cognitive errors, which lead to errors in diagnosis.

One of the major goals of emergency department (ED) providers is to identify and stabilize those patients who have an imminently life-threatening condition in an expedient manner and then provide appropriate disposition for ongoing treatment. This task requires the provider to, first and foremost, rule out worst case scenarios.[1] However, more than any other specialty, emergency providers make new diagnoses from undifferentiated symptoms, such as fever, headache, or abdominal pain, but without the benefit of a prior relationship with, or any knowledge about, the acutely ill and injured patient. This is also the case for many patients who visit the ED for evaluation and management of conditions that are not immediately life-threatening. Furthermore, the ED often serves as the safety net for scores of uninsured and under-insured patients in the United States, further exacerbating the pressures on timely and accurate

[a] Department of Emergency Medicine, Ben Taub General Hospital, 1504 Taub Loop, Houston, TX 77030, USA; [b] Center for Innovations in Quality, Effectiveness and Safety, Michael E. DeBakey Veterans Affairs Medical Center, Baylor College of Medicine, 2002 Holcombe Boulevard 152, Houston, TX 77030, USA; [c] Department of Emergency Medicine, CS Mott Children's Hospital of Michigan, 1540 East Hospital Drive, Room 2-737, SPC 4260, Ann Arbor, MI 48109-4260, USA
* Corresponding author.
E-mail address: Medford.davis@gmail.com

Pediatr Clin N Am 65 (2018) 1097–1105
https://doi.org/10.1016/j.pcl.2018.07.003
0031-3955/18/© 2018 Elsevier Inc. All rights reserved.

pediatric.theclinics.com

diagnostic decision making.[2] As a result, many patients' symptoms have not previously been evaluated by any other physician and follow-up care is not always readily available to reevaluate or iterate a diagnosis initiated in the ED. These factors make accurate and timely diagnosis in the ED both a critical and a challenging task.

DIAGNOSTIC ERROR IN THE PEDIATRIC EMERGENCY DEPARTMENT

Several cases of diagnostic error in the ED have made national news headlines in recent years. When Ebola arrived in the United States in 2014, the first patient diagnosed was sent home from the ED undetected after doctors and nurses did not communicate with each another about his relevant travel history.[3] As a result, the man exposed additional people and ultimately died. In New York City[4] and in England,[5] missed sepsis resulted in the death of 2 children; delayed follow-up of laboratory results played a role in both cases.

Emergency medicine faces many challenges to achieving diagnostic accuracy. Emergency providers have never met patients or their families before and do not have an established rapport. The resulting lack of trust complicates the patient–provider relationship. No universal electronic medical record is available to communicate a detailed past medical history for every patient who walks through the ED doors. An unexpected ED visit is a stressful and rare event for most patients, and their emotional or physical distress limits their ability to communicate their own history clearly and accurately. Although the ED can rapidly diagnose many conditions, tests for rarer conditions (eg, lupus) are not readily available or cannot be completed within the time limits of an emergency visit.[6,7]

In addition to these limitations, the environment is less structured in emergency medicine than other specialties.[7] Providers are under pressure to rapidly diagnose, treat, and provide disposition for a high volume of patients arriving at irregular times throughout the day with an unpredictable variety of illnesses and acuities.[6,8] At any given time, an ED provider is caring, on average, for 6 to 7 patients simultaneously.[9] An ED shift requires hundreds of decisions both about patient treatment and about prioritization of multiple competing patients and tasks.[1] While trying to make these decisions, providers are interrupted every 3 to 6 minutes.[10] All of these competing priorities leave the provider with only a short amount of time available to collect the necessary history to make a diagnosis.

When patients are acutely ill requiring urgent intervention, information gathering and diagnosis are necessarily deferred not only for the acutely ill patient but also for any other patients presenting simultaneously.[7,11] These constraints make it particularly difficult for a provider to engage in slow, deliberate thinking, and make the ED particularly susceptible to diagnostic error.[12] Furthermore, because ED providers rarely see the same patients again or receive any follow-up about what happens to their patients after disposition, if a diagnostic error is made the provider does not have the opportunity to become aware of it or learn from it.[11,13]

Beyond the pressures of any busy ED, pediatric patients present a particular challenge. General EDs do not always have the right-sized supplies, medications, or staff training for the optimal treatment of children.[14] Age and weight-specific vital signs increase the likelihood that a critical illness, such as sepsis or respiratory distress, will be overlooked, and children can deteriorate more rapidly from stable to unstable illness than adults.[14] Younger children cannot reliably communicate their symptoms or complaints. For these reasons, diagnostic error may be even more prevalent in the pediatric ED than in the adult ED, yet data on its epidemiology remain sparse.

THE DIAGNOSTIC PROCESS

To make a diagnosis, the emergency provider uses several cognitive processes. The hypothetico-deductive model of clinical reasoning describes how a provider generates diagnostic hypotheses, refines the list, and finally verifies the diagnosis.[11] Brainstorming of initial hypotheses typically begins as soon as the provider reads the chief complaint recorded by triage. In cases of extreme uncertainty, or when laboratory tests have already returned from the waiting room before the first evaluation, hypotheses may be generated bottom-up based on data instead of top-down based on symptoms.[1]

Refinement of initial hypotheses largely occurs while interviewing the patient to obtain the history of the presenting illness. The provider asks probing questions to rule out a life-threatening illness and to confirm or eliminate different potential hypotheses.[1] For example, to decide whether a D-dimer or computed tomography angiography of the chest is needed to rule out pulmonary embolism, a patient with chest pain might be asked whether they have traveled recently. The process of generating and narrowing down hypotheses has been related to pattern-matching in which a provider seeks to fit the presenting complaints into a pattern of disease they have encountered previously, giving an advantage to more experienced physicians who have seen more cases.[7]

It is important for context to note that while a provider interviews a patient to determine the workup plan and diagnosis, they are simultaneously caring for multiple patients (median 6-7, max 12-16 patients) and more patients may be checking into the waiting room by the minute.[9] This time pressure can explain why after a provider is reasonably certain about the list of potential diagnoses, they typically stop asking questions regardless of whether they have obtained all relevant information.[7] A quick physical examination is then used to confirm or eliminate the hypotheses generated from the history and diagnostic studies are ordered as needed to either further refine or to confirm the hypothesis. Finally, all data gathered are integrated by the provider to determine the diagnosis.[1,7,15]

WHAT IS DIAGNOSTIC ERROR?

When this process goes awry, a diagnostic error may result. There are many places in the diagnostic process vulnerable to mistakes, including gathering relevant information, integrating and interpreting that information, determining the diagnosis, and communicating the diagnosis to the patient (**Fig. 1**).[15]

Diagnostic error has been less studied than other types of medical error, such as medication (eg, wrong dose) or procedural (eg, wrong-site surgery), perhaps because it is more difficult to define and, therefore, often goes unnoticed and unreported. As a result, the exact prevalence remains unknown but most patients will be the victims of at least one diagnostic error in their lifetime.[15] Several nuanced definitions of diagnostic error have been proposed, with some debate around the contributions of timeliness, provider intent, and patient harm:

- Diagnoses that were unintentionally delayed, wrong, or missed[16]
- Mistakes or failure in the diagnostic process[17]
- Misdiagnosis-related preventable harm[18]
- Missed opportunity to make a correct or timely diagnosis based on the available evidence, regardless of patient harm.[19]

Recently, the National Academies of Science, Engineering, and Medicine (NASEM) defined diagnostic error as "a failure to establish an accurate and timely explanation of the patient's health problem(s) or communicate that explanation to the patient."[15]

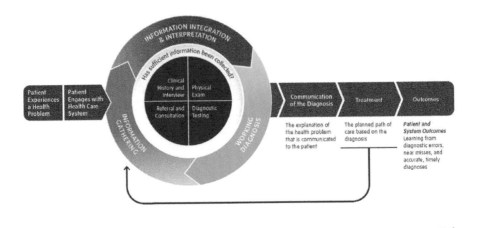

Fig. 1. Where failures in the diagnostic process occur. (*Reprinted with* permission from Improving Diagnosis in Health Care, 2015 the National Academy of Sciences, Courtesy of the National Academies Press, Washington, DC.)

The natural evolution of a patient's symptoms over time makes it difficult to pinpoint the exact time when a diagnosis crosses from being underway to being missed or delayed[7]; however, at some point, most experts will agree that sufficient evidence was available and an opportunity for accurate diagnosis was missed.[19] Many diagnostic errors do not result in patient harm, leading to underrecognition and underreporting; however, most have the potential to cause harm.[20,21] Diagnostic errors generally do not involve malicious intent. Instead, the imperfect nature of the human thought process makes providers susceptible to these errors.

COGNITIVE FACTORS AND PROCESS DYSFUNCTIONS

Cognitive processes, or the way the human brain works, are hypothesized to be a major contributor to diagnostic error. The brain can reason through a problem slowly and sequentially, and is often forced to do so when encountering a new or unfamiliar problem, but it prefers to process information quickly and automatically by relying on shortcuts or heuristics.[22] These 2 methods of thought are referred to as system 1 (automatic and subconscious) and system 2 (slow and methodical).[23] System 1 shortcuts allow people to think more efficiently by relying on patterns and prior experiences but they are susceptible to failures, called cognitive biases. Cognitive biases that can lead to diagnostic error include[15]

- Anchoring bias: Too much weight is assigned to the earliest or most salient features of a patient's history or test results, and other evidence to the contrary is ignored. For example, 1 in 9 patients with ST-segment elevation on electrocardiogram did not have an ST-segment elevation myocardial infarction (STEMI) but received treatment of an STEMI nonetheless.[24]
- Premature closure: After a provider arrives at a plausible diagnosis, they accept it as the best diagnosis and stop asking questions to seek an alternative diagnosis, even if a comprehensive history or workup is not yet complete.[7]

- Confirmation bias: After a provider arrives at a diagnosis, all future evidence aligning with that diagnosis is considered confirmation of its accuracy, whereas any contrary evidence is subconsciously ignored.
- Availability bias: Providers generate hypotheses from diagnoses they have encountered most recently, regardless of whether a diagnosis is rare, or whether it is the most relevant to the current case.
- Overconfidence: Providers' confidence in their diagnosis remains constant regardless of their accuracy.[25] Overconfidence in having a correct diagnosis can lead to a failure to seek assistance, order additional tests, or to consider contrary evidence.
- Affective bias: Unconscious biases based on emotions, countertransference, or stereotypes can distract from factual evidence to the contrary. For example, providers are less likely to refer women and blacks for cardiac testing than men and whites, despite an identical description of symptoms.[26,27]
- Representativeness: Providers make diagnoses based on perceived similarities or stereotypes that are unrelated to the actual probability of the diagnosis.

Unfortunately, even after training in these types of biases, providers have not been able to reliably identify when biases are present in a diagnosis, making them difficult to detect and address.[28] Cognitive forcing strategies have been suggested as interventions to ameliorate cognitive biases. These strategies require a provider to consciously slow down their thinking and systematically evaluate all potential alternatives and mimics before finalizing a diagnosis, effectively forcing themselves to use system 2 thinking.[29] Although system 1 is referred to as fast thinking, the time taken to reach a conclusion is less relevant than the conscious or subconscious method of arriving at it, and actual speed does not predict inaccuracy, so cognitive forcing is more about the thought process than the speed.[30] However, this strategy has not proven to be effective,[31] and fatigue, uncertainty, and stress, all common in the ED, commonly cause people to default back to the fast type of system 1 thinking, which is inherently susceptible to cognitive biases.[32] In summary, cognitive biases are difficult to detect and to address.

NEXT STEPS TO IMPROVE DIAGNOSTIC ERROR IN THE PEDIATRIC EMERGENCY DEPARTMENT

Reflecting on these challenges, diagnostic uncertainty is necessarily more common in the ED than in other specialties. Although an ED provider may view their role as complete when a patient is deemed safe for discharge home, patients have a less nuanced view of physician specialties. They often view ED providers as interchangeable with other outpatient, clinic-based providers, and expect a similar level of diagnostic certainty. Although diagnostic certainty cannot always be achieved in the ED, diagnostic error is defined not only by the accuracy of the diagnosis but also by the appropriateness of the communication of the diagnosis to the patient.[15] Therefore, in cases in which an ED provider cannot fully explain a patient's symptoms at the time of the ED visit, it is important that they communicate their uncertainty to the patient along with a specific plan and timeline for the patient to seek follow-up care to continue the diagnostic process.[33] Research shows that patients are most receptive to an open discussion of their possible differential diagnoses, rather than a simple statement that their diagnosis is unknown.[34]

Beyond the approach to the patient interaction, additional research on diagnostic error in the pediatric ED is required to improve the current state. Although definitions and frameworks exist for the ambulatory population,[35,36] work to comprehensively define, measure the prevalence, track the cause, and develop preventative solutions for diagnostic error in the pediatric ED remains in progress. The effectiveness of potential strategies for improvement cannot be monitored without first agreeing on the baseline. Exact diagnostic error rates in the ED are unknown because existing ED studies of diagnostic error focus on subpopulations of ED patients at higher risk for error.[20,37–40] Diagnostic error is suspected to be high in the pediatric population based on malpractice claims and self-reporting by pediatricians but these pediatric studies are not specific to the ED.[41,42] Extrapolating the 5% diagnostic error rate in the non-ED outpatient adult population,[43,44] which was similar to the rate seen in a single-center pediatric ED study,[40] to the more than 25 million annual pediatric emergency visits in the United States[45] suggests that at least 1 million children experience a diagnostic error each year. Considering the dual constraints of both the ED environment and the pediatric population, and the increased susceptibility to error of each, 5% may be a significant underestimate of true diagnostic error prevalence.[12]

Poor consensus on the exact definition, timing, and cause of diagnostic errors has contributed to the difficulty in establishing prevalence and must be resolved to begin reliably tracking diagnostic errors.[46,47] In the ED, events used to screen for errors have varied from 10-day return ED visit leading to hospitalization[20] to 30-day return ED visit with diagnosis of stroke,[38] missed diagnosis on radiographs,[48] malpractice claims,[37] review of voluntary error reports,[39] and mismatch between ED admitting diagnosis and hospital discharge diagnosis.[40] Other ED quality indicators, such as upgrade to the intensive care unit after admission or call-backs for abnormal results, could also be used to identify a subpopulation at risk for diagnostic error.[49] Searching for these electronic triggers in the electronic medical record is a proven tactic for identifying diagnostic error[20,50,51] but consensus must be reached on the most specific and sensitive triggers for the pediatric ED. Active prospective screening or comprehensive retrospective screening of all presenting ED patients has not been undertaken.

In conclusion, although diagnosis is not always the primary goal in the ED, particularly for patients without immediately life-threatening conditions, emergency medicine can and should take more responsibility for avoiding diagnostic error, through both open patient communication and a targeted research agenda to improve the diagnostic process.

ACKNOWLEDGMENTS

Dr. Singh is supported by the VA Health Services Research and Development Service (CRE12-033; Presidential Early Career Award for Scientists and Engineers USA 14-274), the VA National Center for Patient Safety, the Agency for HealthCare Research and Quality (R01HS022087), the Gordon and Betty Moore Foundation, and in part by the Houston VA HSR&D Center for Innovations in Quality, Effectiveness and Safety (CIN13-413). Views expressed do not represent views of these funding sources, which also had no role in the preparation, review, or approval of the article.

Dr. Mahajan is supported by the Eunice Kennedy Shriver National Institute of Child Health & Human Development of the National Institutes of Health under Award Number R01HD085233, the Agency for Healthcare Research and Quality under award number R01HS024953 and the Health Resources and Services Administration (HRSA), Maternal and Child Health Bureau (MCHB), Emergency Medical Services for Children (EMSC) Network Development Demonstration Program under cooperative agreement U03MC28844. The funding agencies had no role in the preparation, review, or approval of the content. The information or content and conclusions are those of the author and does not represent the official views of the funding agencies and should not be construed as the official position or policy of, nor should any endorsements be inferred by HRSA, HHS or the US Government.

REFERENCES

1. Croskerry P. Achieving quality in clinical decision making: cognitive strategies and detection of bias. Acad Emerg Med 2002;9(11):1184–204.
2. Henry J Kaiser Family Foundation. Health Insurance Coverage of the Total Population. 2013. Available at: http://kff.org/other/state-indicator/total-population/. Accessed September 11, 2015.
3. Bever L. Dallas hospital blames 'flaw' in 'workflow' for release of Ebola patient as a more complete picture of his travel emerges. Washington, DC: Washington Post; 2014.
4. Dwyer J. An Infection, unnoticed, turns unstoppable. New York: The New York Times; 2012.
5. Jha S. To err is homicide in Britain - the case of Dr Hadiza Bawa-Garba. The Health Care Blog 2018. Available at: http://thehealthcareblog.com/blog/2018/01/30/to-err-is-homicide-in-britain-the-case-of-dr-hadiza-bawa-garba/. Accessed January 30, 2018.
6. Fordyce J, Blank FS, Pekow P, et al. Errors in a busy emergency department. Ann Emerg Med 2003;42(3):324–33.
7. Kuhn GJ. Diagnostic errors. Acad Emerg Med 2002;9(7):740–50.
8. Schenkel S. Promoting patient safety and preventing medical error in emergency departments. Acad Emerg Med 2000;7(11):1204–22.
9. Chisholm CD, Weaver CS, Whenmouth L, et al. A task analysis of emergency physician activities in academic and community settings. Ann Emerg Med 2011;58(2):117–22.
10. Chisholm CD, Collison EK, Nelson DR, et al. Emergency department workplace interruptions: are emergency physicians "interrupt-driven" and "multitasking"? Acad Emerg Med 2000;7(11):1239–43.
11. Kovacs G, Croskerry P. Clinical decision making: an emergency medicine perspective. Acad Emerg Med 1999;6(9):947–52.
12. Croskerry P, Sinclair D. Emergency medicine: a practice prone to error? CJEM 2001;3(4):271–6.
13. Schiff GD. Minimizing diagnostic error: the importance of follow-up and feedback. Am J Med 2008;121(5 Suppl):S38–42.
14. Instiute of Medicine. Emergency care for children: growing pains. Washington, DC: The National Academies Press; 2007. 978-0-309-10171-4.
15. Institute of Medicine. National academies of sciences, engineering, medicine. improving diagnosis in health care. Washington, DC: The National Academies Press; 2015. 978-0-309-37769-0.
16. Graber ML, Franklin N, Gordon R. Diagnostic error in internal medicine. Arch Intern Med 2005;165(13):1493–9.
17. Schiff GD, Hasan O, Kim S, et al. Diagnostic error in medicine: analysis of 583 physician-reported errors. Arch Intern Med 2009;169(20):1881–7.
18. Newman-Toker DE, Pronovost PJ. Diagnostic errors–the next frontier for patient safety. JAMA 2009;301(10):1060–2.

19. Singh H. Editorial: helping health care organizations to define diagnostic errors as missed opportunities in diagnosis. Jt Comm J Qual Patient Saf 2014;40(3):99–101.
20. Medford-Davis L, Park E, Shlamovitz G, et al. Diagnostic errors related to acute abdominal pain in the emergency department. Emerg Med J 2016;33(4):253–9.
21. Singh H, Giardina TD, Meyer AN, et al. Types and origins of diagnostic errors in primary care settings. JAMA Intern Med 2013;173(6):418–25.
22. Kahneman D. Thinking, fast and slow. New York: Farrar, Straus and Giroux; 2011.
23. Croskerry P, Singhal G, Mamede S. Cognitive debiasing 1: origins of bias and theory of debiasing. BMJ Qual Saf 2013;22(Suppl 2):ii58–64.
24. Sharkey SW, Berger CR, Brunette DD, et al. Impact of the electrocardiogram on the delivery of thrombolytic therapy for acute myocardial infarction. Am J Cardiol 1994;73(8):550–3.
25. Meyer AN, Payne VL, Meeks DW, et al. Physicians' diagnostic accuracy, confidence, and resource requests: a vignette study. JAMA Intern Med 2013;173(21):1952–8.
26. Schulman KA, Berlin JA, Harless W, et al. The effect of race and sex on physicians' recommendations for cardiac catheterization. N Engl J Med 1999;340(8):618–26.
27. Croskerry P. The cognitive imperative: thinking about how we think. Acad Emerg Med 2000;7(11):1223–31.
28. Zwaan L, Monteiro S, Sherbino J, et al. Is bias in the eye of the beholder? A vignette study to assess recognition of cognitive biases in clinical case workups. BMJ Qual Saf 2017;26(2):104–10.
29. Croskerry P. Cognitive forcing strategies in clinical decisionmaking. Ann Emerg Med 2003;41(1):110–20.
30. Sherbino J, Dore KL, Wood TJ, et al. The relationship between response time and diagnostic accuracy. Acad Med 2012;87(6):785–91.
31. Sherbino J, Kulasegaram K, Howey E, et al. Ineffectiveness of cognitive forcing strategies to reduce biases in diagnostic reasoning: a controlled trial. CJEM 2014;16(1):34–40.
32. Kahneman D, Klein G. Conditions for intuitive expertise: a failure to disagree. Am Psychol 2009;64(6):515–26.
33. Bhise V, Rajan SS, Sittig DF, et al. Defining and measuring diagnostic uncertainty in medicine: a systematic review. J Gen Intern Med 2018;33(1):103–15.
34. Bhise V, Meyer AND, Menon S, et al. Patient perspectives on how physicians communicate diagnostic uncertainty: an experimental vignette study. Int J Qual Health Care 2018;30(1):2–8.
35. Singh H, Giardina TD, Forjuoh SN, et al. Electronic health record-based surveillance of diagnostic errors in primary care. BMJ Qual Saf 2012;21(2):93–100.
36. Singh H, Sittig DF. Advancing the science of measurement of diagnostic errors in healthcare: the safer Dx framework. BMJ Qual Saf 2015;24(2):103–10.
37. Kachalia A, Gandhi TK, Puopolo AL, et al. Missed and delayed diagnoses in the emergency department: a study of closed malpractice claims from 4 liability insurers. Ann Emerg Med 2007;49(2):196–205.
38. Newman-Toker DE, Moy E, Valente E, et al. Missed diagnosis of stroke in the emergency department: a cross-sectional analysis of a large population-based sample. Diagnosis (Berl) 2014;1(2):155–66.
39. Okafor N, Payne VL, Chathampally Y, et al. Using voluntary reports from physicians to learn from diagnostic errors in emergency medicine. Emerg Med J 2016;33(4):245–52.

40. Warrick C, Patel P, Hyer W, et al. Diagnostic error in children presenting with acute medical illness to a community hospital. Int J Qual Health Care 2014; 26(5):538–46.

41. Troxel D. The doctor's advocate. director's forum. diagnostic error in medical practice by specialty. 2014. Available at: https://www.thedoctors.com/the-doctors-advocate/third-quarter-2014/diagnostic-error-in-medical-practice-by-specialty/. Accessed February 6, 2018.

42. Singh H, Thomas EJ, Wilson L, et al. Errors of diagnosis in pediatric practice: a multisite survey. Pediatrics 2010;126(1):70–9.

43. Graber ML. The incidence of diagnostic error in medicine. BMJ Qual Saf 2013; 22(Suppl 2):ii21–7.

44. Singh H, Meyer AN, Thomas EJ. The frequency of diagnostic errors in outpatient care: estimations from three large observational studies involving US adult populations. BMJ Qual Saf 2014;23(9):727–31.

45. Wier LMHY, Owens P, Washington R. Overview of children in the emergency department, 2010. HCUP statistical brief #157. Rockville (MD): Agency for Healthcare Research and Quality; 2010. Available at: https://www.hcup-us.ahrq.gov/reports/statbriefs/sb157.jsp.

46. Zwaan L, Singh H. The challenges in defining and measuring diagnostic error. Diagnosis (Berl) 2015;2(2):97–103.

47. Newman-Toker DE. A unified conceptual model for diagnostic errors: underdiagnosis, overdiagnosis, and misdiagnosis. Diagnosis (Berl) 2014;1(1):43–8.

48. Guly HR. Diagnostic errors in an accident and emergency department. Emerg Med J 2001;18(4):263–9.

49. Schull MJ, Guttmann A, Leaver CA, et al. Prioritizing performance measurement for emergency department care: consensus on evidence-based quality of care indicators. CJEM 2011;13(5):300–9. E328-43.

50. Singh H, Thomas EJ, Khan MM, et al. Identifying diagnostic errors in primary care using an electronic screening algorithm. Arch Intern Med 2007;167(3):302–8.

51. Szekendi MK, Sullivan C, Bobb A, et al. Active surveillance using electronic triggers to detect adverse events in hospitalized patients. Qual Saf Health Care 2006;15(3):184–90.

Recognition, Diagnostics, and Management of Pediatric Severe Sepsis and Septic Shock in the Emergency Department

Raina Paul, MD

KEYWORDS

• Sepsis • Severe sepsis • Septic shock • Resuscitation

KEY POINTS

- Treatment of pediatric sepsis is predicated on early recognition and timely delivery of appropriate fluids, empiric broad-spectrum antibiotics, and vasoactive agents.
- Identifying severe sepsis patients for research is difficult and *International Classification of Disease* codes alone should not be relied on.
- Evidence for many national guidelines have been extrapolated from adult data. Well-designed pediatric sepsis studies are sparse; hence, further studies are needed to support consensus-based best practices.
- Performance gaps exist in ideal care of the pediatric septic shock patient. Quality-improvement initiatives have emerged to help translate recommendations into actual care to improve outcomes.

INTRODUCTION

Timely recognition, evaluation, and treatment of pediatric sepsis are crucial when considering the pediatric patient who presents in shock. The national and international guidelines and their supporting literature are unanimous in their recommendations that early recognition and timely therapeutics are necessary for improved survival and decreased morbidity. The literature, however, is less concrete in defining how emerging advances in the field, such as biomarkers, timing of antibiotics, and various vasoactive agents, can be used to aid in time-sensitive care of these patients. The following is a summary of the recent literature as it pertains to the initial presentation of severe sepsis and septic shock in the pediatric patient within the emergency department (ED).

Disclosure Statement: The author has no disclosures or conflicts of interest.
Pediatric Emergency Department, Division of Emergency Medicine, Advocate Children's Hospital, 1700 Luther Lane, Park Ridge, IL 60068, USA
E-mail address: Raina.paul@advocatehealth.com

Pediatr Clin N Am 65 (2018) 1107–1118
https://doi.org/10.1016/j.pcl.2018.07.012
pediatric.theclinics.com

EPIDEMIOLOGY

Severe sepsis is one of the leading causes of pediatric mortality worldwide, accounting for more than 8 million deaths annually.[1] From 2004 to 2012, pediatric severe sepsis prevalence in the United States increased (3.7% to 4.4%), with an associated 176,000 hospitalizations and mortality of 8.2% (11,000 deaths) in 2012.[2] The prevalence of sepsis, severe sepsis, and septic shock in epidemiologic studies varies, however, based on definitions used and the source of the sampled cohorts. Furthermore, mortality statistics do not account for variability in recognition and delivery of care.[2–4] True estimates of the burden of septic shock in the pediatric population remain ambiguous.

Early recognition and rapid treatment are crucial to improving outcomes for children with severe sepsis and septic shock. Han and colleagues[5] studied children presenting to community hospital EDs, noting an association between use of pediatric advanced life support (PALS) and American College of Critical Care Medicine (ACCM) guidelines and mortality, with mortality decreasing to 38% from 8% with early application of the guidelines. Paul and colleagues[6] noted that after implementation of a quality-improvement initiative to improve recognition, rapid intravenous (IV) access, initiation of IV fluids, and timely antibiotic and vasoactive agent delivery, mortality decreased from 4.0% to 1.7%. Similarly, Karapinar and colleagues noted achievement of best practice outcomes with a 28-day mortality rate of 3% for fluid refractory shock patients when the 2002 guidelines were implemented.[7]

In 2017 the American College of Critical Care Medicine provided updated guidelines for the hemodynamic support of the neonatal and pediatric septic shock patient; however, there are few changes in the current guidelines compared with prior updates from 2002 and 2007.[8] There are now strong recommendations to assess these patients at the institutional level with early cross-collaborations between the referral hospital, transport, emergency services, and ICU. Additionally, there is a strong focus on bundle implementation, a practice endorsed by the Institute for Healthcare Improvement, a quality-improvement and health care delivery organization.[9] Bundles are a series of interventions relating to a treatment or process. They demand all-or-none thinking and measurement that aid in provider recollection and implementation of the bundle. They facilitate identifying failures once the bundle is implemented, and these failures are actively used to redesign the process. Bundles should be applied at the recognition, resuscitation, and performance optimization stages to ensure enhanced adherence to recommended care.[9] An example of a bundle includes the 5-point bundle for ideal sepsis care as part of a quality-improvement initiative in the Boston Children's Hospital ED (**Fig. 1**).[6]

RECOGNITION

Recognition of pediatric severe sepsis is fraught with a dynamic and often obscure presentation. There is no single diagnostic test that can aid an ED clinician yet early recognition is the crucial step in initiating timely therapies to improve outcomes. The first clinical sign is often hypothermia or hyperthermia as well as altered capillary refill. Peripheral vasodilation (warm shock) is often indicated by a capillary refill of less than 2 seconds whereas vasoconstriction (cold shock) usually presents with a capillary refill of greater than 2 seconds. Many studies, however, have demonstrated this assessment is marred by inaccuracies. One study demonstrated that 66% of children thought to have "cold shock," as determined by experienced clinicians, were actually vasodilated during concurrent invasive monitoring.[10]

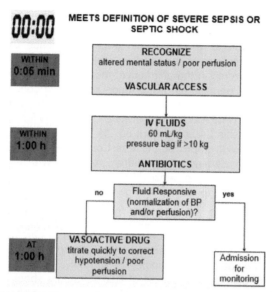

Fig. 1. Example of bundled elements for ideal sepsis care in the Boston Children's Hospital ED quality-improvement initiative. (*Adapted from* Paul R, Neuman MI, Monuteaux MC, et al. Adherence to PALS sepsis guidelines and hospital length of stay. Pediatrics 2012;130(2):e274; with permission; and *Modified from* Pediatric Advanced Life Support Manual, American Heart Association.)

Other clinical signs that can aid in recognition include altered mental status, which is difficult to determine in the chronic medical condition population where caregiver input is crucial, especially as mortality is higher in this group.[3]

Tachycardia can be a sign of pain, anxiety, and dehydration in the pediatric patient and thus must evaluated in context with other clinical parameters. Scott and colleagues[11] examined 40,356 visits to the ED and noted that 81% whom had vitals consistent with systemic inflammatory response syndrome, as defined by Goldstein and colleagues,[12] were discharged from the ED without IV fluids or readmission in 72 hours. Hyperthermia, often present in severe sepsis, can result in tachycardia; thus, some investigators advocate the use of temperature-corrected heart rates to optimize the specificity of this vital sign. Two studies have examined the expected tachycardia in a patient with fever, generally noting an increase in heart rate by 5 beats per minute for every 1°F above 100°F.[13,14] Cruz and colleagues[15] applied this concept to a best practice alert (BPA) for septic shock patients in a tertiary-care ED. The tool was 81% sensitive and 89% specific in identifying the 210 patients with shock. Positive predictive values and negative predictive values were 4% and 99.9%, respectively. The BPA did not alert for 40 children with shock. Of these, 11 did not receive vital signs in triage because they were being actively resuscitated on arrival. Of the remaining 29 patients, 23 were tachycardic within the temperature correction range and 6 presented with normal vital signs but subsequently decompensated in the ED after receiving antibiotics.[15]

Optimizing the sensitivity and specificity of a BPA is critical, as described by Balamuth and colleagues.[16] This BPA, which has been adopted by several tertiary children's hospitals in the country, initially flags a triage provider if the heart rate or blood pressure is out of range. This provider is then prompted to consider if the patient has a fever or signs and symptoms of infection. If so, assessment of capillary refill, mental status, and presence of a high-risk condition that would increase the risk of developing sepsis (such as a neutropenic patient, presence of asplenia, those <2 months of age, or presence of an indwelling line) is determined. If 1 of these specificity questions is answered in the affirmative, the clinician determines whether the sepsis pathway should be initiated. If the triage provider is concerned without the BPA alerting, a bedside huddle and pathway initiation can occur as well. In this study, using vital signs within the BPA alone, sensitivity and specificity for identifying a patient within severe sepsis within 24 hours were 86.2% and 99.1%, respectively. Adding clinician judgment markedly improved these test characteristics, identifying 43 additional electronic sepsis alert–negative children, resulting in a sensitivity of 99.4% and specificity 99.1% for severe sepsis.[16] Other sometimes referred to as trigger tools, have been developed to aid the emergency medicine clinician in rapid identification of these patients (**Fig. 2**).

Recognizing pediatric septic shock requires an understanding of how presentation can differ from adult counterparts. Contrary to adults, low cardiac output (CO), as opposed to low systemic vascular resistance (SVR), is known to be associated with higher mortality in pediatric septic shock.[17–28] Ceneviva and colleagues[26] demonstrated that 58% of children in a cohort of fluid refractory shock patients had low CO and high SVR, whereas 22% had low CO and low SVR. It has also been shown that although in adults oxygen consumption is primarily related to oxygen delivery, in children oxygen extraction is the primary determinant.[19] The dilemma of the ED provider, however, is that currently there are only rudimentary methods with which to

Septic Shock Trigger/Identification Tool

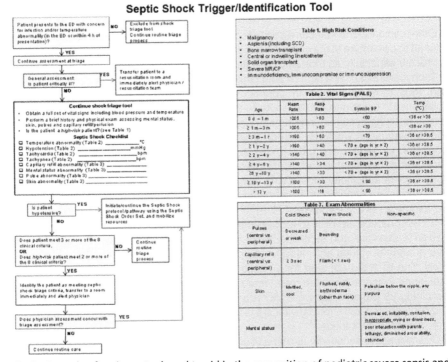

Fig. 2. Example of a trigger tool used to aid in the recognition of pediatric severe sepsis and septic shock. (*Courtesy of* the Pediatric Septic Shock Collaborative (PSSC) Septic Shock Trigger Tool of the American Academy of Pediatrics, Itasca, IL; with permission.)

evaluate CO and SVR in real time. Placement of a central line with measurements of central venous pressure and mixed venous saturation can aid in determining these diagnostic states; however, with the advent of the intraosseous needle, additional access is rarely needed during the first critical hours of sepsis resuscitation. Doppler ultrasonography is a tool that is accessible and used often by many ED providers for other conditions and should be used more frequently to assess hemodynamic parameters, including CO and measurement of the internal vena cava to determine intravascular volume status in an objective way.[28]

Biomarkers also can be used as adjuncts in determination of the severe sepsis state. The most commonly used is lactic acid. Although lactic acid in the adult sepsis population is used consistently, it has less predictive value in pediatrics if normal. Scott and colleagues[29] noted that if the lactic acid level was greater than 4.0 mmol/L, patients had a 5.5 relative risk of developing organ dysfunction at 24 hours. However, 4% of the normal lactate population also went on to develop organ dysfunction. Recently, the same investigators have shown that in a population of 1299 pediatric patients, an elevated lactate was significantly associated with 30-day mortality (adjusted odds ratio of 3.26).[30] An elevated lactate level, however, had a sensitivity for 30-day mortality of only 20%. Conclusions from these and other studies are that lactic acid can be helpful in determining propensity of developing organ dysfunction and mortality but clinicians should not be reassured if the value is normal. Another biomarker helpful in the risk stratification of the severe sepsis patient includes troponin. Blood troponin levels correlate well with poor cardiac function and response to inotropic support.[31–33]

In recent years, research regarding protein and mRNA biomarkers for sepsis has emerged.[34,35] Biomarkers have potential utility in risk stratification of patients who may have sepsis, patients who are more likely to have worse outcomes, and patients who may benefit from certain therapeutics. Thus far, however, no one set of biomarkers is routinely recommended for clinical practice despite steady progress in identifying those with optimized sensitivity and specificity. Procalcitonin, an amino acid peptide, has been shown to identify sepsis more consistently than C-reactive protein in critically ill patients. There has been a wide range of sensitivities and specificities reported, however, and in less sick populations, such as those in the ED, procalcitonin has not been reliably shown to differentiate between sepsis and systemic inflammatory response syndrome.[36] Procalcitonin has also shown benefit in guiding duration of antibiotic course, allowing for earlier cessation of antibiotics when procalcitonin levels decrease.[37]

More recently a collection of biomarkers, collectively labeled the pediatric sepsis biomarker risk model (PERSEVERE) and PERSEVERE–XP, has shown tremendous promise in risk stratifying pediatric patients with sepsis. PERSEVERE is a collection of 12 biomarkers, selected from proteins directly related to 80 genes associated with mortality in septic shock. PERSEVERE–XP combines the previous set with 4 mRNA biomarkers and has been shown clinical promise in risk stratification for those with septic shock as well as hypothesizing a pathophysiologic reason for disparate mortality outcomes in this population.[35,38]

RETROSPECTIVE IDENTIFICATION OF PEDIATRIC PATIENTS WITH SEVERE SEPSIS AND SEPTIC SHOCK

Many studies have relied on the International Consensus Conference Guidelines by Goldstein and colleagues for the identification of pediatric patients with severe sepsis and septic shock.[11] Applying these definitions retrospectively can be problematic. These guidelines were initially developed for research purposes and can be problematic for application to quality-improvement initiatives as well as initial recognition by frontline providers. The SPROUT (Sepsis, Prevalence, Outcomes and Therapies) study group showed that in a pediatric ICU, 31% of patients identified as having severe sepsis or septic shock by the treating provider did not meet definitions as described by Goldstein and colleagues[12] yet still had a 17% mortality rate.[39] Balamuth and colleagues[2,40] noted that *International Classification of Disease, Ninth Revision*, codes and the strategy defined by Angus and colleagues (infection plus organ dysfunction coding strategies)[41] had limitations as well in their sensitivity and specificity when retrospectively identifying those with severe sepsis. As more quality-improvement efforts are emerging locally and nationally to evaluate process and outcome measures in pediatric sepsis care, the limitations of current identification strategies must be understood.

FLUID MANAGEMENT

The first clinical question that often arises with regard to fluid management of the pediatric patient with septic shock is the type of fluid recommended, specifically colloid versus crystalloid. Maitland and colleagues[42] in a randomized controlled trial noted a reduction in malarial septic shock mortality from 18% to 4% with use of albumin versus crystalloid IV fluids. Similarly, the Saline versus Albumin Fluid Evaluation trial noted there was a trend toward improved outcomes with albumin resuscitation versus crystalloid; however, this study targeted the intensive care population.[43] In contrast, the study by Carcillo and colleagues that generated tremendous initial favor for rapid resuscitation used a combination of crystalloid and colloid, although this was not the primary question in this case series.[44] Weiss and colleagues performed a matched analysis comparing those who had received normal saline only, those receiving lactated Ringer solution only, and those receiving a combination of both.[45] Use of lactated Ringer solution was not found superior to that of normal saline, and the combined group, after risk stratification, was found to have a longer length of stay in the hospital. Further prospective trials are needed to evaluate the noninferiority and efficacy of alternate fluid–type resuscitation for septic shock. The ACCM and PALS guidelines continue to recommend normal saline as a first-line fluid, particularly in the first hour of resuscitation.[46–49]

A second equally important question relates to volume and timeliness of fluid delivery. Again PALS recommends 60 mL/kg of IV normal saline within 60 minutes of development of severe sepsis or septic shock, whereas the 2002 ACCM guidelines recommended a more aggressive approach of 20 mL/kg IV fluid boluses over 5 minutes.[46–49] Regardless, frequent reassessments are critical to assess for not only fluid responsiveness and normalization of hemodynamic parameters but also signs of fluid overload, such as rales or hepatomegaly. The latter should prompt earlier use of vasoactive agents.[46–49] This recommendation, however, is supported by few studies. Carcillo and colleagues, in the aforementioned study noted better outcomes with rapid resuscitation whereas Paul and colleagues[50] demonstrated improved hospital and ICU length of stay when 60 mL/kg of fluids were given within 60 minutes versus over a longer time period.[50] Adherence to these guidelines is technically feasible, as noted in the study by Stoner and colleagues,[51] who demonstrated that 20 mL/kg of IV fluids can be pushed over 5 minutes through a peripheral IV catheter of various gauge sizes, including a 22-gauge catheter. Given the relative paucity of pediatric data as well as recent adult data demonstrating better outcomes with less volume resuscitation, the optimal strategy for pediatric septic shock resuscitation is in question.[52–54] Investigators are currently addressing this issue in a prospective trial (the SQUEEZE trial) in Canada, comparing usual care with a fluid-sparing strategy. Conclusions of this anticipated study are not yet published.[55]

ANTIBIOTIC DELIVERY

PALS septic shock guidelines have had a consistent recommendation regarding antibiotic delivery for more than a decade.[46–48] In particular, it is recommended that antibiotics be delivered within 60 minutes from onset of severe sepsis or septic shock. These recommendations have permeated current pathways endorsed by several national groups; however, the evidence for delivery within an hour is limited. Kumar and colleagues,[56] in the adult severe sepsis population, demonstrated that for every hour delay in delivery of antibiotics, survival fraction decreased. Multiple other adult studies exist demonstrating this association but the data for pediatrics are severely limited. Weiss and colleagues[57] noted that in 130 severe sepsis patients, with a mortality of 12%, 18% received antibiotics in the first hour. After risk stratification, it was noted that delivery of antibiotics after 3 hours was associated with fewer organ failure–free days. Median time to antimicrobial delivery was 140 minutes. On the contrary, van Paridon and colleagues,[55] in their study of 79 children in a single-institution pediatric ICU, failed to demonstrate an association between timing of antimicrobial administration and outcomes, including ICU length of stay and 1-year mortality. In this study, 25% received antimicrobials in the first hour, and mortality was 6% overall, with a median time to antimicrobial administration of 115 minutes. Similarly, Creedon and colleagues[58] noted no association between timing of antibiotic delivery and outcomes. Until further studies emerge, national guidelines continue to recommend antibiotic delivery within the first critical hour of resuscitation.

VASOPRESSORS AND INOTROPES

Several vasoactive agents can be used in the initial management of severe sepsis and septic shock, including dobutamine, dopamine, norepinephrine, and epinephrine.[8] If the exact CO state is known, such as decreased contractility of the heart by echocardiography, then dobutamine can be initiated safely. This information is often not apparent to an ED provider, however, and thus the first agents recommended at presentation include epinephrine, dopamine, and norepinephrine. In prior national recommendations, dopamine was suggested as a first-line agent for cold or undifferentiated shock.[47,48] In recent years, however, data have emerged that epinephrine may be a more beneficial initial agent for certain shock states.[8,49] There has been 1 randomized controlled trial examining the outcomes with use of dopamine versus epinephrine, conducted in a Brazil pediatric ICU.[59] This was a single-center study of 120 children who had persistent hypoperfusion after 40 mL/kg of fluid resuscitation who were then randomized to receive epinephrine or dopamine. Dopamine or epinephrine was administered via the intraosseous or peripheral route while central access was obtained, and there were no extravasation events noted. Mortality rate was lower in the epinephrine versus dopamine group (7% vs 14%; $P = .033$). The odds ratio of death for those patients in the dopamine group versus the epinephrine group was 6.5 (95% CI, 1.1–37.8). More hyperglycemia was seen in the epinephrine group given its known endocrine stress response.[59] The current guidelines recommend norepinephrine for warm shock and epinephrine for cold or undifferentiated shock, although there are few data to support these recommendations.[60–67] Warm shock indicates a vasodilatory state with a low SVR for which norepinephrine is a more effective initiating agent. Deep and colleagues[28] noted, however, that using a noninvasive ultrasound CO monitor device to measure ongoing hemodynamics and presence of warm or cold shock often presented heterogeneously and was dynamic, requiring frequent alterations of vasoactive agent.

CORTICOSTEROIDS

National guidelines continue to recommend use of corticosteroids in fluid and vasoactive agent refractory shock.[48,49] Again, there are few studies to support this unanimous use and data are emerging that suggest there is a subset of sepsis patients who may not benefit from its administration. Wong and colleagues[68] noted that in children with septic shock who did receive corticosteroids, the adaptive immune response was down-regulated versus those who did not receive corticosteroids, raising concerns that they may suppress adaptive immunity in this population. Further study is warranted to investigate this further.

QUALITY-IMPROVEMENT COLLABORATIVES

In recent years there has been a tremendous effort to improve adherence to ideal standard of care for pediatric septic shock. Multiple institutions have demonstrated that delivering timely fluids and antibiotics is possible in a heterogeneous cohort of patients using robust quality-improvement methodology and is associated with improved outcomes. Using bundled care has shown to aid in provider adherence to recommended best practices.[6,69] There is still a significant gap in delivering optimal care to these patients. Recently completed and ongoing quality-improvement collaboratives have attempted to harness the power of multi-institutional sharing of best practice process interventions to change provider behavior and improve systems for detection and timely treatment, ultimately improving outcomes. These collaboratives, including the 2012 Children's Hospital Association rapid cycle collaborative,[70] the American Academy of Pediatrics Pediatric Septic Shock Collaborative, and the Improving Pediatric Sepsis Outcomes, have addressed and will continue to address the performance gap for some of the most critically ill ED patients.

SUMMARY

In summary, the literature supporting use of fluids, antibiotics, and vasoactive agents in the resuscitation of the pediatric septic shock patient is both at once robust and inconclusive. This is a heterogeneous population with innate and disparate patient-level components that make studying outcomes difficult, leading to ambiguity within the current literature. These patient-level factors make it of utmost importance to continue pathophysiologic study. As further bench-to-bedside research addressing these gaps is awaited, expert consensus-based guidelines can be relied on in determining best practice and standard of care. Point-of-care clinical judgment must be kept forefront in decision making, however, and recommended therapies delivered with caution. The first critical hour of resuscitation often occurs in EDs; thus, ED providers have a unique chance to alter the devastating consequences of unrecognized and inadequately treated severe sepsis and septic shock.

REFERENCES

1. Black RE, Cousens S, Johnson HL, et al. Global, regional, and national causes of mortality in 2008: a systematic analysis. Lancet 2010;375(9730):1969–87.
2. Balamuth F, Weiss SL, Neuman MI, et al. Pediatric severe sepsis in U.S. children's hospitals. Pediatr Crit Care Med 2014;15(9):798–805.
3. Watson RS, Carcillo JA, Linde-Zwirble WT, et al. The epidemiology of severe sepsis in children in the United States. Am J Respir Crit Care Med 2003; 167(5):695–701.

4. Gaieski DF, Edwards JM, Kallan MJ, et al. Benchmarking the incidence and mortality of severe sepsis in the United States. Crit Care Med 2013;41(5):1167–74.

5. Han YY, Carcillo JA, Dragotta MA, et al. Early reversal of pediatric-neonatal septic shock by community physicians is associated with improved outcome. Pediatrics 2003;112:793–9.

6. Paul R, Melendez E, Stack A, et al. Improving adherence to PALS septic shock guidelines. Pediatrics 2014;133:e1358–66.

7. Karapinar B, Lin JC, Carcillo JA. ACCM guidelines use, correct antibiotic therapy, and immune suppressant withdrawal are associated with improved survival in pediatric sepsis, severe sepsis, and septic shock. Crit Care Med 2004; 32(12 Suppl 3):A161.

8. Davis AL, Carcillo JA, Rajesh AK, et al. American College of critical care medicine clinical practice parameters for hemodynamic support of pediatric and neonatal septic shock. Crit Care Med 2017;45(6):1061–93.

9. Available at: www.ihi.org/Topics/Bundles/Pages/default.aspx. Accessed October 9, 2017.

10. Ranjit S, Aram G, Kissoon N, et al. Multimodal monitoring for hemodynamic categorization and management of pediatric septic shock: A pilot observational study*. Pediatr Crit Care Med 2014;15(1):e17–26.

11. Scott HF, Deakyne SJ, Woods JM, et al. The prevalence and diagnostic utility of systemic inflammatory response syndrome vital signs in a pediatric emergency department, academic emergency medicine. Acad Emerg Med 2015;22(4): 381–9.

12. Goldstein B, Giroir B, Randolph A, et al. International Consensus Conference on Pediatric Sepsis. International pediatric sepsis consensus conference: definitions for sepsis and organ dysfunction in pediatrics. Pediatr Crit Care Med 2005;6:2–8.

13. Hanna CM, Greenes DS. How much tachycardia in infants can be attributed to fever? Ann Emerg Med 2004;43:699–705.

14. Davies P, Maconochie I. The relationship between body temperature, heart rate and respiratory rate in children. Emerg Med J 2009;26:641–3.

15. Cruz AT, William EA, Graff JM, et al. Test characteristics of an age- and temperature-adjusted tachycardia alert in pediatric septic shock. Pediatr Emerg Care 2012;28(9):889–94.

16. Balamuth F, Alpern ER, Abbadessa MK, et al. Improving recognition of pediatric severe sepsis in the emergency department: contributions of a vital sign–based electronic alert and bedside clinician identification. Ann Emerg Med 2017;70(6): 759–68.

17. Pollack MM, Fields AI, Ruttimann UE, et al. Sequential cardiopulmonary variables of infants and children in septic shock. Crit Care Med 1984;12:554–9.

18. Pollack MM, Fields AI, Ruttimann UE, et al. Distributions of cardiopulmonary variables in pediatric survivors and nonsurvivors of septic shock. Crit Care Med 1985;13:454–9.

19. Carcillo JA, Pollack MM, Ruttimann UE, et al. Sequential physiologic interactions in pediatric cardiogenic and septic shock. Crit Care Med 1989;17:12–6.

20. Monsalve F, Rucabado L, Salvador A, et al. Myocardial depression in septic shock caused by meningococcal infection. Crit Care Med 1984;12:1021–3.

21. Mercier JC, Beaufils F, Hartmann JF, et al. Hemodynamic patterns of meningococcal shock in children. Crit Care Med 1988;16:27–33.

22. Simma B, Fritz MG, Trawöger R, et al. Changes in left ventricular function in shocked newborns. Intensive Care Med 1997;23:982–6.

23. Walther FJ, Siassi B, Ramadan NA, et al. Cardiac output in newborn infants with transient myocardial dysfunction. J Pediatr 1985;107:781–5.

24. Ferdman B, Jureidini SB, Gale G, et al. Severe left ventricular dysfunction and arrhythmias as complications of gram-positive sepsis: Rapid recovery in children. Pediatr Cardiol 1998;19:482–6.

25. Feltes TF, Pignatelli R, Kleinert S, et al. Quantitated left ventricular systolic mechanics in children with septic shock utilizing noninvasive wall-stress analysis. Crit Care Med 1994;22:1647–58.

26. Ceneviva G, Paschall JA, Maffei F, et al. Hemodynamic support in fluid-refractory pediatric septic shock. Pediatrics 1998;102:e19.

27. Brierly J, Thiruchelvan T, Peters MJ, et al. Hemodynamics of early pediatric fluid resistant septic shock using non-invasive cardiac output (USCOM) distinct profiles of CVC infection and community acquired sepsis. Crit Care Med 2006;33. 171-T.

28. Deep A, Goonasekera CD, Wang Y, et al. Evolution of haemodynamics and outcome of fluid-refractory septic shock in children. Intensive Care Med 2013; 39:1602–9.

29. Scott HF, Donoghue AJ, Gaieski DF, et al. The utility of early lactate testing in undifferentiated pediatric systemic inflammatory response syndrome. Acad Emerg Med 2012;19:1276–80.

30. Scott HF, Brou L, Deakyne SJ, et al. Association between early lactate levels and 30-day mortality in clinically suspected sepsis in children. JAMA Pediatr 2017; 171(3):249–55.

31. Fenton KE, Sable CA, Bell MJ, et al. Increases in serum levels of troponin I are associated with cardiac dysfunction and disease severity in pediatric patients with septic shock. Pediatr Crit Care Med 2004;5:533–8.

32. Briassoulis G, Narlioglou M, Zavras N, et al. Myocardial injury in meningococcus-induced purpura fulminans in children. Intensive Care Med 2001;27:1073–82.

33. Thiru Y, Pathan N, Bignall S, et al. A myocardial cytotoxic process is involved in the cardiac dysfunction of meningococcal septic shock. Crit Care Med 2000;28: 2979–83.

34. Langley RJ, Wong HR. Early diagnosis of sepsis: is an integrated omics approach the way forward? Mol Diagn Ther 2017;21(5):525–37.

35. Wong HR, Cvijanovich NZ, Anas N, et al. Improved risk stratification in pediatric septic shock using both protein and mRNA biomarkers. PERSEVERE-XP. Am J Respir Crit Care Med 2017;196(4):494–501.

36. Tang BM, Eslick GD, Craig JC, et al. Accuracy of procalcitonin for sepsis diagnosis in critically ill patients: systematic review and meta-analysis. Lancet Infect Dis 2007;7:210–7.

37. Hochreiter M, Kohler T, Schweiger AM, et al. Procalcitonin to guide duration of antibiotic therapy in intensive care patients: a randomized prospective controlled trial. Crit Care 2009;13:R83.

38. Kaplan JM, Wong HR. Biomarkers discovery and development in critical care medicine. Pediatr Crit Care Med 2011;12(No. 2):165–73.

39. Weiss SL, Fitzgerald JC, Maffei FA, et al, SPROUT Study Investigators and Pediatric Acute Lung Injury and Sepsis Investigators Network. Discordant identification of pediatric severe sepsis by research and clinical definitions in the SPROUT international point prevalence study. Crit Care 2015;19:325.

40. Balamuth F, Weiss SL, Hall M, et al. Identifying pediatric severe sepsis and septic shock: accuracy of diagnosis codes. J Pediatr 2015;167:1295–300.e4.

41. Angus DC, Linde-Zwirble WT, Lidicker J, et al. Epidemiology of severe sepsis in the United States: analysis of incidence, outcome, and associated costs of care. Crit Care Med 2001;29:1303–10.

42. Maitland K, Pamba A, English M, et al. Randomized trial of volume expansion with albumin or saline in children with severe malaria: Preliminary evidence of albumin benefit. Clin Infect Dis 2005;40:538–45.

43. Finfer S, Bellomo R, Boyce N, et al, SAFE Study Investigators. A comparison of albumin and saline for fluid resuscitation in the intensive care unit. N Engl J Med 2004;350:2247–56.

44. Carcillo JA, Davis AL, Zaritsky A, et al. Role of early fluid resuscitation in pediatric septic shock. JAMA 1991;266:1242–5.

45. Weiss SL, Keele L, Balamuth F, et al. Crystalloid Fluid Choice and Clinical Outcomes in Pediatric Sepsis: A Matched Retrospective Cohort Study. J Pediatr 2017;182:304–10.

46. Zaritzky AL, Nadkarni VM, Kickey RW, et al. Pediatric advanced life support manual. Dallas (TX): American Heart Association; 2002.

47. Ralston M, Hazinski MF, Zaritsky AL, et al. Pediatric advanced life support manual. Dallas (TX): American Heart Association; 2006.

48. Kleinman ME, Chameides L, Schexnayder SM, et al. Pediatric advanced life support: 2010 America Heart Association. Guidelines for cardiopulmonary resuscitation and, emergency cardiovascular care. Circulation 2010;126(5):e1361–99.

49. Brierley J, Carcillo JA, Choong K, et al. Clinical practice parameters for hemodynamic support of pediatric and neonatal septic shock: 2007 update fromthe American College of Critical Care Medicine. Crit Care Med 2009;37(2):666–88.

50. Paul R, Neuman MI, Monuteaux MC, et al. Adherence to PALS sepsis guidelines and hospital length of stay. Pediatrics 2012;130:e273–80.

51. Stoner MJ, Goodman DG, Cohen DM, et al. Rapid fluid resuscitation in pediatrics; testing the ACCM guidelines. Crit Care Med 2005;33:A68.

52. Hjortrup PB, Haase N, Wetterslev J, et al. Effects of fluid restriction on measures of circulatory efficacy in adults with septic shock. Acta Anaesthesiol Scand 2017; 61(4):390–8.

53. Rhodes A, Evans LE, Alhazzani W, et al. Surviving sepsis campaign: international guidelines for management of sepsis and septic shock: 2016. Intensive Care Med 2017;43(3):304–77.

54. Parker MJ, Thabane L, Fox-Robichaud A, et al, Canadian Critical Care Trials Group and the Canadian Critical Care Translational Biology Group. A trial to determine whether septic shock-reversal is quicker in pediatric patients randomized to an early goal-directed fluid-sparing strategy versus usual care (SQUEEZE): study protocol for a pilot randomized controlled trial. Trials 2016; 17(1):556.

55. van Paridon BM, Sheppard C, G GG, et al. Alberta Sepsis Network: Timing of antibiotics, volume, and vasoactive infusions in children with sepsis admitted to intensive care. Crit Care 2015;19:293.

56. Kumar A, Roberts D, Wood KE, et al. Duration of hypotension before initiation of effective antimicrobial therapy is the critical determinant of survival in human septic shock. Crit Care Med 2006;34(6):1589–96.

57. Weiss SL, Fitzgerald JC, Balamuth F, et al. Delayed antimicrobial therapy, increases mortality and organ dysfunction duration in pediatric sepsis. Crit Care Med 2014;42:2409–17.

58. Creedon J, Vargas A, et al. Peds emergency care, in press.

59. Ventura AM, Shieh HH, Bousso A, et al. Double-Blind Prospective Randomized Controlled Trial of dopamine versus epinephrine as firstline vasoactive drugs in pediatric septic shock. Crit Care Med 2015;43:2292–302.

60. Redl-Wenzl EM, Armbruster C, Edelmann G, et al. The effects of norepinephrine on hemodynamics and renal function in severe septic shock states. Intensive Care Med 1993;19:151–4.

61. Sakr Y, Reinhart K, Vincent JL, et al. Does dopamine administration in shock influence outcome? Results of the Sepsis Occurrence in Acutely Ill Patients (SOAP) Study. Crit Care Med 2006;34:589–97.

62. Meadows D, Edwards JD, Wilkins RG, et al. Reversal of intractable septic shock with norepinephrine therapy. Crit Care Med 1988;16:663–6.

63. Desjars P, Pinaud M, Potel G, et al. A reappraisal of norepinephrine therapy in human septic shock. Crit Care Med 1987;15:134–7.

64. Morimatsu H, Singh K, Uchino S, et al. Early and exclusive use of norepinephrine in septic shock. Resuscitation 2004;62:249–54.

65. Hall LG, Oyen LJ, Taner CB, et al. Fixed-dose vasopressin compared with titrated dopamine and norepinephrine as initial vasopressor therapy for septic shock. Pharmacotherapy 2004;24:1002–12.

66. Lampin ME, Rousseaux J, Botte A, et al. Noradrenaline use for septic shock in children: Doses, routes of administration and complications. Acta Paediatr 2012;101:e426–30.

67. Tourneux P, Rakza T, Abazine A, et al. Noradrenaline for management of septic shock refractory to fluid loading and dopamine or dobutamine in full-term newborn infants. Acta Paediatr 2008;97(2):177–80.

68. Wong HR, Cvijanovich NZ, Allen GL, et al. Corticosteroids are associated, with repression of adaptive immunity gene programs in pediatric septic shock. Am J Respir Crit Care Med 2014;189:940–6.

69. Han YY, Kissoon N, Carcillo JA, et al. The Global Pediatric Sepsis Initiative. Pediatr Crit Care Med 2014;15(suppl):15–6.

70. Paul R, Melendez E, Wathen B, et al. A quality improvement collaborative for pediatric sepsis: lessons learned. Pediatric Patient Safety and Quality 2018;3(1): e051.

Critical Care in the Pediatric Emergency Department

Kristen A. Smith, MD, MS, Heidi R. Flori, MD*

KEYWORDS

- TBI • Seizure • Respiratory failure • Metabolic • Cardiac • Critical care

KEY POINTS

- Acute respiratory failure and pediatric acute respiratory distress syndrome must be identified and precisely managed in the emergency department.
- A large number of patients with congenital heart disease, either before or after surgery, will return to emergency department with both cardiac and medical illnesses requiring specific and aggressive attention.
- Management of pediatric traumatic brain injury may include intracranial pressure monitor placement and management of intracranial hypertension with hyperosmolar therapy, sedation and analgesia, ventilator management, and consultation with pediatric neurosurgery.
- After the initial 1-hour management in pediatric status epilepticus, general anesthesia with midazolam infusion is recommended as next-tier therapy.
- Presentation of inborn errors of metabolism may be severe yet vague and require time-sensitive and specific management.

INTRODUCTION

The pediatric intensive care unit (PICU) shares a symbiotic and complementary relationship with the pediatric emergency department (ED). Efficient management on one end will inevitably benefit efficient care and throughput on the other. This is particularly relevant for ED patients being transported to a PICU at another institution and/or if high census in the receiving PICU requires a transient delay in the ED to PICU transfer. Accordingly, many clinical practice guidelines for some of our most common diagnoses involve phases of care that greatly benefit from critical care management that commences in the ED.

Disclosure Statement: Neither Dr K.A. Smith nor Dr H.R. Flori has any relationships with commercial entities with direct financial interest in the subject matter or materials discussed or with companies making competing products.
Pediatric Critical Care Medicine, University of Michigan School of Medicine, 1500 East Medical Center Drive, SPC 5243, Ann Arbor, MI 48109-5243, USA
* Corresponding author.
E-mail address: heidiflo@med.umich.edu

This article is broken down into critical illness categories based on primary organ system involved (respiratory, neurologic, cardiovascular, and metabolic) and focuses on "beyond the first hour" strategies in selected disease processes for each category. The management of septic shock is covered in the Raina Paul's article, "Recognition, Diagnostics and Management of Pediatric Severe Sepsis and Septic Shock in the Emergency Department," elsewhere in this issue of *Pediatric Clinics of North America*. Basics of resuscitation are not covered.

ACUTE RESPIRATORY FAILURE

Respiratory emergencies account for a great proportion of all ED visits. The vast majority of patients will be evaluated and managed without need for critical care interventions; however, a significant minority will require advanced respiratory care before transfer to a PICU can be accomplished. For patients in overt respiratory failure, intubation and mechanical ventilation are required. There has been a dramatic increase in the use of noninvasive respiratory support such as continuous positive airway pressure/biphasic positive airway pressure and heated high-flow nasal cannula (HHFNC) with data supporting these modalities decreasing the need for intubation.[1] The availability of these technologies coupled with the expertise of our pediatric respiratory therapists in the manipulation of these modalities has allowed expanded use in ED environments.[1–3]

HEATED HIGH-FLOW NASAL CANNULA

HHFNC have been successfully implemented in all age groups: from neonate through adulthood.[4,5] This success is multifactorial. The added humidity of the flow provides excellent mucolysis. HHFNC provides improved ventilation and "wash out" of physiologic dead space in the upper airways. The increased flow provides support to the increasing minute ventilation needs of the pediatric patient with increasing respiratory distress. Usual HHFNC rates often supply a bit of end-expiratory pressure that can stent the closing airway. This feature can be the biggest liability to this modality as well, because the provider must be clear to assess whether the patient is "flow starved" and therefore will respond nicely to HHFNC, or whether the patient is "pressure starved" in which case use of HHFNC will be inappropriate and the provider risks delaying the needed transition to positive pressure strategies such as continuous positive airway pressure/biphasic positive airway pressure or invasive mechanical ventilation. The HHFNC "dose" required to reduce the effort of breathing has been recently determined to be approximately 1.5 to 2.0 L/kg/min.[6] Flows are not usually greater than 8 LPM in infants with variable rates used in children but usually less than 20 LPM, and up to 50 LPM in adults.[4] Research predicting patients at increased risk of HHFNC failure is limited, but some authors have identified failure to have improvement in oxygenation indices (SpO_2/Fio_2 ratio of <200) within 1 hour after initiation portends the need for more invasive support.[7]

HHFNC systems that experience acute increases in pressure from a kinking of the tubing, for example, will "pop-off" with cessation of forward flow to the patient. Unless the system is reset with this occurrence, the patient will have nasal prongs in place with no flow of gas, resulting in partial occlusion of the airway. Risks of delayed escalation of care or unidentified equipment failure can be best mitigated by the use of operationalized guidelines that include appropriate initiation strategies and distinct reassessment by qualified providers to ensure patient tolerance and improvement. Finally, some HHFNC systems are not portable, which may mean use of an alternate modality of respiratory support when transferring the patient from the ED to a different location in the hospital.

PEDIATRIC ACUTE RESPIRATORY DISTRESS SYNDROME IN THE EMERGENCY DEPARTMENT

Acute respiratory distress syndrome (ARDS) was first described by David Ashbough in 1966[8] in a case series of 12 patients with a syndrome consisting of acute hypoxemia, poor lung compliance, and bilateral infiltrates on chest radiograph. Interestingly, 4 of those 12 patients were between 11 and 19 years of age. Since that time, definitions have changed and included hypoxemia assessments based on oxygen saturation rather than arterial blood gas.

The *1994 American European Consensus Conference*[9] determined the minimal oxygenation defect required for the diagnosis of ARDS to be a Pao_2/Fio_2 of less than 300. Biomarker studies in children, as in adults, have confirmed alveolar epithelial and vascular endothelial injury even in the earliest days of hypoxemia and, in about 25% of cases, before invasive mechanical ventilation was started.[10] The mission of the National Institutes of Health–funded Prevention and Early Treatment of Acute Lung Injury network (available from: http://petalnet.org) includes partnering intensive care units (ICUs) with EDs for earlier diagnosis and initiation of supportive measures.

In 2015, the Pediatric Acute Lung Injury Consensus Conference[11] determined new, specific definitions for patients with pediatric ARDS (PARDS) (**Table 1**). Patients who are invasively mechanically ventilated or on full face mask biphasic positive airway pressure may qualify for PARDS. Further, patients with comorbidities, such as cyanotic heart disease, chronic lung disease, and left ventricular dysfunction, now have specific criteria enabling a PARDS diagnosis. The Pediatric Acute Lung Injury Consensus Conference also defined an at-risk group as those patients with a milder acute hypoxemia, acute pulmonary disease on chest radiography—whether unilateral or bilateral—and an associated diagnosis within 7 days of this clinical presentation. The preferred assessment of oxygenation defect for PARDS should be oxygenation index if arterial blood gas available or oxygenation saturation index if no arterial blood gas available.

- Oxygenation index = $(Fio_2 * \text{Mean airway pressure} * 100)/Pao_2$
- Oxygenation saturation index = $(Fio_2 * \text{Mean airway pressure} * 100)/SaO_2$

Why is earlier diagnosis, even when in the ED, relevant? Mechanistic studies in both adults and children have indicated that ARDS pathophysiology starts far before

Table 1
2015 PALICC definition of PARDS

Age	Excludes Perinatal Lung Disease
Timing	Within 7 d of known ARDS risk factor
Pulmonary edema etiology	Not cardiac or fluid overload based
Oxygenation defect: mild PARDS	$4 \leq OI < 8$ or $5 \leq OSI < 7.5$
Oxygenation defect: moderate PARDS	$8 \leq OI < 16$ or $7.5 \leq OSI < 12.3$
Oxygenation defect: severe PARDS	$OI \geq 16$ or $OSI \geq 12.3$

Abbreviations: ARDS, acute respiratory distress syndrome; OI, oxygenation index; OSI, oxygenation saturation index; PALICC, Pediatric Acute Lung Injury Consensus Conference; PARDS, pediatric acute respiratory distress syndrome.

mechanical ventilation is initiated.[10] Even recent studies indicate that many patients with ARDS are not identified as such early in their course and sometimes are never properly diagnosed. Although therapies do not exist to reverse existing ARDS, it is well-known that improperly applied mechanical ventilation, fluid resuscitation, and/or sedation that results in improper patient/ventilator synchrony can quickly result in worsened ventilator-induced lung injury physiology. To date, randomized, controlled trials in adults and large observational studies in children have endorsed lung protective mechanical ventilation,[12] attainment of a euvolemic fluid balance (after shock has been reversed),[13–15] and goal-directed, nurse-implemented sedation.[16] Some of the recent Pediatric Acute Lung Injury Consensus Conference recommendations for ventilation in patients with PARDS[11] include physiologic tidal volume 3 to 8 mL/kg, increased positive end-expiratory pressure (PEEP) (up to 15 in severe ARDS) limiting plateau pressure to 28 cm H_2O, targeting saturations of 88% to 97%, targeting pH 7.15 to 7.30, and use of cuffed endotracheal tubes to maintain mean airway pressure and PEEP.

NEUROLOGIC EMERGENCIES

Pediatric neurocritical care focuses on timely recognition and stabilization of conditions that threaten central and peripheral nervous function. The recognition process begins in the ED. This section focuses on the advances in evaluation and management of pediatric traumatic brain injury and status epilepticus (SE). Routine ABCs and Advanced Trauma Life Support guidelines are not covered.

Traumatic Brain Injury

Traumatic brain injury (TBI) is the leading cause of death and disability in children in the United States, accounting for nearly 500,000 ED visits annually. The rate of injury after a fall is increasing and there remains a paucity of evidence on improving long-term neurologic outcomes.[17] For this reason, we prioritize immediate stabilization to prevent secondary injury—the primary goal of ED and ICU care. This begins and continues with ongoing vigilance of airway, breathing, and circulation. Secondary insults like hypoxia and hypotension have devastating effects on the injured brain.

Airway

Neuroprotective goals of airway management include prevention of hypoxia and hypercarbia. To accomplish this goal, ensure the patient has a patent airway and adequate level of consciousness to allow for adequate respiration. An experienced provider should intubate any patient with a Glasgow Coma Score of 8 or less, unstable facial fractures, and/or hemodynamic instability. Field intubations should be avoided unless performed by experienced personnel.[18] Oral intubation should be performed with attention to maintaining alignment of the cervical spine. Modified rapid sequence induction is recommended with additional support immediately available.

Evidence on optimal rapid sequence induction agents for trauma patients remains lacking.[19] Etomidate and a short-acting nondepolarizing agent such as rocuronium remain safe options for minimizing effects on hemodynamics and intracranial pressure (ICP), but concerns regarding the potential for adrenal insufficiency with repeated use remain. A narcotic with benzodiazepine plus neuromuscular blockade remains another option with the risk of hypotension, but the benefit of analgesia and anxiolysis. Ketamine is relatively contraindicated[20] out of concern for elevating the ICP, but recent evidence suggests this may be unfounded. Propofol should be avoided owing to dose-related hypotension,[19] with resultant hypoperfusion related secondary brain injury.

Breathing

Patients with TBI are at risk for lung injury from aspiration, pulmonary contusion, or neurogenic pulmonary edema after injury, requiring vigilance in ventilation and oxygenation strategies. Further, disordered control of breathing is common after TBI. The following are recommendations for neuroprotective strategies when mechanically ventilating patients with TBI.

- The use of end-tidal carbon dioxide capnometry is the standard of care in trauma resuscitation. Goal-directed ventilation aims for $Paco_2$ of 35 to 40 mm Hg, using end-tidal carbon dioxide as a surrogate.[21] Values of greater than 40 are associated with increased cerebral blood volume and resultant increases in ICP. Values of less than 35 increase the risk for long-term cerebral ischemia.
- Pulse oximetry should be used to achieve SpO_2 of 90% to 98%. Hyperoxia can cause additional free radical damage to the injured brain and should be avoided.
- The use of PEEP is controversial owing to increased intrathoracic pressure causing increased ICP. Generally, PEEP of 5 to 10 cm H_2O is safe.[22]
- Tidal volumes of 6 to 8 mL/kg are recommended.
- There is no evidence supporting superiority or inferiority of any single mode of ventilation.

Circulation

The primary aim in TBI resuscitation is to provide adequate blood supply to the injured brain by balancing cerebral blood volume with ICP. Hypotension should be addressed rapidly with crystalloid in 20 mL/kg aliquots. Once a patient has received 40 to 60 mL/kg of crystalloid, consider colloid resuscitation to prevent crystalloid toxicity. Targeted blood pressure (BP) management is aimed at maintaining an adequate cerebral perfusion pressure (CPP; **Table 2**). If vasoactive agents are needed to maintain CPP, norepinephrine remains the first-line agent.[23] Beware of hypotension without an increase in the heart rate, which is concerning for neurogenic shock and spinal cord injury; imaging should be obtained and neurosurgery contacted immediately.

Cerebral perfusion pressure

CPP is based on arterial BP monitoring or central venous pressure and ICP. Until the ICP monitor is placed, however, clinicians must rely on noninvasive BP and estimation of ICP. Discussions are ongoing regarding the appropriate CPP for age in children because the cerebral metabolic rate and cerebral blood flow vary from infancy to adolescence and adult standards may be inappropriate. Most pediatric trauma centers use an age-based guideline (see **Table 2**).

Table 2	
Cerebral perfusion pressure goals by age	
Age	**mm Hg**
0–5 y	>40
6–17 y	>50
>18 y	50–60

Data from Allen BB, Chiu YL, Gerber LM, et al. Age-specific cerebral perfusion pressure thresholds and survival in children and adolescents with severe traumatic brain injury*. Pediatr Crit Care Med 2014;15(1):62–70.

Radiologic evaluation

Emergent neuroimaging is indicated in all TBI.[24] Computed tomography scanning is the preferred modality because it will identify fracture, blood, midline shift, and cerebral edema. MRI is not indicated emergently, because most lesions with an acute intervention can be identified on computed tomography scans, which can be obtained more rapidly without need for anesthesia.

Invasive neuromonitoring

ICP monitoring is indicated for all patients with Glasgow Coma Score of 8 or less. Different types of monitors are available with the ultimate determination residing in the hands of the neurosurgeon. Externalized ventricular drains have the added benefit of cerebral spinal fluid drainage in addition to monitoring, whereas parenchymal monitors can only transduce pressure. Goal-directed management targets an age-based ICP and CPP (see **Table 2**).[25] A CPP of less than 40 mm Hg is associated with increased mortality and worse functional outcomes. Because not all systems are compatible, if the patient is to be transferred to another facility after monitor placement, it is imperative to ensure that the receiving facility can transduce ICP using the chosen modality.

Acute management of intracranial hypertension

The diagnosis of ICH is based on vital signs (bradycardia, hypertension, irregular respirations, pupillary examination, posturing) until invasive monitoring in place. As shown in **Fig. 1**, early management options including elevation of the head of the

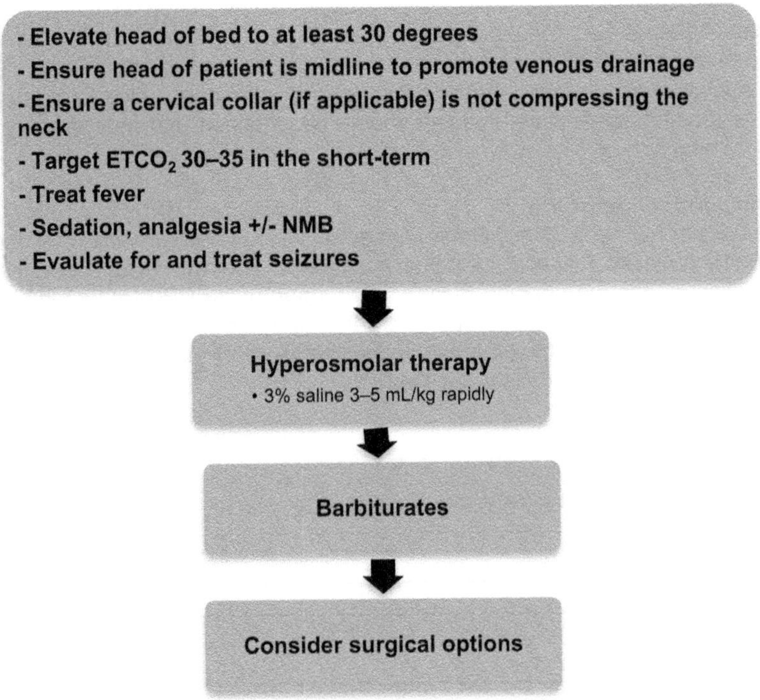

Fig. 1. Acute management of intracranial hypertension. $ETCO_2$, end-tidal carbon dioxide; NMB, neuromuscular blockade.

bed, placing the head midline, avoiding neck compression from a cervical collar, and mild hyperventilation. All can be performed at the bedside with minimal assistance and yet are brain saving. Other management options are vital, but require some coordination and planning and are reviewed herein.

Temperature regulation

Fever should be prevented in all patients with TBI. Normothermia is the goal, because hypothermia has no proven benefit. Begin with antipyretics, if no contraindication is present; however, cooling devices may be required.[26] If so, invasive temperature monitoring is needed and neuromuscular blockade should be used to prevent shivering. If your unit is unfamiliar with the use of cooling devices, seek an expert opinion.

Sedation

Adequate sedation and analgesia are the standard of care in trauma. Not only does this measure control symptoms associated with trauma, but also appropriate level of sedation will reduce cerebral metabolic rate and reduce ICP. Neuromuscular blockade should be used if ICP remains elevated despite adequate sedation and analgesia.

Seizures

Patients should be evaluated with electroencephalography (EEG) as clinically indicated. Seizures should be treated aggressively because they increase the cerebral metabolic rate and elevate the ICP. Prolonged seizures are associated with poor outcomes.

Hyperosmolar therapy

Hyperosmolar therapy is a mainstay in management of ICH, but the agent of choice is controversial. Hypertonic (3%) saline is more proven and recommended in the 2012 TBI guidelines.[27] Dosing for 3% saline is 3 to 5 mL/kg given rapidly, aiming for a goal sodium of 145 to 155 mmol/L. Patients may only require bolus dosing, but infusions are also helpful.[28] Mannitol is as effective, but carries significantly more risk, especially acutely. Mannitol has been associated with abrupt hypotension, which is increased in the presence of hypovolemia in trauma patients and can cause renal crystallization and acute kidney injury.[28]

Barbiturates

Barbiturates are extremely effective in decreasing the cerebral metabolic rate and ICP.[27] They carry significant risk, however. Barbiturates can cause diminished cardiac output, hypotension, and increased intrapulmonary shunting. They should not be used without invasive BP and ICP monitoring and expert consultation.

Surgical options

Decompressive craniectomy (DC) has been suggested for ICH refractory to maximal medical management. However, the utility remains controversial. Recently, 2 randomized controlled trials proved that early DC improves ICP and ICU duration of stay, but results in worse functional outcomes. The DECRA trial showed DC resulted in lower ICP, fewer interventions to control ICP, and a duration of shorter ICU stay, but increased mortality and worse functional outcomes.[29] The RESCUEICP trial showed that DC resulted in reduced mortality but increased incidence of vegetative state.[30]

STATUS EPILEPTICUS

SE is a continuous seizure for greater than 5 minutes or 2 or more discrete seizures between which there is incomplete recovery of consciousness. After 30 minutes without recovery of consciousness, the brain suffers irreversible excitotoxicity.[31] Thus, it is within this window where we focus treatment efforts. The basics of management, including airway, breathing, and circulation, are not reviewed herein.

Etiology

SE is one of the most common neurologic emergencies in children. It is encountered in nearly 20 per 100,000 children-years[32] and more common in children less than 12 months of age.[33] In first-time seizures, 12% present in SE.[34] The most common causes of SE in children are infection with fever, low medication levels, and remote symptomatic causes.[35] Mortality of SE is less than 10%, but higher in cases of bacterial meningitis, metabolic disorders, and progressive neurodegenerative conditions.[32] If left untreated, cases of refractory SE carry the highest morbidity and mortality (16%–32%).[36]

Neurologic Monitoring

EEG is recommended for all patients in SE. For patients with refractory SE and other select patients, continuous EEG is preferred. Nearly one-half of patients who no longer have clinical seizures remain in nonconvulsive SE, so prolonged EEG should be considered.[37]

Imaging is deferred until seizures are controlled.[38–40] Once stable for imaging, MRI is preferred unless seizures are related to trauma. Cytotoxic edema from seizure can mimic acute stroke on MRI, so neuroradiology should be consulted. Emergent neuroimaging is reserved for patients with histories and physical examinations consistent with trauma or intracranial mass, but cessation of seizure activity takes priority.

Management

Antiepileptic drugs

A summary guideline is found in **Fig. 2**. For antiepileptic drug dosing and side effects, see **Table 3**. Children on existing antiepileptic drugs may not follow a traditional guideline because they may be dosed with medications they are already on, because they have been effective for these children in their past. Consult your pediatric neurologist for assistance.

The initial treatment of SE with benzodiazepines at 5 minutes remains the mainstay of treatment.[41] The dose may be repeated at 10 minutes (see **Fig. 2**). No single benzodiazepine has been found to be more effective than others, so give what is available by any mode available (intravenous, intramuscular, per rectum, etc). Intramuscular midazolam is as effective as intravenous for the cessation of seizures, preventing hospitalization, and preventing ICU admission.[42]

Refractory status epilepticus

After seizure has persisted for 20 to 30 minutes without return to baseline, 10% to 25% of SE becomes refractory.[43] This is also when disordered control of breathing becomes apparent. Early intubation is warranted if apnea, desaturation, or the inability to protect one's airway is present. The most commonly used agents in refractory SE are phenobarbital, fosphenytoin, valproic acid, and levetiracetam (see **Table 3**). Phenobarbital has falling out of favor in children less than 1 year of age owing to concerns for long-term cognitive impairment. Fosphenytoin is effective, but not without risk. It can cause arrhythmia, hypotension, and apnea. Additionally, to avoid cardiovascular collapse, it needs to be run over 30 to 60 minutes. Valproic acid is effective in aborting seizures but contraindicated in patients less than 2 years of age, those with hepatic dysfunction, and those with mitochondrial disorders. Levetiracetam

1st Tier: Status Epilepticus	
Within 5–20 min of seizure onset	
If IV access: • Lorazepam 0.1 mg/kg IV (Max 4 mg) • Diazepam 0.2 mg/kg IV (Max 10 mg) • Midazolam 0.2 mg/kg IV (Max 10 mg) May repeat once after 5 min	If no IV access: • Midazolam IN, buccal, or IM 0.2 mg/kg (Max 10 mg) • Diazepam PR 0.2–0.5 mg/kg (Max 20 mg) May repeat once after 5–10 min
2nd Tier: Refractory Status Epilepticus	
Within 20–30 min of seizure onset **Alert critical care team for ICU admission** **Consult pediatric neurology and initiate EEG monitoring**	

Children 1 – 12 mo
 • Phenobarbital 20–30 mg/kg IV
     o May repeat 10 mg/kg after 10 min
 • Levetiracetam 60 mg/kg IV
	Children > 12 mo
	 • Fosphenytoin 20 mg PE/kg IV or IM (Max 1500 mg PE)
	     o May repeat 10 mg PE/kg after 10 min
	 • Levetiracetam 60 mg/kg IV (Max 2500 mg)
	 • Valproic Acid 20–40 mg/kg IV (No Max)

3rd Tier: Super-refractory Status Epilepticus	
Within 30–60 min of seizure onset Proceed with endotracheal intubation	

Begin general anesthesia with a continuous infusion
 Target cessation of seizure for 24–48 h
 • Midazolam: Titrate infusion until cessation of seizure
     o Bolus 0.2 mg/kg IV (Max 10 mg)
     o Infusion start at 100–200 mcg/kg/hr
 • If no cessation of seizure:
     o Repeat bolus 0.2 mg/kg (Max 10 mg) AND
     o Increase infusion by 50–100 mcg/kg/hr
 • Dosing range 400–2000 mcg/kg/hr	

4th Tier: Super-refractory Status Epilepticus, continued	
Beyond 60 min If not intubated, intubate now	

Continue general anesthesia with a different agent
 Target burst suppression for 24–48 h
 • Pentobarbital
     o Bolus 5 mg/kg (No Max)
     o Infusion start at 0.5 mg/kg/hr
 • If no burst suppression
     o Repeat bolus 2–5 mg/kg (No Max) AND
     o Increase infusion by 0.5 mg/kg/hr
 • Monitor for bradycardia, hypotension, intestinal ischemia, and paralytic ileus	

Fig. 2. Treatment Algorithm of Status Epilepticus in Children. EEG, electroencephalography; ICU, intensive care unit; IM, intramuscularly; IN, intranasally; IV, intravenously; PE, phenytoin equivalents; PR, per rectum.

has the best side effect profile and is becoming most providers' first agent after benzodiazepines.

Superrefractory status epilepticus

If seizure persists despite first- and second-line therapies, the child has superrefractory SE and general anesthesia is indicated.[44] Two commonly used agents to induce general anesthesia are administered intravenously—midazolam and pentobarbital. Both require a stable airway and continuous EEG monitoring. Arterial

Table 3
Antiepileptic agents for treatment of status epilepticus

Drug	Dose	Route	Side Effects
Lorazepam	0.1 mg/kg (maximum 4 mg)	IV	Respiratory depression
Diazepam	0.2 mg/kg (maximum 10 mg)	IV, PR	Cardiovascular compromise
Midazolam	0.2 mg/kg (maximum 10 mg)	IV, IN, Buccal, IM	
Phenobarbital	20–30 mg/kg	IV	Respiratory depression Cardiovascular compromise
Levetiracetam	60 mg/kg	IV	Somnolence
Fosphenytoin	20 mg PE/kg (maximum 1500 mg PE)	IV, IM	Respiratory depression Cardiovascular compromise Arrhythmia
Valproic Acid	20–40 mg/kg	IV	Contraindicated in patients <2 y and those with known hepatic failure or mitochondrial disease
Midazolam infusion	Starting dose 100–200 μg/kg/h	IV	Respiratory depression Cardiovascular compromise
Pentobarbital	Starting dose 0.5 mg/kg/h	IV	Respiratory depression Dose-related hypotension Bradycardia Paralytic ileus Intestinal ischemia
Propofol	Consult an expert	IV	PRIS Pain with injection Dose-related hypotension
Ketamine	Consult an expert	IV	Tachycardia Hypertension
Isoflurane	Consult an expert		Cardiovascular compromise Infection DVT Paralytic ileus

Abbreviations: DVT, deep venous thrombosis; IM, intramuscular; IN, intranasal; INH, inhaled; IV, intravenous; PE, phenytoin equivalents; PR, per rectum; PRIS, propofol infusion syndrome.

BP monitoring is recommended because they both can cause cardiovascular compromise.

Midazolam is generally accepted to be the first-line anesthetic agent. It works by enhancing the affinity at the gamma-amino butyric acid A (GABA$_A$) receptor, causing opening of chloride-gated channels. Once channels are open, the postsynaptic membrane is hyperpolarized, which renders the postsynaptic neuron resistant to excitation.[45] Midazolam at anesthetic doses is as effective in aborting SE as other intravenous anesthetic agents, yet has a lower mortality.[46] High-dose infusions control seizures in more than one-half of patients with refractory SE.[47,48] The use of high-dose infusions carries a similar side effect profile as low-dose infusions, but are superior in the cessation of seizure activity. Side effects include dose-related hypotension but at a lesser incidence (8%) than with other agents (71%).[49] Vasopressors are occasionally needed and epinephrine is the preferred agent.

Pentobarbital acts by binding the GABA$_A$ receptor and potentiating activity at chloride-gated channels, hyperpolarizing the postsynaptic membrane and making the postsynaptic neuron less excitable—similar to midazolam. It is as effective at aborting seizures as midazolam,[45] but has a worse side effect profile. In addition to a higher incidence of hypotension, patients on pentobarbital require more days of mechanical ventilation and have an increased incidence of ventilator-associated pneumonias, bowel ischemia, and intestinal ileus.[50]

Other agents used to treat SE include propofol and ketamine infusions and inhaled anesthetics. These agents should not be used without consultation with anesthesia and intensive care. Propofol is a general anesthetic with direct activity at $GABA_A$ receptors. It is a potent anticonvulsant with a rapid onset and metabolism.[51,52] Dose-related hypotension is a known side effect and vasopressors are often needed. Propofol infusion syndrome is a life-threatening complication associated with prolonged propofol use. Propofol infusion syndrome was first described in children and is caused by mitochondrial dysfunction. Clinically, it presents as lactic acidosis, rhabdomyolysis, renal failure, and cardiovascular collapse. If present, propofol should be stopped immediately. Owing to the risk profile of propofol, it is not commonly used to manage SE in children.

Ketamine is an N-methyl D-aspartate antagonist that inhibits glutamate and limits neuronal excitation,[52] thus treating SE. Onset is rapid and patients suffer less hemodynamic instability than with other agents. Owing to its effect on the sympathetic nervous system, hypertension can occur. However, data on long-term exposure are limited and evidence on efficacy is lacking, so it is not commonly used.[53]

Inhaled anesthetics require consultation with pediatric anesthesia, the use of specialized equipment and personnel, and the presence of an endotracheal tube and arterial line. Although effective in controlling seizures, the impact of prolonged exposure is unknown and significant cardiovascular compromise can occur. Additionally, there remain logistical issues with administration and scavenging of gas, so it must be delivered in an operating room or the ICU.[54–56]

CARDIOVASCULAR EMERGENCIES IN PATIENTS WITH CONGENITAL HEART DISEASE

The Centers for Disease Control and Prevention report that congenital heart disease (CHD) affects 1% of births per year in the United States.[57–59] Twenty-five percent of patients born with CHD require surgery or other procedures in their first year of life. Prenatal diagnosis has drastically decreased the number of infants presenting to the ED in cardiogenic shock after closure of ductal-dependent lesions. However, nearly 1.5 million children are living in the United States with CHD and more than 20,000 patients with CHD are operated on annually; 55% are infants and 38% are children less than 18 years of age. The tremendous volume of CHD births, and those patients undergoing surgery, inherently results in these patients coming to EDs for intercurrent illnesses, and/or complications or worsening of their underlying disease processes. It is imperative for pediatric ED clinicians to accurately identify these patients, and to initiate and maintain appropriate care until the patient can be admitted to their destination PICU.

International data indicate that patients with CHD seeking ED care most often present sub acutely with acute respiratory illness, dysrhythmia, worsening cyanosis or heart failure, and other less frequent conditions.[59,60,61] For patients with palliated conditions, such as cavopulmonary anastomoses or Fontan physiology, any respiratory illness can be life threatening. These physiologies are predicated on passive return of venous blood flow to the right heart and, therefore, any condition that would increase transpulmonary pressure can result in severe cyanosis and death. These patients require aggressive, inpatient management of any pneumonic process, pleural effusions, and pulmonary edema. Similarly, these patients do not tolerate a supine position or positive pressure ventilation. For patients with cyanotic heart disease, the hemoglobin should be checked because excessive hypoxemia may be mitigated with transfusion. Patients presenting with worsening cyanosis with underlying history of shunt physiology require immediate echocardiography to identify obstruction to blood flow that may also require urgent surgical or procedural attention. The patient and family should be queried about anticoagulation use at home and possible lapses in dosing, as well as intercurrent risk factors for acute dehydration that may also place the patient at risk for a hypercoagulable state.

Older children with a history of CHD surgery may often present to EDs with syncopal-type events owing to arrhythmias—whether heart block or, more commonly, atrial tachyarrhythmias, such as atrial flutter, because atrial enlargement over time after these surgeries may result in distortion of the conduction systems.

Finally, patients with CHD may have altered immune function,[61] whether asplenia (especially in complete atrioventricular canal and pulmonary atresia) or polysplenia (seen most commonly in interrupted inferior vena cava and total anomalous pulmonary venous return) as well as altered lymphocyte function in patients with DiGeorge syndrome or similar genetic abnormalities. Therefore, all ED clinicians managing patients with a history of CHD and presentation consistent with sepsis, even in its mildest forms, must have a high index of suspicion for the risk of bacterial sepsis and should aggressively diagnose and presumptively apply broad spectrum antibiotics until culture results are ascertained and an accurate history of the potential immunocompromised state is determined.

METABOLIC EMERGENCIES

The acute presentation of neonates and children with inborn errors of metabolism remains an important and anxiety-provoking consideration for both ED and PICU providers.[62,63] Certain inborn errors present most prominently in the neonatal period (amino acid disorders, organic acidemias, urea cycle defects, mitochondrial defects, peroxisomal defects, etc), whereas other patients who retain residual activity of deficient enzymes may present at a later age. Many of these diagnoses are autosomal recessive in inheritance. Fortunately, there are increasing numbers of treatment opportunities available, including but not limited to enzyme replacement therapy, special diets, substrate inhibitors, and even organ transplantation.

These patients often have an acute-on-chronic course heralded by recurrent "attacks" precipitated by fever, fasting, medications, and so on. Each inborn error can present with a variety of vague symptoms such as altered level of consciousness, seizures, hypoglycemia, sepsis, liver failure, and cytopenias, that can lead the practitioner down a primary pathway appropriate for that presentation (ie, antibiotics and cultures for presumed sepsis) but without prompt diagnosis of the underlying cause—the inborn error itself.

Common red flags on laboratory studies include an anion gap metabolic acidosis, presence or absence of lactic acidosis, presence or absence of ketosis, and hyperammonemia in some. If missed, persistent hyperammonemia can be a life-threatening complication soon after the ED presentation, because these patients must be quickly triaged to a PICU that can offer immediate hemodialysis and have access to metabolic disease specialists and pharmacies that can supply alternate hyperammonemia management such as sodium benzoate. In addition, sending blood and urine for quantitative amino acids and qualitative urine organic acids while in the ED is often imperative for proper diagnosis of the patient because these derangements will be less evident as the patient convalesces.

Fortunately, more advanced diagnostics are also becoming standard of care, as is the newborn screening process,[64] so more of these patients are diagnosed before their first catastrophic presentation. More centers are being established as Pediatric Metabolic Disease Centers of Excellence providing structured programs and ED based guidelines for more efficient management. The family may be able to arrive to the ED in crisis but with their specific disease documentation in hand to quickly triage these patients to their appropriate therapeutic regimen.[65]

Management

- Manage the overt presentation (ie, antibiotics and cultures for presumed sepsis).
- Diagnose and manage the inborn error itself (as discussed).
  - NPO pending further deterioration.
    - Enteral feeds may be contributing to metabolic toxicity.
    - Start intravenous glucose and electrolytes.
- Contact a metabolic disease specialist and the PICU immediately.

REFERENCES

1. Wing R, James C, Maranda LS, et al. Use of high-flow nasal cannula support in the emergency department reduces the need for intubation in pediatric acute respiratory insufficiency. Pediatr Emerg Care 2012;28(11):1117–23.

2. Long E, Babl FE, Duke T. Is there a role for humidified heated high-flow nasal cannula therapy in paediatric emergency departments? Emerg Med J 2016;33(6):386–9.

3. Slain KN, Shein SL, Rotta AT. The use of high-flow nasal cannula in the pediatric emergency department. J Pediatr (Rio J) 2017;93(Suppl 1):36–45.

4. Mikalsen IB, Davis P, Oymar K. High flow nasal cannula in children: a literature review. Scand J Trauma Resusc Emerg Med 2016;24:93.

5. Hernandez G, Roca O, Colinas L. High-flow nasal cannula support therapy: new insights and improving performance. Crit Care 2017;21(1):62.

6. Weiler T, Kamerkar A, Hotz J, et al. The relationship between high flow nasal cannula flow rate and effort of breathing in children. J Pediatr 2017;189:66–71.

7. Kamit Can F, Anil A, Anil M, et al. Predictive factors for the outcome of high flow nasal cannula therapy in a pediatric intensive care unit: is the SpO2/FiO2 ratio useful? J Crit Care 2018;44:436–44.

8. Ashbaugh D, Bigelow D, Petty T, et al. Acute respiratory distress in adults. Lancet 1967;Aug 12:319–23.

9. Bernard G, Artigas A, Brigham K, et al. The North American-European consensus conference on ARDS. Am J Respir Crit Care Med 1994;149:818–24.

10. Sapru A, Flori H, Quasney M, et al, Pediatric Acute Lung Injury Consensus Conference Group. Pathobiology of acute respiratory distress syndrome. Pediatr Crit Care Med 2015;16(5Suppl):S6–22.

11. Pediatric Acute Lung Injury Consensus Conference Group. Pediatric acute respiratory distress syndrome: consensus recommendations from the Pediatric Acute Lung Injury Consensus Conference. Pediatr Crit Care Med 2015;16(5):428–39.

12. Acute Respiratory Distress Syndrome Network, Brower RG, Matthay MA, Morris A, et al. Ventilation with lower tidal volumes as compared with traditional tidal volumes for acute lung injury and the acute respiratory distress syndrome. N Engl J Med 2000;342(18):1301–8.

13. Flori HR, Church G, Liu KD, et al. Positive fluid balance is associated with higher mortality and prolonged mechanical ventilation in pediatric patients with acute lung injury. Crit Care Res Pract 2011;2011:854142.

14. Valentine SL, Sapru A, Higgerson RA, et al. Fluid balance in critically ill children with acute lung injury. Crit Care Med 2012;40(10):2883–9.

15. Wiedemann HP, Wheeler AP, Bernard GR, et al. Comparison of two fluid-management strategies in acute lung injury. N Engl J Med 2006;354(24):2564–75.

16. Curley MA, Wypij D, Watson R, et al. Protocolized sedation vs usual care in pediatric patients mechanically ventilated for acute respiratory failure: a randomized clinical trial. JAMA 2015;313(4):379–89.

17. Centers for Disease Control and Prevention National Center for Injury Prevention and Control. Traumatic brain injury and concussion data and statistics. 2016. Available at: https://www.cdc.gov/TraumaticBrainInjury/data/index.html. Accessed November 6, 2017.

18. Stockinger ZT, McSwain NE Jr. Prehospital endotracheal intubation for trauma does not improve survival over bag-valve-mask ventilation. J Trauma 2004; 56(3):531–6.

19. Flower O, Hellings S. Sedation in traumatic brain injury. Emerg Med Int 2012; 2012:637171.

20. Zeiler FA, Teitelbaum J, West M, et al. The ketamine effect on ICP in traumatic brain injury. Neurocrit Care 2014;21(1):163–73.

21. Coles JP, Fryer TD, Coleman MR, et al. Hyperventilation following head injury: effect on ischemic burden and cerebral oxidative metabolism. Crit Care Med 2007; 35(2):568–78.

22. Cooper KR, Boswell PA, Choi SC. Safe use of PEEP in patients with severe head injury. J Neurosurg 1985;63(4):552–5.

23. Di Gennaro JL, Mack CD, Malakouti A, et al. Use and effect of vasopressors after pediatric traumatic brain injury. Dev Neurosci 2010;32(5–6):420–30.

24. Ashwal S, Holshouser BA, Tong KA. Use of advanced neuroimaging techniques in the evaluation of pediatric traumatic brain injury. Dev Neurosci 2006;28(4–5): 309–26.

25. Allen BB, Chiu YL, Gerber LM, et al. Age-specific cerebral perfusion pressure thresholds and survival in children and adolescents with severe traumatic brain injury*. Pediatr Crit Care Med 2014;15(1):62–70.

26. Adelson PD, Wisniewski SR, Beca J, et al. Comparison of hypothermia and normothermia after severe traumatic brain injury in children (Cool Kids): a phase 3, randomised controlled trial. Lancet Neurol 2013;12(6):546–53.

27. Kochanek PM, Carney N, Adelson PD, et al. Guidelines for the acute medical management of severe traumatic brain injury in infants, children, and adolescents–second edition. Pediatr Crit Care Med 2012;13(Suppl 1):S1–82.

28. Burgess S, Abu-Laban RB, Slavik RS, et al. A systematic review of randomized controlled trials comparing hypertonic sodium solutions and mannitol for traumatic brain injury: implications for emergency department management. Ann Pharmacother 2016;50(4):291–300.

29. Cooper DJ, Rosenfeld JV, Murray L, et al. Decompressive craniectomy in diffuse traumatic brain injury. N Engl J Med 2011;364(16):1493–502.

30. Hutchinson PJ, Kolias AG, Timofeev IS, et al. Trial of Decompressive Craniectomy for Traumatic Intracranial Hypertension. N Engl J Med 2016;375(12):1119–30.

31. Fujikawa DG, Itabashi HH, Wu A, et al. Status epilepticus-induced neuronal loss in humans without systemic complications or epilepsy. Epilepsia 2000;41(8): 981–91.

32. Asadi-Pooya AA, Poordast A. Etiologies and outcomes of status epilepticus in children. Epilepsy Behav 2005;7(3):502–5.

33. DeLorenzo RJ. Epidemiology and clinical presentation of status epilepticus. Adv Neurol 2006;97:199–215.

34. Shinnar S, Berg AT, Moshe SL, et al. The risk of seizure recurrence after a first unprovoked afebrile seizure in childhood: an extended follow-up. Pediatrics 1996;98(2 Pt 1):216–25.

35. DeLorenzo RJ, Hauser WA, Towne AR, et al. A prospective, population-based epidemiologic study of status epilepticus in Richmond, Virginia. Neurology 1996;46(4):1029–35.

36. Eriksson KJ, Koivikko MJ. Status epilepticus in children: aetiology, treatment, and outcome. Dev Med Child Neurol 1997;39(10):652–8.

37. DeLorenzo RJ, Waterhouse EJ, Towne AR, et al. Persistent nonconvulsive status epilepticus after the control of convulsive status epilepticus. Epilepsia 1998; 39(8):833–40.

38. Grant PE. Imaging the developing epileptic brain. Epilepsia 2005;46(Suppl 7): 7–14.

39. Scott RC, Gadian DG, King MD, et al. Magnetic resonance imaging findings within 5 days of status epilepticus in childhood. Brain 2002;125(Pt 9):1951–9.

40. Scott RC, King MD, Gadian DG, et al. Hippocampal abnormalities after prolonged febrile convulsion: a longitudinal MRI study. Brain 2003;126(Pt 11): 2551–7.

41. Treiman DM, Meyers PD, Walton NY, et al. A comparison of four treatments for generalized convulsive status epilepticus. Veterans Affairs Status Epilepticus Cooperative Study Group. N Engl J Med 1998;339(12):792–8.

42. Prasad M, Krishnan PR, Sequeira R, et al. Anticonvulsant therapy for status epilepticus. Cochrane Database Syst Rev 2014;(9):CD003723.

43. Berg AT, Levy SR, Novotny EJ, et al. Predictors of intractable epilepsy in childhood: a case-control study. Epilepsia 1996;37(1):24–30.

44. Riviello JJ Jr, Claassen J, LaRoche SM, et al. Treatment of status epilepticus: an international survey of experts. Neurocrit Care 2013;18(2):193–200.

45. Claassen J, Hirsch LJ, Emerson RG, et al. Treatment of refractory status epilepticus with pentobarbital, propofol, or midazolam: a systematic review. Epilepsia 2002;43(2):146–53.

46. Gilbert DL, Gartside PS, Glauser TA. Efficacy and mortality in treatment of refractory generalized convulsive status epilepticus in children: a meta-analysis. J Child Neurol 1999;14(9):602–9.

47. Claassen J, Hirsch LJ, Emerson RG, et al. Continuous EEG monitoring and midazolam infusion for refractory nonconvulsive status epilepticus. Neurology 2001; 57(6):1036–42.

48. Fernandez A, Lantigua H, Lesch C, et al. High-dose midazolam infusion for refractory status epilepticus. Neurology 2014;82(4):359–65.

49. Lampin ME, Dorkenoo A, Lamblin MD, et al. [Use of midazolam for refractory status epilepticus in children]. Rev Neurol (Paris) 2010;166(6–7):648–52.

50. Holmes GL, Riviello JJ Jr. Midazolam and pentobarbital for refractory status epilepticus. Pediatr Neurol 1999;20(4):259–64.

51. Indra S, Haddad H, O'Riordan MA. Short-term propofol infusion and associated effects on serum lactate in pediatric patients. Pediatr Emerg Care 2017;33(11): e118–21.

52. Reznik ME, Berger K, Claassen J. Comparison of intravenous anesthetic agents for the treatment of refractory status epilepticus. J Clin Med 2016;5(5) [pii:E54].

53. Zeiler FA, Teitelbaum J, West M, et al. The ketamine effect on intracranial pressure in nontraumatic neurological illness. J Crit Care 2014;29(6):1096–106.

54. Zeiler FA, Zeiler KJ, Teitelbaum J, et al. Modern inhalational anesthetics for refractory status epilepticus. Can J Neurol Sci 2015;42(2):106–15.

55. Manatpon P, Kofke WA. Toxicity of inhaled agents after prolonged administration. J Clin Monit Comput 2018;32(4):651–66.

56. Ikeda KM, Connors R, Lee DH, et al. Isoflurane use in the treatment of super-refractory status epilepticus is associated with hippocampal changes on MRI. Neurocrit Care 2017;26(3):420–7.

57. Centers for Disease Control and Prevention (CDC). Congenital heart disease data and statistics. CDC 24/7: saving lives, protecting people. 2016. Available at: https://www.cdc.gov/ncbddd/heartdefects/data.html. Accessed October 30, 2017.

58. Congenital Heart Public Health Consortium. Congenital Heart Public Health Consortium fact sheet - long version. 2012. Available at: www.aap.org. Accessed October 30, 2017.

59. Judge P, Meckler Mshs G. Congenital heart disease in pediatric patients: recognizing the undiagnosed and managing complications in the emergency department. Pediatr Emerg Med Pract 2016;13(5):1–28.

60. Lee YS, Baek JS, Kwon BS, et al. Pediatric emergency room presentation of congenital heart disease. Korean Circ J 2010;40(1):36–41.

61. Dalton H, Bakerman P, Biswas S. Cardiovascular critical care. In: Society of Critical Care Medicine, editor. Self-assessment in pediatric multiprofessional critical care. Mount Prospect (IL): Society of Critical Care Medicine; 2010. p. 10–32.

62. Reid Sutton V. Inborn errors of metabolism: metabolic emergencies. Alphen aan den Rijn (The Netherlands): Wolters Kluwer; 2017.

63. Ezgu F. Inborn errors of metabolism. Advances in Clinical Chemistry 2016;73: 195–249.

64. Ezgu F. Recent advances in the molecular diagnosis of inborn errors of metabolism. Clin Biochem 2014;47(9):759–60.

65. Zand DJ, Brown KM, Lichter-Konecki U, et al. Effectiveness of a clinical pathway for the emergency treatment of patients with inborn errors of metabolism. Pediatrics 2008;122(6):1191–5.

Child Abuse and Conditions That Mimic It

Elaine S. Pomeranz, MD[a,b,]*

KEYWORDS

- Child abuse • Sexual abuse • Inflicted injury • Mimics of abuse

KEY POINTS

- Abusive head trauma (AHT) is the most lethal form of child abuse and should be considered in the differential diagnosis of any infant with altered mental status, even without signs of trauma.
- Although abdominal trauma secondary to abuse is less common than accidental abdominal trauma, it is associated with a higher likelihood of hollow organ injury, morbidity, and mortality.
- Bruising or skeletal injury in nonambulatory children is suspicious for abuse. The younger the infant, the higher the index of suspicion should be.
- Even when child abuse can be diagnosed clinically, pertinent laboratory studies should be considered to rule out conditions that mimic child abuse.
- Most child sexual abuse leaves no physical evidence. A normal anogenital examination should be well documented, but does not rule out abuse.

INTRODUCTION

Few diagnostic dilemmas confronting emergency physicians are as fraught as evaluating children for possible child abuse.[1] Histories may be misleading or absent; serious injuries may be missed in the absence of outward signs of trauma, and family members may be emotional for more than the usual reasons. Additionally, either missing it or overdiagnosing it can lead to serious consequences for the child and family. Ensuing physician court testimony may also be a deterrent to making the diagnosis. Nevertheless, it is a legal and moral obligation that all physicians share.

Child abuse has been recognized as a medical issue since 1962 when C. Henry Kempe wrote about the battered child syndrome.[2] In the next decade, national databases were created to track and analyze the problem, leading to a burgeoning of

[a] Department of Pediatrics and Communicable Diseases, University of Michigan, 1540 Hospital Drive, CW 2-737, Ann Arbor, MI 48109, USA; [b] Department of Emergency Medicine, University of Michigan, 1540 Hospital Drive, CW 2-737, Ann Arbor, MI 48109, USA
* Department of Pediatrics and Communicable Diseases, University of Michigan, 1540 Hospital Drive, CW 2-737, Ann Arbor, MI 48109.
E-mail address: pomeranz@med.umich.edu

Pediatr Clin N Am 65 (2018) 1135–1150
https://doi.org/10.1016/j.pcl.2018.07.009
0031-3955/18/© 2018 Elsevier Inc. All rights reserved.

pediatric.theclinics.com

research and the development of a group of experts, while physicians became mandated reporters. Primary care and emergency physicians are on the front lines for suspecting child abuse and for ruling out medical conditions that may mimic abuse.

Because children account for almost one-third of emergency department visits, it is crucial for emergency physicians and primary care physicians to understand the various forms that child abuse takes, the warning signs to recognize, and how to evaluate it in the emergency department setting so that the right thing can be done for the most vulnerable patients.

ABUSIVE HEAD TRAUMA OF INFANCY

Abusive head trauma (AHT) of infancy is current terminology for what has been known by various names including shaken baby syndrome. AHT is the preferred term, as it does not imply a mechanism that may be difficult to prove. AHT is the most lethal form of inflicted childhood trauma in children younger than 4 years of age and most commonly affects infants in the first year of life, for whom the incidence is greater than 20 cases per 100,000 population.[3,4] Many survivors have serious long-term neurologic sequelae, including blindness, deafness, and profound neurocognitive impairment.

Classic findings in AHT are subdural and/or subarachnoid hemorrhages, with or without skull fracture, scalp hematoma, or other external signs of trauma. Retinal hemorrhages are found in most cases[5] and are usually more extensive than any found in minor trauma.[6] Therefore, a dilated eye examination should be obtained in cases of suspected AHT, preferably documented by an ophthalmologist (**Fig. 1**).

Posterior rib fractures are also commonly associated with AHT, and rarely seen in babies with accidental trauma. A skeletal survey should be part of the evaluation of any child under the age of 2 years with suspected abuse. Because rib fractures can be difficult to detect initially and are quite specific for AHT,[7] repeat skeletal imaging 2 weeks after the initial presentation is recommended for its forensic value if the initial skeletal survey obtained at time of presentation is negative (**Fig. 2**).

Although AHT crosses all demographic lines, it is more likely to occur with young parents, chaotic family situations, and if there is an unrelated adult in the household.[8] Perpetrators are most often fathers, followed by mothers' boyfriends, with babysitters and mothers less likely according to a study by Starling and colleagues.[9]

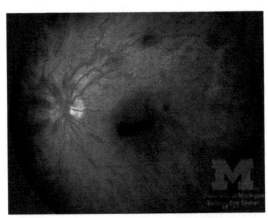

Fig. 1. Extensive retinal hemorrhages. (*Courtesy of* University of Michigan Kellogg Eye Institute.)

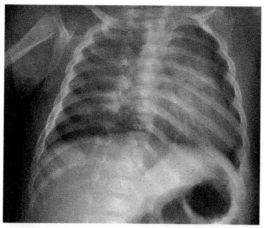

Fig. 2. Multiple healing rib fractures. (*Courtesy* of Peter Strouse, MD.)

A retrospective analysis of the medical records of 173 children identified as having been victims of AHT[10] revealed that the children had been evaluated by medical providers an average of 2.8 times previously, resulting in an average 1 week delay in diagnosis. More than 30% of cases were missed on the initial visit. The younger the baby was, the more nonspecific the presenting findings (eg, vomiting, irritability) and the less likely the diagnosis was to be made. This seminal study underscores the difficulty in diagnosing AHT in children and in ascertaining its true prevalence.

Brain Imaging

There are well developed guidelines for brain imaging children with mild and moderate head injury.[11] However, these algorithms rely on an accurate history of the injury and may not be applicable for children with AHT and unreliable medical history.

Common presenting complaints for infants with AHT include changes in behavior, seizures, vomiting, and apnea. Sometimes, trauma is disclosed, but its severity is minimized. The decision to obtain a computed tomography (CT) scan is easier when patients have obvious signs of injury or abnormal neurologic examination but more difficult if the complaint is a vague one such as vomiting or irritability. Brain imaging should be considered if the physical examination reveals bruising, abrasions, scars suggestive of physical abuse, oral injuries including labial or lingual frenulum tears, or any history that is inconsistent with physical examination findings.

If brain imaging is indicated, CT is fast and easy to obtain in the emergency department. It will detect brain injury, but MRI is the current gold standard for evaluating AHT, as it provides more sensitive and specific information. MRI offers details valuable in directing further care and in the forensic investigation. It is also a better imaging tool for detecting subtle cervical spine injuries that may be present but not clinically apparent or detectable with plain films or CT. When MRI cannot be obtained at the time of presentation, it should be obtained as soon as possible thereafter (**Fig. 3**).

How a physician making the initial diagnosis of AHT takes a history is critical. A timeline of what occurred when, who saw the child last when he or she looked well, who was present at the time of discovery of the injury, details of the mechanics of any alleged fall or other injury, and what the child's health was like prior to this event are some of the key questions to ask. It is also important not to suggest a mechanism

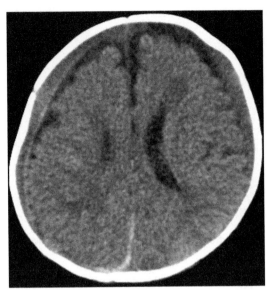

Fig. 3. Brain CT with old and new subdural hemorrhages. (*Courtesy* of Peter Strouse, MD.)

to the person providing the history, such as asking about shaking the baby, as the story may then change over time.

Differential Diagnosis

Once head injury is confirmed with imaging, further workup should include careful examination and skeletal survey, looking for subtle injuries often associated with AHT, as well as testing for conditions such as coagulopathies like severe hemophilia and metabolic diseases like glutaric aciduria type 1 that can present with brain hemorrhage. Babies who do not receive vitamin K at birth are also at risk for intracranial hemorrhage.

Abnormalities of coagulation can occur as a result of serious brain injury, so cause and effect may need to be teased out later. Hymel and colleagues[12] found in a study of abused babies that prolonged PT may be related to parenchymal brain injury. Disseminated intravascular coagulation and venous sinus thrombosis may be associated with severe head injury, but can also occur in the setting of serious medical illness.

Although subdural hematomas were found in 8% of 111 term newborns in 1 study,[13] they were all completely asymptomatic and resolved by 4 weeks of age. For neonates, it is therefore important to get a good birth history to rule out occult birth trauma, as complicated deliveries like vacuum extractions and forceps use can result in occult hemorrhages that are often blamed for the trauma in court.

When a child presents in critical condition, the emotional climate can make it easy to forget to get a detailed history, perform a detailed examination, and obtain studies to generate an appropriate differential diagnosis that includes occult trauma. In fatal cases, it is valuable to have a conversation with the medical examiner discussing concerns and determining which studies should be done in the emergency department as opposed to during the autopsy so that important evidence is not lost. Having such a protocol in place ahead of time can be valuable.

OTHER BATTERED CHILD PRESENTATIONS
Abdominal Trauma

Although abdominal trauma accounts for less than 1% of child abuse cases,[14] it has a high mortality and was found in 14% of child abuse autopsies.[15] Babies and toddlers are most likely to endure such abuse, and their inability to communicate contributes to the lethality, along with the delayed presentation and detection resulting from absence of history of trauma or external evidence of trauma. Consequently, the American Academy of Pediatrics guidelines for the evaluation of suspected abuse[16] include screening for abdominal injury. When abdominal trauma cases were looked at by Ledbetter and colleagues,[17] 11% overall were considered the result of abuse, but that figure jumped to 44% in children younger than 4 years. Single solid organ injury is more common in accidental abdominal trauma of children whereas multiple hollow organ injuries are more common in abuse cases.

Bruising

Bruises were shown by Sugar and colleagues[18] to be rare in nonambulatory infants ("those who don't cruise rarely bruise"), but common in active toddlers and children, therefore making them more challenging to diagnose as the result of abuse in that age group. Although it was believed that bruises could be dated by a sequence of colors that change as the hemoglobin breaks down, further research showed this to be unreliable. In a review of the literature on bruising by Maguire and colleagues[19] the accuracy of dating of bruises by physicians was less than 40%, and reliability between observers was low. Another review published in the forensic literature[20] found that even bruises caused by the same mechanism at the same time on the same individual had different appearances at different times during their resolution. In addition, bruises can be difficult to detect in children with darker skin.

In addition to the importance of correlating bruises with developmental age, where on the body they are located may also help distinguish accidental from inflicted injury. The Maguire review found that whereas accidental bruises are solitary, small and appear over bony prominences, abusive ones are more likely to be found in groups, and tend to be larger and not necessarily related to bony prominences. Bruises on buttocks, trunk and back are unusual in accidental trauma. When bruises have a specific outline or pattern, they may reveal a mechanism of injury as in the case of loop marks, handprints or grab marks, or repetitive linear marks (**Fig. 4**).

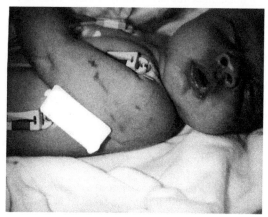

Fig. 4. Linear bruises (grab marks) on arm of baby with abusive head trauma of infancy, personal file.

Differential Diagnosis

There are several normal findings and medical conditions that can mimic abusive bruising and must be ruled out.

Dermal melanosis (Mongolian spots) are not bruises but may appear to be. They are blue-gray birthmarks often found near the gluteal cleft. They are most common in African Americans, but can occur in any race. The key to differentiating these from bruises is that they do not fade in the days to weeks that true bruises do. It is helpful when they are already documented on early well child visits.

Acquired conditions often cause bruises in unusual locations initially suspicious for abuse. These include idiopathic thrombocytopenic purpura, Henoch-Schonlein purpura, and leukemia. Bleeding disorders like von Willebrand disease should also be considered, and appropriate laboratory studies obtained.

Normal laboratory studies will not rule out Henoch Schonlein purpura, because it is a problem of platelet function rather than of number, but this purpuric rash is often clustered over the buttocks and lower extremities and may be accompanied by joint swelling, pain, testicular swelling, and kidney involvement not seen in simple bruising.

There are also other conditions with normal laboratory studies that can mimic abusive bruising, such as phytophotodermatitis caused by sun exposure after certain plants come in contact with the skin, citrus fruits being the most common culprits. Cultural practices such as cupping and coining can also result in transient skin lesions that mimic abuse, a reminder of the importance of a good history.

SKELETAL INJURY

When a child presents with multiple fractures in the absence of a history of major trauma, battering must be considered. One of the earliest reports of child abuse was Tardieu's landmark description of children with multiple inflicted fractures published in 1860.[21] Much later, Caffey described fractures in infants with subdural hemorrhage and suggested that they were the result of abuse.[22] Tardieu and Caffey are credited with leading the way to Kempe's 1962 description of the battered child syndrome.[2]

When babies and toddlers are abused, they often present with multiple fractures, whereas accidental fractures are rare in this age group. Worlock and colleagues[23] concluded that 80% of abusive fractures occur in children 18 months or younger, compared with 2% of accidental fractures. Many of these abusive fractures are occult. Therefore, it is crucial to obtain a skeletal survey for children under 2 years of age suspected of being abused. It may also be important for older children with disabilities who are unable to disclose abuse and who have a high incidence of maltreatment.[24]

Skeletal surveys consist of at least 2 dedicated views of each area of the body, resulting in approximately 20 images. Guidelines for obtaining these images from the American College of Radiology and the Society for Pediatric Radiology are available online.[25] Although it is time consuming to obtain all these images in the emergency department, occult fractures are often subtle and easily hidden under casts or splints used for previously identified fractures. For example, the child placed in a spica cast for a recognized femur fracture may also have smaller unrecognized metaphyseal avulsion fractures. Although these may not be clinically important, they may be key to making the diagnosis of abuse.

In addition to multiple fractures in a child without a documented or easily confirmed history of major trauma, there are other findings on plain films that should raise suspicion for abuse, as they are rarely seen in accidental injury. These include but are not limited to those listed in **Box 1**.

> **Box 1**
> **Findings consistent with child abuse**
>
> - Metaphyseal avulsion fractures of the long bones, also known as classic metaphyseal lesions
> - Rib fractures, especially posterior rib fractures, which often accompany abusive head trauma
> - Comminuted or complex skull fractures (not simple linear ones that are asymptomatic and may result from a minor fall in young children)
> - Any long bone fracture in a baby not yet walking
> - Any skeletal injury not consistent with the history provided
> - Any fracture without a history except for a tibial toddler's fracture in the appropriate age group
> - Unusually high number of previous injuries originally thought to be accidental

Classic metaphyseal fractures are the result of high-energy rotational forces on the ends of long bones. They are often seen in conjunction with abusive head trauma, as the extremity may be held during a shaking process. Such forces shear the metaphysis and can appear as a corner avulsion or as a bucket handle, depending upon the plane of the x-ray beam in relation to the bone. They were described in Kempe's original report of the battered child syndrome (**Fig. 5**).

Some other red flags include delay in seeking care for an obvious fracture, blaming a sibling or dog for the injury, and the absence of the caretaker who witnessed the injury, circumstances unusual in young children with accidental skeletal injury.

Dating fractures is an important component of identifying abuse, as well as being helpful in a forensic investigation to determine who was with the child at the time that it occurred. Again, a discrepancy between history offered and date of fracture suggested by imaging may support the diagnosis of abuse, as does the finding of multiple fractures in different stages of healing. Although it is relatively straightforward in the hands of radiology experts[26–28] to date many long bone fractures, this is not true of skull fractures. Likewise, metaphyseal fractures may be dated, but they do not heal in the same way as diaphyseal fractures.

Radiology input is also helpful in considering whether any type of imaging aside from plain films would be helpful. For instance, a nuclear bone scan may be useful, but these are often difficult to interpret in children with active growth plates and therefore warrant prior discussion.

Differential Diagnosis

As in other forms of abuse, there are medical conditions that may mimic the findings of abusive skeletal injury. Likewise, they may need to be ruled out with laboratory or other evidence for forensic reasons even when they can be clinically excluded.

Osteogenesis imperfecta (OI) is often invoked as a cause of fractures by the defense in the courtroom, but is much less common than child abuse and can usually be diagnosed by family history and physical examination and radiologic findings. There are many different types, and it is important for any physician testifying in a case of suspected abusive fractures to be familiar with the 4 major ones. Children with type 1 OI have blue sclerae, and these families often have dentinogenesis imperfecta and/or early onset hearing loss. Children with type 1I OI have bones that appear osteopenic on radiographs, often with bowing of the long bones and accessory wormian bones of the skull. Type 2 is lethal in the perinatal or neonatal period, and therefore not usually

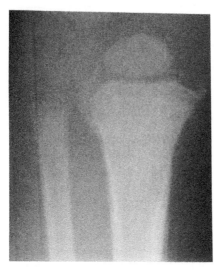
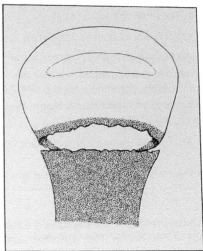
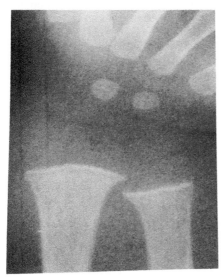

Fig. 5. Bucket handle fractures. (*Data from* Finkel MA. In: Reece RM, Christian CW, editors. Child abuse: medical diagnosis and management. 3rd edition. American Academy of Pediatrics; 2009. p. 128–9; with permission.)

confused with abuse. However, types 3 and 4 may be mistaken for abuse, as they can arise from new mutations not apparent from family history. Type 4 can present the biggest diagnostic dilemma as there may not be the other findings mentioned previously; however, this type is rare. Indeed, OI is extremely rare (less than 3 cases per 1,000,000 population)[29] without family history for OI, abnormal teeth or wormian bones on skull radiograph.[30] Other medical conditions to be considered include osteopenia of prematurity, rickets, scurvy, secondary hyperparathyroidism, Menkes kinky hair syndrome, as well as some skeletal dysplasias, malignancies, neuromuscular disorder,s or other diseases that result in osteopenia because of limited mobility.[1]

ABUSIVE SKIN FINDINGS OTHER THAN BRUISING
Burns

Infant skin is only half as thick as adult skin, and consequently is much more sensitive to burn injury. As children reach school age, their skin achieves adult depth, but very young children can sustain severe burns very rapidly and are therefore the most vulnerable to this type of abuse, as well to accidental burn injuries.

Scalds are common in both abusive and accidental burn injury. It takes only a few seconds for a child to sustain a third-degree burn if the water is hot enough. A burn that takes 10 minutes of immersion at 120° F takes only 3 seconds at 140° F.[30] Therefore, it often takes a scene investigator measuring the temperature of the hot water to know whether the history of an accidental scald injury is plausible. It is also necessary to know the developmental level of the patient. In a study conducted by Allasio and Fischer,[31] healthy children 10 to 18 months were observed trying to get into an empty bathtub placed in a clinic. Parental predictions were unreliable and even some of the 10-month old infants were successful.

Some burn characteristics that help a clinician decide whether a scald is likely to be the result of abuse include the absence of splash marks, a clear stocking glove line of demarcation suggesting the child was held still in the water, bilateral symmetry of burns, and sparing of areas such as buttocks and perineum that suggest the child was already held down as the water flowed around him or her in the tub (**Fig. 6**).

The most common accidental scald pattern seen in toddlers is one in which hot liquid is spilled on them when they pull down a pot or bowl or when they collide with someone carrying a container of hot liquid. These tend to be on the head, neck, shoulder and chest and are less deep as they run downwards and the liquid cools.

Thermal burns may have a pattern that tells their story. The sharper the pattern, the more concern there is for abuse. In accidental injury, the child is usually moving when he or she comes into contact with the hot object. For example, accidental cigarette burns are single and have indistinct margins as the child brushes by, whereas abusive ones tend to be in groups and have a round appearance with a deep sharp edged circumference and a diameter of 7 to 10 mm. Hair dryers, curling irons, and fabric irons are other household items that have been implicated in both accidental and abusive burns. As in bruises, body location may help distinguish accidents from abuse. A study

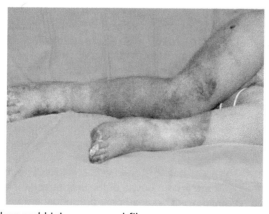

Fig. 6. Stocking glove scald injury, personal file.

of accidental curling iron burns presenting to emergency departments found they were on the hands of toddlers and preschoolers in 58% of the cases, but in other places, such as near the eyes, of older children.[32]

Differential Diagnosis

The appearance of burns evolves over time, and their various appearances can be mimicked by other conditions such as staphylococcal infection or the previously described phytophotodermatitis caused by various plants coming in contact with the skin prior to sun exposure. As with bruises, some cultural practices such as cupping are similar to acupuncture and meant to protect or heal children but can cause burns.

SEXUAL ABUSE

Ideally, the evaluation of a child for alleged sexual abuse should be a rare occurrence in the emergency department. Disclosures are usually delayed,[33] and interviewing the child victim is best done by professionals with special training who can take their time gently drawing the child out, a process ill-suited to the emergency setting. Moreover, because most child sexual abuse does not follow the rape model, few children will present with acute injuries immediately following sexual contact.[34] Usually, when children present to the emergency department for alleged sexual abuse, it is the disclosure that is the family emergency, not the physical condition of the child.

Therefore, the role of the emergency department physician in these situations should be to conduct a physical examining of the entire body to look for acute injury and document any positive signs of physical trauma as well as any spontaneous utterances the child makes about what happened, and then to refer him or her to the appropriate expert and legal agency for follow up. If the child is unable to cooperate with the examination, it should be deferred to another time and place so as not to repeat the psychological trauma unless there are acute injuries requiring medical attention. In those cases, the examination should be done in the operating room under anesthesia.

Evidence collection is generally indicated if the most recent sexual assault has occurred in the preceding 72 hours, although a study by Christian and colleagues[35] of 273 prepubertal children who presented to an emergency department within 44 hours of their assault concluded that the first 24 hours are when 90% of the positive evidence is found. Moreover, 64% of this evidence was collected from clothing and linens. They concluded that swabbing the child's body is not useful beyond the first 24 hours.

With male victims, the genital examination is straightforward and should be able to be accomplished in the context of a routine head to toe examination. However, victims are more often female, and their genital examination requires time and patience. A prepubertal girl should be examined first in the supine frog leg position. Gentle traction on the labia majora makes it easier to expose the vestibule. If possible, it is helpful to follow this with an examination in the prone knee-chest position as gravity works in favor of the examiner by allowing the anterior vaginal wall and any redundant tissue to fall open. However, this position is awkward and may be more threatening to the child as she is facing away from the examiner when prone. For older girls, the usual lithotomy position may work (**Figs. 7** and **8**).

If swabs are used, they should be moistened with sterile (but not bacteriostatic) saline or water, as the nonestrogenized mucosa of the prepubescent is very sensitive to dry touch. A speculum should never be used on a prepubescent unless the examination is occurring under anesthesia.

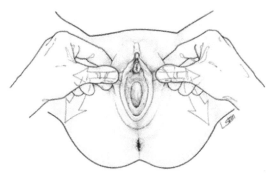

Fig. 7. Supine labial traction examination method. (*From* Finkel MA. Medical evaluation of child sexual abuse. 2nd edition. Finkel MA, Giardino AP, editors. Sage Publications; 2002. p. 62.)

Any genital examination should include an anal examination. This can be done in the prone knee chest, the lateral decubitus, or the supine position with the knees pulled up to the chest. Perianal erythema is not specific for abuse, and venous dilatation and dependent pooling may be confused with bruising. More concerning is a loss of elasticity of the anal sphincter, and, of course, any acute signs of trauma.

Most forms of child sexual abuse are perpetrated by someone the child knows, often repeatedly over a prolonged period, and the trauma inflicted may be more psychological than physical. Positive genital and/or anal findings may be subtle. Therefore, it is valuable to have a child abuse expert examine a child when there is a concern for repeated sexual abuse.

Documentation of examinations for sexual abuse should be as specific as possible and requires familiarity with the anatomy of prepubescent genitalia (**Fig. 9**).

There is much mythology about the hymen and a misconception that it can be either intact if there is no sexual intercourse or broken if there has been, thereby serving as a litmus test for abuse in a prepubescent girl. In reality, the hymen is an elastic membrane with an opening in the center that may be stretched. There are many natural variations in both its size and shape. The only situation in which there is no opening in this membrane is in the medical condition known as imperforate hymen, usually discovered at menarche, when blood builds up behind the hymen, forming a bulging mass. Therefore, a genital examination should not use terminology such as intact, but should carefully describe what is seen using specific anatomic terms.

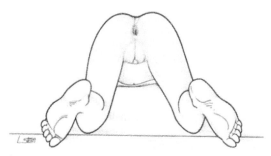

Fig. 8. Prone knee chest examination position. (*From* Finkel MA. Medical evaluation of child sexual abuse. 2nd edition. Finkel MA, Giardino AP, editors. Sage Publications; 2002. p.6.)

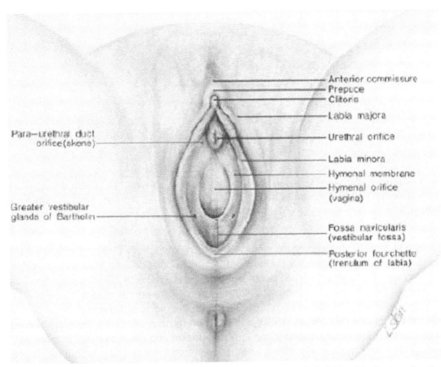

Fig. 9. Normal female prepubescent external genitalia. (*From* Finkel MA. Medical evaluation of child sexual abuse. 2nd edition. Finkel MA, Giardino AP, editors. Sage Publications; 2002. p.46.)

Mimics of Sexual Abuse

Accidental straddle injuries can be mistaken for abuse. If the child is verbal and can describe what happened, it is very helpful. When that is not possible, it is important to bear in mind that accidental injuries to the genital area are rarely bilaterally symmetric and often involve bruising of the inner thighs and/or labia majora. There may also be small lacerations or hematomas of the labia minora or posterior fourchette. It is rare in accidental injury for the relatively protected area within the vestibule to show signs of trauma without external signs.

Nonspecific irritation of the anogenital area is not uncommon in infants and toddlers still in diapers as well as in young children who may not have good toileting hygiene or when children have a diarrheal illness.

Infections such as group A beta-hemolytic *Streptococcus* can cause vaginitis severe enough to cause skin breakdown and bleeding, as can other common pathogens. Although vaginal discharge is not commonly found in sexually abused girls, culturing it when present may help differentiate ordinary infections from sexually transmitted diseases concerning for abuse in children **Table 1**.

The list of medical conditions that can mimic the appearance of sexual abuse is long, but some of the more common ones include Crohn disease, Behcet syndrome, molluscum contagiosum, human papilloma virus (HPV), or herpes simplex virus (HSV), which may be acquired from the hands of caretakers during diaper changes. Urethral or anal prolapse may also be mistaken for sexual abuse findings.

Table 1
Implications of commonly encountered sexually transmitted diseases for the diagnosis and reporting of sexual abuse of infants and prepubertal children

Sexually Transmitted Disease Confirmed	Sexual Abuse	Suggested Action
Gonorrhea[a]	Diagnostic[b]	Report[c]
Syphilis[a]	Diagnostic	Report
HIV infection[d]	Diagnostic	Report
C trachomatis infection[a]	Diagnostic[b]	Report
T vaginalis infection	Highly suspicious	Report
C acuminata infection[a] (anogenital warts)	Suspicious	Report
Herpes simplex (genital location)	Suspicious	Report[e]
Bacterial vaginosis	Inconclusive	Medical follow-up

[a] If not perinatally acquired and rare nonsexual vertical transmission is excluded.
[b] Although the culture technique is the "gold standard," current studies are investigating the use of nucleic acid-amplification tests as an alternative diagnostic method in children.
[c] To the agency mandated in the community to receive reports of suspected sexual abuse.
[d] If not acquired perinatally or by transfusion.
[e] Unless there is a clear history of autoinoculation.
From Kellogg N. The evaluation of sexual abuse in children. Pediatrics 2005;116(2):509; with permission.

MEDICAL CHILD ABUSE, ALSO KNOWN AS MUNCHAUSEN SYNDROME BY PROXY

Medical child abuse is a form of abuse in which a parent, usually the mother,[36] convinces medical providers to subject the child to repeated medical evaluation and treatment based on a history of a medical problem that is either fabricated by or caused by that parent. It is difficult to detect for several reasons, the first and foremost being that it is hard to believe a parent would intentionally carry out such a carefully planned and intentional form of abuse.

Although perpetrators are biological mothers in 90% of known cases, anyone acting in the parent role can be the abuser, with adoptive mothers,[37] fathers,[38] and babysitters[39] also reported.

Victims are usually infants and young children unable to disclose the abuse. As they get older, younger siblings may become the new victims. Children who survive this form of abuse often have serious physical problems as a result of the induction of symptoms or as a result of the many medical procedures to which they have been subjected. All the survivors suffer severe psychological damage as a result of the betrayal of the person they should have been able to trust to protect them.[40] Some older children may take on the false symptoms and develop Munchausen syndrome themselves.[41]

Because we are only aware of the deceptions that fail, the actual incidence of Munchausen syndrome by proxy (MSBP) is unknown, although cases have been reported from countries around the globe.

Perpetrators usually appear to be very concerned and sometimes claim to have revived their child repeatedly after they stop breathing or have cardiac arrest. They often ingratiate themselves by almost obsequiously listening to the clinician caring for their child, and then stage events to convince the clinician to order more and more testing and procedures.

This form of abuse is difficult to recognize unless a clinician detects the pattern of never seeing the problem him or herself and never having any caregiver other than the perpetrator witness it after the mother brings the child in repeatedly. Thus, it is an especially challenging diagnosis for an emergency physician to make, as he or she may see the child only once or twice. To make it even more difficult to detect, MSBP perpetrators often doctor shop, going from 1 provider and 1 emergency room to another so that the pattern is not as obvious. As these perpetrators escalate, they present their children to primary care providers, then local emergency departments, and then specialists and subspecialists at large tertiary care centers, often coming through those emergency departments also.

Presenting complaints cover an enormous range, but apnea, seizures, feeding problems, vomiting, and fever are among the most common ones.

Other parental conditions may result in a child brought in repeatedly for medical care that cannot be confirmed, such as an overanxious or hypochondriacal parent, vulnerable child syndrome, or a parent who has another psychiatric diagnosis like psychosis. These are different from medical child abuse in that there is a genuine concern for the child as opposed to the deliberate attempt to deceive the medical provider and subject the child to unnecessary procedures and treatment as seen in MSBP.

Physicians should consider MSBP in their differential diagnosis if a child is repeatedly presented by the same caretaker for a condition that only occurs in the care of that provider, physical examination shows no evidence of it, and work-up does not result in any explanation of the reported problem. If it is suspected, it should be discussed with a child abuse expert without revealing such a suspicion to the likely perpetrator so as not to encourage her to escalate her abuse in an attempt to prove to the medical provider that the medical condition is real. Proving such cases requires painstaking study of all the child's medical records and is extremely time consuming. There are few child protective services workers with expertise in this type of abuse, so it usually falls to a child abuse expert with experience to definitively make the diagnosis.

SUMMARY

Child abuse can be difficult to diagnose, as the history is often misleading; even some of its most severe forms are often not accompanied by external signs of trauma. It can take many forms, ranging from a few facial bruises or a torn frenulum in an infant to fatal intracranial or intraabdominal hemorrhage. When there are external signs, they may be subtle, but the location and pattern of any skin findings may be helpful in differentiating accidental from inflicted injury. Any physical findings should be well documented, with photography when possible. It is important to be familiar with medical conditions that can mimic abuse and to rule these out in a forensically defensible way. Although it is an uncomfortable diagnosis to make and court phobia may make it tempting to ignore the warning signs, making the diagnosis may save a child's life, and is the physician's moral and legal imperative.

REFERENCES

1. Child abuse: medical diagnosis and management. 3rd edition. American Academy of Pediatrics; 2009.
2. Kempe CH, Silverman FN, Steele BF, et al. The battered-child syndrome. JAMA 1962;181:17–24.
3. Keenan HT, Runyan DK, Marshall SW, et al. A population-based study of inflicted traumatic brain injury in young children. JAMA 2003;290(5):621–6.
4. Barlow KM, Minns RA. Annual incidence of shaken impact syndrome in young children. Lancet 2000;356(9241):1571–2.

5. Duhaime AC, Alario AJ, Lewander WJ, et al. Head injury in very young children: mechanism, injury types, and ophthalmologic findings in 100 hospitalized patients younger than 2 years of age. Pediatrics 1992;90:179–85.
6. Gilles EE, McGregor ML, Levy-Clarke G. Retinal hemorrhage asymmetry in inflicted head injury: a clue to pathogenesis? J Pediatr 2003;143(4):494–9.
7. Barsness KA, Cha ES, Bensard DD, et al. The positive predictive value of rib fractures as an indicator of nonaccidental trauma in children. J Trauma 2003;54(6): 1107–10.
8. Schnitzer PG, Ewigman BG. Child deaths resulting from inflicted injuries: household risk factors and perpetrator characteristics. Pediatrics 2005;116:e87–693.
9. Starling SP, Holden JR, Jenny C. Abusive head trauma: the relationship of perpetrators to their victims. Pediatrics 1995;95(2):259–62.
10. Jenny C, Hymel KP, Ritzen A, et al. Analysis of missed cases of abusive head trauma. JAMA 1999;281(7):621–6.
11. Kupperman N, Holmes JF, Dayan PS, et al. Identification of children at very low risk for clinically important brain injuries after head trauma: a prospective cohort study. Lancet 2009;374:1160–70.
12. Hymel KP, Abshire TC, Luckey DW, et al. Coagulopathy in pediatric abusive head trauma. Pediatrics 1997;99(3):371–5.
13. Whitby EH, Griffiths PD, Rutter S, et al. Frequency and natural history of subdural haemorrhages in babies and relation to obstetric factors. Lancet 2004;363(9412): 846–51.
14. Cooper A, Floyd T, Barlow B, et al. Major blunt abdominal trauma due to child abuse. J Trauma 1988;28(10):1483–7.
15. Pollanen MS, Smith CR, Chiasson DA, et al. Fatal child abuse-maltreatment syndrome. A retrospective study in Ontario, Canada, 1990-1995. Forensic Sci Int 2002;126(2):101–4.
16. Christian CW, Committee on Child Abuse and Neglect, American Academy of Pediatrics. The evaluation of suspected child physical abuse. Pediatrics 2015; 135(5):e1337–54.
17. Ledbetter DJ, Hatch El Jr, Feldman KW, et al. Diagnostic and surgical implications of child abuse. Arch Surg 1988;123:1101–5.
18. Sugar NF, Taylor JA, Feldman KW. Bruises in infants and toddlers: those who don't cruise rarely bruise. Puget Sound Pediatric Research Network. Arch Pediatr Adolesc Med 1999;153(4):399–403.
19. Maguire S, Mann MK, Sibert J, et al. Can you age bruises accurately in children? A systematic review. Arch Dis Child 2005;90(2):187–9.
20. Langlois NE, Gresham GA. The aging of bruises: a review and study if the color changes with time. Forensic Sci Int 1991;50:227–38.
21. AT. Etude medio-legale sur les services et mauvais traitements exerces surdes enfants. Ann Hyg Publ Med Leg 1860;13:361–8.
22. Caffey J. Multiple fractures in the long bones of infants suffering from chronic subdural hematoma. Am J Roentgenol 1946;56:163–73.
23. Worlock P, Stower M, Barbor P. Patterns of fractures in accidental and non-accidental injury in children: a comparative study. Br Med J 1986;293:100–2.
24. RJ G. Child abuse and developmental disabilities. Washington, DC: U.S. Department of Health, Education and Welfare; 1980.
25. Radiology ACoR-SfP. Practice Parameter for the performance and interpretation of skeletal surveys in children. 2016.
26. O'Connor JF, CJ. Dating fractures. 2nd edition. St Louis (MO): Mosby; 1998.

27. Prosser I, Maguire S, Harrison SK, et al. How old is this fracture? Radiologic dating of fractures in children: a systematic review. AJR Am J Roentgenol 2005;184(4):1282–6.

28. Chapman S. The radiologic dating of injuries. Arch Dis Child 1992;67:1063–5.

29. Taitz LS. Child abuse and metabolic bone disease: are they often confused? Br Med J 1991;302:1244.

30. Moritz AR, Henriques FC. Studies of Thermal Injury, II: the relative importance of time and surface temperature in the causation of cutaneous burns. Am J Pathol 1947;23:695–720.

31. Allasio D, Fischer H. Immersion scald burns and the ability of young children to climb into a bathtub. Pediatrics 2005;115:1419–21.

32. Qazi K, Gerson LW, Christopher NC. Curling iron related injuries presenting to US emergency departments. Acad Emerg Med 2001;8:395–7.

33. Elliott DM, BJ. Forensic abuse evaluations of older children: disclosures and symptomatology. Behav Sci Law 1994;12:261–77.

34. Finkel MA. In: Reece RM, Christian CW, editors. Child abuse: medical diagnosis and management. 3rd edition. American Academy of Pediatrics; 2009. p. 270.

35. Christian CW, Lavelle JM, De Jong AR, et al. Forensic evidence findings in prepubertal victims of sexual assault. Pediatrics 2000;106(1 Pt 1):100–4.

36. Sheridan MS. The deceit continues: an updated literature review of Munchausen syndrome by proxy. Child Abuse Negl 2003;27:431–51.

37. MW. A mother's trial. New York: Bantam Books; 1984.

38. Makar AF, Squier PJ. Munchausen syndrome by proxy: father as perpetrator. Pediatrics 1990;85:370–3.

39. Richardson GF. Munchausen syndrome by proxy. Am Fam Physician 1987;36:119–23.

40. McGuire TL, Feldman KW. Psychological morbidity of children subjected to Munchausen syndrome by proxy. Pediatrics 1989;83:289–92.

41. Conway SP, Pond MN. Munchausen syndrome by proxy abuse: a foundation for adult Munchausen. Aust N Z J Psychiatry 1995;29:504–7.

Recent Advances in Pediatric Concussion and Mild Traumatic Brain Injury

Andrea Ana Almeida, MD[a], Matthew Thomas Lorincz, MD, PhD[a],
Andrew Nobuhide Hashikawa, MD, MS[b],*

KEYWORDS

- Pediatric • Concussion • Traumatic brain injury • Sports injury • Children
- Adolescent • Head injury

KEY POINTS

- Pediatric concussions remain common and are increasingly being managed by primary care physicians.
- Concussion is a clinical diagnosis despite the availability of ancillary tests such as computerized neuropsychological testing, advanced imaging, and blood biomarkers.
- After 1 to 2 days of complete rest, light activity that stays below cognitive and physical activity symptom threshold has been found to be beneficial during the acute phase of injury and lessen symptom burden.
- Investigation and treatment of comorbidities, such as injuries to the vestibular or cervical musculoskeletal system and mood disorders, are important and may help decrease the duration of symptoms in a subset of patients.
- Current evidence does not indicate that children who participate in contact and collision sports are at risk for long-term neurologic or psychiatric consequences.

INTRODUCTION

Concussion or mild traumatic brain injury (mTBI) is defined as the immediate and transient functional disturbance of the brain caused by either a direct blow to the head, neck, or body with forces that are then transmitted to the head.[1,2] These forces result

Disclosure Statement: None of the authors have any relevant commercial or financial conflicts of interest to disclose and do not have any relevant funding sources to report.
[a] Department of Neurology, Michigan Medicine, Michigan NeuroSport, 2301 Commonwealth Boulevard, Suite 1022, Ann Arbor, MI 48105, USA; [b] Department of Emergency Medicine, Children's Emergency Services, Michigan Medicine, North Campus Research Complex, University of Michigan Injury Center, 2800 Plymouth Road, Suite G080, NCRC Building 10, Ann Arbor, MI 48105, USA
* Corresponding author.
E-mail address: Drewhash@med.umich.edu

in a rapid onset of neurologic functional impairment with or without loss of consciousness evolving over minutes to hours with spontaneous resolution over a period of hours to days.[3] Amnesia or loss of consciousness is not included in the definition of concussion. Traditional neuroimaging (computed tomography [CT] or MRI) available in emergency departments (ED) do not reveal whether a patient has sustained a concussion; rather, concussion remains a clinical diagnosis based on examination findings and patient-reported acute symptoms that cannot be explained by medications, alcohol, cervical injury, or other coexisting comorbidities.[3,4] Over the past 30 years, there has been substantial variation in the way mTBI was defined, but the Centers for Disease Control and Prevention (CDC), the World Health Organization, and the US Department of Defense have developed a working definition of mTBI (**Box 1**).[3] **Table 1** shows TBI grading of severity, mild, moderate, and severe as outlined by the CDC.[5] Between 80% and 90% of all TBI in the United States are estimated to be in the mild category or concussions.[3]

EPIDEMIOLOGY

In the United States, concussions are the most common neurologic injury occurring in recreational and sports activities and are now recognized as a major public health problem globally.[1] The CDC estimates that every year there are up to 3.8 million sports-related TBI, with the majority being concussions.[6] TBIs result in more than 2.5 million visits to the ED for all ages, most of which are mTBI.[3] Among children and adolescents between 0 and 19 years of age, more than one-half million ED visits are for TBI.[7] In the outpatient setting, more than 50% of the 750,000 patients diagnosed with concussions were estimated to be pediatric patients.[8] Since 2000, there has been a significant increase in the number of pediatric patients evaluated for and diagnosed with concussions in both the outpatient and inpatient setting.[9,10] Playground-related TBI treated in the ED among children under 15 years of age increased significantly between 2005 and 2013, with an ED visit rate of 53.5 per 100,000 for children ages 5 to 9 years, with the majority (96%) of all children treated and released from the ED.[11] Sports-related TBI ED visits increased 57% between 2001 and 2009 and the overall continued increase in ED and outpatient visits is multifactorial, in part because of the increased public awareness, states' legislation surrounding mTBI, and the requirement for medical evaluation before returning to

---

Box 1
Definition of mild traumatic brain injury

Mild traumatic brain injury is the occurrence of injury to the head arising from blunt trauma or acceleration or deceleration forces with one or more of the following:
Any period of observed or self-reported:
- Impaired consciousness, disorientation, or transient confusion
- Memory dysfunction surrounding injury time
- Loss of consciousness for less than 30 minutes
Other observed signs of neuropsychological or neurologic dysfunction:
- Seizures acutely after head injury
- Presence of lethargy, irritability, or vomiting after head injury, especially in infants and younger children
- Presence of headache, dizziness, irritability, poor concentration, fatigue, especially in older children or adults.

Adapted from McCrea MA, Nelson LD, Guskiewicz K. Diagnosis and management of acute concussion. Phys Med Rehabil Clin N Am 2017;28(2):273; with permission.

Table 1
Criteria for traumatic brain injury severity classification

	Mild	Moderate	Severe
Glasgow Coma Scale	13–15	9–12	3–8
Structural imaging	Normal	Normal or abnormal	Normal or abnormal
Loss of consciousness	<30 min	30 min - 24 h	>24 h
Posttraumatic amnesia	0-1 d	>1 and <7 d	>7 d
Abbreviated Injury Scale Score (Head)	1–2	3	4–6

Adapted from Centers for Disease Control and Prevention. Report to Congress on Traumatic Brain Injury in the United States: epidemiology and rehabilitation. Atlanta (GA): National Center for Injury Prevention and Control; Division of Unintentional Injury Prevention; 2015. Available at: https://www.cdc.gov/traumaticbraininjury/pdf/tbi_report_to_congress_epi_and_rehab-a.pdf.

sports activities. All 50 states now have passed legislation for management of sports-related concussions in children.[12,13] Reliance on ED-based data alone likely underestimates the incidence of concussion in children; recent data suggest increasing health care use for initial and follow-up concussion in primary care clinics.[14,15]

CLINICAL SYMPTOMS OF CONCUSSION

The clinical symptoms of concussion vary substantially, but include the physical, emotional, cognitive, and sleep-related symptoms listed in **Box 2**.[16] These nonspecific symptoms are often seen in other health disorders, including mood disorders, learning disabilities, and developmental disorders, and so must be taken into the context of the acute injury. For patients who sustain any TBI, the ED is where the vast majority of patients are medically evaluated, but more than 90% of patients with TBI are discharged home from the ED.[3] The Pediatric Emergency Care Applied Research Network validated prediction rules for identifying very low-risk children who would not need neuroimaging were first published in 2009 and have become a valuable decision tool for reducing unnecessary radiation exposure in the pediatric population.[17] The Pediatric Emergency Care Applied Research Network algorithm is divided into 2 age groups, less than 2 years of age and 2 years of age or older, and is provided in **Fig. 1**.[17,18]

Pediatric patients in the low-risk category group do not require neuroimaging. Patient in the middle risk group can be observed depending on physician experience,

---

Box 2
Symptoms of concussion

- Physical (10): Headache, nausea, vomiting, balance problems, dizziness, visual problems, fatigue, sensitivity to light, sensitivity to noise, numbness/tingling

- Cognitive (4): Feeling mentally foggy, feeling slowed down, difficulty concentrating, difficulty remembering

- Emotional (4): Irritability or moodiness, sadness, decreased interest in hobbies, nervousness

- Sleep (4): Drowsiness, sleeping less than usual, sleeping more than usual, trouble falling asleep

Adapted from Centers for Disease Control and Prevention (CDC). Heads up to health care providers: tools for providers. Available at: https://www.cdc.gov/headsup/providers/tools.html; with permission. Accessed August 21, 2018.

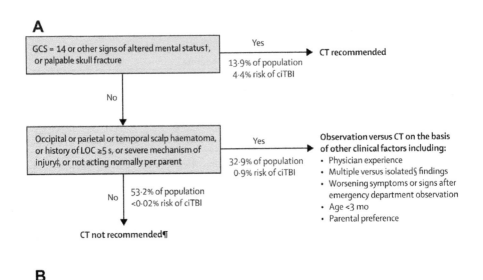

A

GCS = 14 or other signs of altered mental status†, or palpable skull fracture

→ Yes → CT recommended
13·9% of population
4·4% risk of ciTBI

↓ No

Occipital or parietal or temporal scalp haematoma, or history of LOC ≥5 s, or severe mechanism of injury‡, or not acting normally per parent

→ Yes →
32·9% of population
0·9% risk of ciTBI

Observation versus CT on the basis of other clinical factors including:
- Physician experience
- Multiple versus isolated§ findings
- Worsening symptoms or signs after emergency department observation
- Age <3 mo
- Parental preference

No | 53·2% of population
<0·02% risk of ciTBI

↓

CT not recommended¶

B

GCS = 14 or other signs of altered mental status†, or signs of basilar skull fracture

→ Yes → CT recommended
14·0% of population
4·3% risk of ciTBI

↓ No

History of LOC, or history of vomiting, or severe mechanism of injury‡, or severe headache

→ Yes →
28·8% of population
0·8% risk of ciTBI

Observation versus CT on the basis of other clinical factors including:
- Physician experience
- Multiple versus isolated§ findings
- Worsening symptoms or signs after emergency department observation
- Parental preference

No | 57·2% of population
<0·05% risk of ciTBI

↓

CT not recommended¶

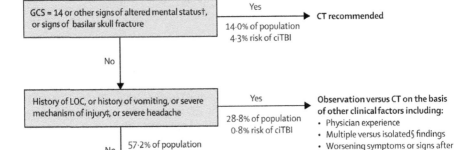

Fig. 1. Suggested CT algorithm for children younger than 2 years (*A*) and for those aged 2 years and older (*B*) with GCS scores of 14–15 after head trauma. (*Reprinted from* The Lancet, Volume 374 Issue 9696, Nathan Kupperman, James F Holmes, Peter S Dayan, et al. Identification of children at very low risk of clinically-important brain injuries after head trauma: a prospective cohort study. p. 1160–70. Copyright 2009, with permission from Elsevier.)

parental comfort, clinical symptoms, and other comorbid injuries. The vast majority of children presenting with mTBI can be discharged home with home observation if they meet certain criteria, including a Glasgow Coma Scale of 15, normal neurologic examination, no significant symptoms, no history of prolonged loss of consciousness or loss of consciousness with normal head CT, normal findings on CT if obtained, reliable family, and no suspicion of nonaccidental trauma.[7]

CONCUSSION DIAGNOSIS

Concussion is a clinical diagnosis and is best made using clinical expertise. Given the varied nature of the presentation of concussion, a comprehensive yet flexible approach depending on the venue and clinician experience is imperative. Although a variety of tools have been used to aid in concussion diagnosis, the venue and clinician experience are significant factors in determining which tools are chosen to aid in diagnosis and management. At athletic practices or competitions, a main consideration is whether an athlete can immediately return to participation. The initial evaluation should first exclude serious injury requiring immediate emergency evaluation at the nearest hospital (**Box 3**).[19]

If the provider has any concern for concussion, the athlete should be removed from participation immediately and, if there are clear signs of concussion, these individuals should be removed from participation and not be allowed to return to participation until cleared by a medical provider with expertise in concussion. If the diagnosis of concussion is uncertain, additional evaluation should be performed, preferably in a quiet environment away from athletic competition. Initial concussion assessment should include a history that includes a description of injury mechanism and a determination of loss of consciousness, amnesia, and associated symptoms. A balance assessment and examination of cognition should also be performed.[4]

The Sport Concussion Assessment Tool (SCAT) has been developed and validated as a relatively rapid screen, taking approximately 10 to 15 minutes to perform, to aid in assessment of concussion.[20] The most recent version, the SCAT5, includes sections focusing on prior history, red flags, observable signs, a sport memory assessment, the Glasgow Coma Scale, cervical spine assessment, symptoms checklist, cognitive screen (Standard Assessment of Concussion), and a neurologic screen including balance (modified Balance Error Scoring System). There is also a child SCAT5 that, in addition to the sections of the adult SCAT5, contains a child- and parent-specific symptom checklist.[21] Serial evaluation is important to identify those suspected of concussion who do not initially manifest clinical symptoms or signs. Diagnostic sensitivity and specificity of the SCAT drops with time so that by days 3 to 5 after injury, the SCAT is no longer useful in making a concussion diagnosis and limits its use in recovery decisions.[20] The SCAT5 symptom checklist has consistently shown usefulness in symptom tracking during recovery, with higher scores predicting longer recovery.[22] An increasing number of potential sideline aids in concussion diagnosis, including the King-Devick test and wearable impact sensors, are not currently recommended.[23]

Computerized Neuropsychological Testing

Computerized neuropsychological testing has become widely used in concussion assessment. Computerized neuropsychological testing has been used both in concussion diagnosis and recovery determination. Postinjury testing is either compared with an individual's preparticipation results or with population normative data. In children, computerized neuropsychological testing, when used after injury, is not sensitive or specific to concussion diagnosis.[24,25] A significant limitation to

---

Box 3
Initial signs requiring immediate emergency evaluation

Transportation to the nearest hospital for any of the following signs and symptoms:
- Glasgow Coma Score of less than 13
- Prolonged period of loss of consciousness (>1 minute)
- Focal neurologic deficit
- Repetitive emesis
- Persistently worsening mental status or other focal neurologic symptoms
- Potential spine injury

Data from NCAA and Sport Science Institute Consensus: diagnosis and management of sport-related concussion best practices. 2016. Available at: http://www.ncaa.org/sport-science-institute/concussion-diagnosis-and-management-best-practices. Accessed August 21, 2018.

computerized neuropsychological testing in children is the ongoing cognitive development, so that an individual's "baseline" is naturally always in flux. Pediatric population norms rely heavily on high school-aged males and may not be representative. Computerized neuropsychological testing is also influenced by factors that may be dissimilar before participation and after injury, including motivation, test setting, sleep, and mood. These concerns, among others, have led to a recent systematic review recommendation that baseline computerized neuropsychological testing should not be used routinely in children and adolescents and that further research is required to clarify the use of computerized neuropsychological testing in pediatric concussion diagnosis and management.[24] Computerized neuropsychological testing can be part of a multimodal assessment of concussion, but should not be used in isolation to make a diagnosis of concussion or in determination of recovery. A comprehensive individualized clinical evaluation should be relied on to make a diagnosis of concussion.

ANTICIPATORY GUIDANCE

Most patients are expected to achieve complete recovery between 1 and 3 weeks after the concussion, but recovery rates vary and are affected by many factors including injury severity, age, gender, and presence of other comorbidities such as depression, attention deficit hyperactivity disorder, and migraines. Referral to a medical provider who is both knowledgeable and comfortable in acute concussion management within 3 to 7 days is highly recommended for concussion symptom management and decisions regarding when return-to-play (RTP) and return-to-learn activities should begin. All 50 states and the District of Columbia have passed legislation surrounding concussions and sports, although there is variability regarding training and requirements for providers who clear athletes to return to sports.[13] Anticipatory guidance must include when patients need to return to the ED for evaluation for severe and rapidly progressive neurologic symptoms including severe alterations in mental status or severe progressive headache or vomiting, seizures, or focal neurologic deficits (**Box 4**).[16]

Box 4
Symptoms for which patients should return to the emergency department

- Severe headache that worsens
- Seizures
- Severe neck pain
- Drowsy, cannot be awakened
- Repeated vomiting
- Slurred speech
- Cannot recognize people or places
- Increasing confusion
- Weakness or numbness in arms or legs
- Unusual behavior change
- Increasing irritability
- Loss of consciousness

Data from Centers for Disease Control and Prevention (CDC). Heads up to health care providers: tools for providers. Available at: https://www.cdc.gov/headsup/providers/tools.html. Accessed August 21, 2018.

OUTPATIENT MANAGEMENT OF SUSPECTED CONCUSSION

A medical provider's first priority is to obtain a complete injury history and its course, which should include mechanism of injury, whether there was loss of consciousness or loss of memory of the injury, and elicitation of initial symptoms and how long they took to develop. History should then focus on symptom evolution. It is common for symptoms to have a delayed presentation after a concussive injury, with symptoms developing minutes, hours, or even the next day. However, development of initial symptom more than 24 hours should prompt a search for an alternative diagnosis.

The Post-Concussion Symptom Score can be used to gauge initial severity of injury and track recovery. A symptom checklist should not be a substitute for an individualized history. Following the clinical course of core concussion symptoms can be useful to aid in tracking concussion recovery. Core clinical concussion symptoms include headache, dizziness, lightheadedness, behavioral abnormalities, difficulties with sleep, visual abnormalities, psychiatric symptoms including anxiety and depression, and issues with cognition and memory. In the initial days after a concussive injury, symptoms typically are fairly constant and become more severe with cognitive or physical exertion. With normal recovery, symptoms should gradually improve, becoming episodic and less prominent with cognitive and physical exertion. Symptoms then typically progress to being present only with periods of provoked cognitive and physical exertion, followed by complete resolution of symptoms even with intense cognitive or physical exertion.

Symptoms associated with concussion are not specific. Differentiation of symptoms present before injury is important in determination of recovery from concussion. A significant proportion of the population may report symptoms consistent with a concussion without suffering a concussive injury.[22] Normal clinical recovery has been defined as less than 30 days in the pediatric population and less than 14 days in adults.[4] **Box 5** lists factors believed to be associated or not associated with prolonged recovery. Emerging evidence suggests that, in some, physiologic recovery may occur after clinical recovery.[22]

Although symptoms lasting longer than the current definitions would not be considered abnormal, medical providers clinically should elicit a history that allows an understanding of what may be driving symptoms and then develop an individualized rehabilitation plan to address ongoing symptoms. Once more serious injuries have

---

Box 5
Symptoms associated or not associated with prolonged concussion recovery

Factors associated with prolonged recovery
- Initial symptom burden
- Female gender
- Age less than 18 years, with ages 13 to 17 being at greatest risk for prolonged recovery
- History of mental health issues
- Concurrent cervical involvement
- Convergence insufficiency

Factors not consistently associated with prolonged recovery
- History of migraine
- History of a neurobehavioral or attention disorder, that is, attention deficit hyperactivity disorder or attention deficit disorder
- Loss of consciousness

Data from Iverson GL, Gardner AJ, Terry DP, et al. Predictors of clinical recovery from concussion: a systematic review. Br J Sports Med 2017;51(12):941.

been excluded and routine examination completed, the outpatient physical examination can be focused on the identification of abnormalities that aid in the diagnosis of concussion and rehabilitation decisions (**Box 6**).[26]

The optimal timing to initiate active rehabilitation strategies is unknown. Emerging evidence suggests that early active rehabilitation strategies, including implementation of cognitive and physical activity, may facilitate recovery.[27] Concussion symptoms can become more diverse when there is a concurrent injury to the cervical spinal muscles and peripheral vestibular system. Individuals with prominent dizziness/vestibular involvement may benefit from an early course of vestibular physical therapy. Similarly, individuals with concurrent mild cervical musculoskeletal injury (whiplash) are likely to benefit from cervical physical therapy. These injuries are sometimes overlooked and may be the leading cause to prolonged recovery.

Clinicians should consider alternative diagnoses in those with a concern for concussion. Patients with a migraine or headache history can have worsening headache frequency after recovery from a concussion and medical providers may find it challenging to differentiate preexisting headaches from concussion. Worsening of headache with exertion can be helpful in differentiating concussive headache from migrainous headache. Patients with a history of preexisting anxiety or depression can experience a clinical worsening of their symptoms.[28] Implementation of acute therapy, such as psychotherapy and/or cognitive–behavioral therapy aimed at treating anxiety and depression, should be considered. For individuals with an atypical course or a prolonged recovery, referral to a specialty clinic with additional expertise and resources in the management of concussion should be considered.

For patients with persistent psychiatric or prominent cognitive symptoms, referral for comprehensive neuropsychometric testing can identify issues associated with prolonged symptoms that may or may not be related to concussion and be valuable in clinical management. Prolonged cognitive deficits after a concussion are uncommonly found to be directly caused by concussion, but may be amenable to treatments for disorders such as depression, anxiety, sleep problems, or unrecognized attention disorders.

Box 6
Outpatient concussion examination areas of emphasis

Mental status
- Level of consciousness
- Orientation
- Concentration
- Memory

Cranial nerves
- Eyes: pupils, extraocular movements, convergence (normal 4 inches), pursuit eye movement, saccades, nystagmus
- Motor
- Strength

Coordination
- Balance and coordination
- Complex balance maneuvers (tandem and single leg eyes closed and eyes open stance)
- Vestibular system: Vestibular Oculomotor Screen 2[6]

Cervical musculoskeletal examination
- Palpation of upper back and superior cervical muscles
- Tests of range of motion
- Elicitation of pain or stiffness

Previously, complete physical and cognitive rest was the mainstay of treatment for concussion. Physical activity was not implemented until symptoms had fully resolved. Rest was prescribed to minimize brain energy demands after a concussive injury. With the advent of new research, light activity has been found to be beneficial during the acute phase of injury and has been shown to lessen symptom burden.[27] Currently, only a brief period (1–2 days) of complete rest is recommended. Research has shown that patients benefit from increasing activity levels gradually and progressively while staying below cognitive and physical activity threshold, which is the level where symptoms return or worsen.[4] The exact amount and duration of activity that may be beneficial or harmful in recovery of concussion is still unknown and requires further research.

During the acute phase of injury, the individual should be instructed to avoid cognitive and physical activity that heightens symptoms. A main emphasis in therapy should be placed on hydration (especially if lightheadedness is present), nutrition, and sleep. Pharmacotherapy can be used to alleviate symptoms during this time and treatment options should be guided by symptom burden. In the acute setting (0–6 hours), certain medications that alter mental status should be avoided (ie, narcotics, opioids, benzodiazepines). In approximately the first 24 hours, acetaminophen can be used to treat headache and/or neck pain. After approximately 24 hours, ibuprofen or naproxen are usually more efficacious than acetaminophen. Continuous use of nonsteroidal anti-inflammatory drugs should be transitioned as needed for severe pain as soon as possible. Antiemetics can be considered for severe nausea and/or vomiting with caution owing to potential side effects and mental status changes. Melatonin has been commonly used to aid with sleep difficulty. Importantly, primary medical providers should have patients wean off any medication that may mask symptoms while the individual progresses through the RTP/activity protocol. Long-term prescription medications are usually unnecessary because most symptoms usually resolve within 2 weeks. However, with a prolonged symptom course, prescribed medications for the specific symptoms may be required. The choice of medication and/or therapy will depend on the patient's comorbidities, history, and present symptoms.

RETURN-TO-LEARN FOR THE CONCUSSED PATIENT

The literature regarding academic reintegration is limited and variable. It is estimated that 47% to 70% of US school districts lack formal guidelines to assist concussed students returning to school.[29–31] Return to full cognitive activity should occur in a stepwise fashion and each plan should be individualized. The process of transitioning back to the classroom after a concussive injury is known as Return-to-Learn (RTL). During the acute phase of the injury, individuals should refrain from cognitive and physical activity that worsen symptoms. Therefore, the RTL process should include accommodations (eg, reducing time spent engaging in cognitive activities; taking breaks during classes; attending classroom lectures but not engaging in note taking, homework, or studying; using additional time for assignments and/or examinations) to help transition back to school. These accommodations should be developed in collaboration with school personnel, physicians, and the associated medical team, as well as athletic trainers, when available. The goal of these accommodations is to maintain the pace in the classroom activities and provide a smooth transition and return to full attendance and participation in all school activities. For a comprehensive list of academic accommodations and modifications, see **Box 7**.

Individuals may experience changes in peer status and social isolation, which can lead to depressed mood and anxiety during the recovery period. Therefore, it is

---

Box 7
Academic accommodations after a concussion

- Notify school of concussion.
- Develop plan for gradual return-to-school demands.
- Provide waiver for missed assignments or examinations.
- Plan to assist/support completion of missing assignments.
- Provide rest time/breaks during school day.
- Consider exemption from upcoming standardized tests.
- Excuse activities requiring rigorous physical activity.
- Reduce homework assignments.
- Reschedule, coordinate, or pace examinations during times when student asymptomatic.
- Negotiate timing of large assignments.
- Assign a counselor.
- Preferential seating for noise reduction and teacher monitoring.
- Allow test taking in distraction-free environment.
- Allow extended time for examinations and assignments.
- Using dedicated notetaker.

Data from Kirk JW, Slomine B, Dise-Lewis JE. School-based management. In: Kirkwood MW, Yeates KO, editors. Mild traumatic brain injury in children and adolescents. New York: Guilford Press; 2012. p. 321–40 and Kirkwood MW, Yeates KO, Wilson PE. Pediatric sport-related concussion: a review of the clinical management of an oft-neglected population. Pediatrics 2006;117(4):1359–71.

---

extremely important to attend to the psychological aspects of the injury and provide psychological intervention when needed. School teachers should be informed about concussions so appropriate accommodations can be made when necessary. In a survey that examined teacher knowledge and classroom management of student concussions, most teachers were found to be fairly knowledgeable about concussion symptoms, but only one-half of the teachers indicated that a concussion might cause difficulty for a student returning to school.[32] Additionally, more than 80% of respondents reported they needed more information on how to manage students with concussions. The study authors concluded there was substantial need for improved training of teachers regarding concussions and classroom management strategies.[32]

RETURN TO PLAY FOR SPORT-RELATED CONCUSSION

An individual should not be allowed to return to play on the same day of a suspected injury. Although light physical activity during recovery of concussion is encouraged, the return-to-play (RTP) progression should not start until symptoms have resolved and the individual has returned to their baseline without medications. An RTP algorithm should be completed before full return to sport. Making RTP decisions can be complex; therefore, it is essential to understand the sport in question as well as the risks it carries.[33] This progression should only be started with the guidance of a health care provider trained in the evaluation and management of concussion. The algorithm is a stepwise protocol that places specific demands on the brain to help determine if the individual is ready to return to sport. RTP guidelines help to decrease the risk of secondary concussions or other types of injury, prematurely engaging in unsafe physical activity, and/or aggravating symptoms.[34] The individual must complete each stage without symptoms before progressing to the next stage. The protocol consists of 5 gradual steps to help safely return an individual to sports (**Table 2**).

Initially, one must start with basic cardiovascular activity, progressing to sport-specific but noncontact activity, followed by contact-related activity, with the final goal to return to competition. A minimum of 24 hours between each stage is recommended, but it has been suggested that a slower, more conservative approach may be used for children.[35–38] The individual should not progress to the next level if they experience symptoms during or after the activity. If symptoms return at any step, an athlete should stop these activities because this may be a sign the individual is not fully recovered. At that point, rest is recommended and, when the individual is once again not experiencing symptoms for a minimum of 24 hours, they should start at the previous asymptomatic level.

Importantly, there is limited literature regarding management and RTP algorithms for specific age groups. A brief period of physical rest followed by gradual resumption of activity is recommended.[4,24] More research is necessary to determine appropriate progression through the RTP protocol and child and adolescent age-specific

Table 2
Graduated return-to-sports algorithm

Stage of Activity	Activity	Stage Objective
Relative rest	Symptom-limited activities of daily living; light walking.	Gradual reintroduction of activities involved with daily living and school/work.
Cardiovascular activity	Light to moderate aerobic exercise without resistance training on stationary bike or walking (treadmill).	Increase cerebral blood flow and heart rate.
Sport-specific noncontact exercise	Progressive aerobic exercise with sports-specific activity (drills) without head impact. May start progressive resistance training.	Interval training by adding fluctuations in heart rate and adding cognitive activity while increasing movement.
Noncontact training practice	Complex training drills, conditioning drills (can add limited controlled contact drills [eg, pushing or hitting sleds or dummies]).	Increase cognitive demand and assess processing speed and coordination. Assess for recurrence of symptoms after adding limited controlled magnitude afforce.
Unrestricted training	Full participation in training activity only after medical clearance.	Assess for recurrence of symptoms. Assess functional skills by coaching staff. Ensure self-confidence and readiness to play.
Full return to play	Participation in full activity without restrictions	Full game-day participation.

An initial period of 24 to 48 hours of both relative physical rest and cognitive rest is recommended before beginning the return to sport progression.

There should be at least 24 hours for each step of the progression. If any symptoms worsen during exercise, the athlete should go back to the previous step. Resistance training should be added only in the later stages (stage 3 or 4 at the earliest). If symptoms are persistent (eg, >10–14 days in adults or >1 month in children), the athlete should be referred to a health care professional who is an expert in the management of concussion.

paradigms should be created. Experts agree that, until children and adolescents have successfully returned to school, they should not return to sport.[4]

NEW RESEARCH AND RECOMMENDATIONS

Incorporating both in-person training of primary care providers on recommended best practices for concussion management concussion guidelines and the integration of a clinical decision making tool into an existing electronic health record system may increase behavior around concussion care. One large, geographically widely distributed pediatric health care network incorporated vestibular oculomotor examination and RTP and RTL guidelines into the electronic health record-based clinical decision support tool and increased documentation for examination and RTL/RTP from 1.8% and 19% before the intervention to 71% and 73% after the intervention.[14]

Evidence-based guidelines for retiring or medically disqualifying an athlete from sport after mTBI and are based on expert opinion.[38] When considering retirement, an individualized approach should be taken and all factors for each case should be considered. It is imperative to take the entire clinical history and psychosocial factors involved into account. Retirement should not be based solely on the number of concussions. If an athlete shows objective evidence of persistent cognitive deficits, a decreased threshold for injury, or unexplained progressively prolonged recovery, retirement from contact or high-risk sports should be encouraged.[35,39,40] Negative downstream consequences can occur if premature retirement is suggested.

Any type of structural injury to the skull or brain indicates a more severe type of brain injury. The decision whether or not to retire after a potentially life-threatening brain injury should be made by a care team with experience in managing moderate to severe TBI, including neurosurgery, neurology, physiatry, and neuropsychology.[40]

BIOMARKERS

Biomarkers that could reliably be used to stratify risk, diagnose, aid in management and inform long-term complications of concussions are likely to improve patient care. Fluid biomarker studied in concussion diagnosis, management, and long-term complications include S100 calcium binding protein B, glial fibrillary acidic protein, αII-spectrin N-terminal fragment, neuron-specific enolase, and neurofilament light. Other biomarkers that have been studied include MRI (functional MRI, diffusion tensor imaging, susceptibility weighted imaging), electroencephalography and quantitative electroencephalography, magnetic resonance spectroscopy, transcranial magnetic stimulation, cerebrovascular reactivity, cerebrospinal fluid biomarkers, and genetic testing. McCrea and colleagues[41] representing the Concussion in Sport Group stated that the level of evidence for neuroimaging, electroencephalography, and fluid biomarkers was low and that their role was best suited for characterizing the pathophysiology of concussion as opposed to clinical use.

LONG-TERM COMPLICATIONS

There is a growing concern that concussions or repetitive head impacts not severe enough to cause concussion (subconcussive blows) may cause or be a risk factor for the development of long-term complications. It is clear, primarily from studies of retired boxers, that some individuals seem to have developed neurologic problems secondary to repetitive mild head trauma in their boxing careers.[42] Researchers subsequently discovered microscopic brain changes in individuals exposed to repetitive mild head trauma, chronic traumatic encephalopathy.[43] Chronic traumatic encephalopathy is a pathologic diagnosis and the consequences of chronic traumatic encephalopathy pathology in life are unknown.[44] The important issue of risk of long-term consequences in children who participate in contact and collision sports has been addressed in epidemiologic studies that did not identify long-term neurologic or psychiatric consequences.[45,46]

SUMMARY

Concussions after a head injury in the pediatric population continues to be a substantial public health concern in the United States with upward trends reported for patients sustaining head injuries from sports or recreation-related activities. Although the majority of pediatric patients and families seek care in the ED, an increasing number of mTBI or concussions are being seen initially by primary care physicians because all 60 states have passed legislation for concussion management for the pediatric athlete. The continued identification of pediatric patients with mTBI using the validated Pediatric Emergency Care Applied Research Network by primary care and ED physicians decreases the need for head CTs and radiation exposure.

Although a number of computerized neuropsychological tests are available and may be used as an adjunct to clinical assessment, the individualized clinical evaluation should be relied on most to make a diagnosis of concussion in the pediatric population. Primary care providers should use a comprehensive RTP and RTL approach that includes specific school-based accommodations tailored for each individual. Use of evidenced based concussion decision making tools incorporated into the outpatient electronic health record along with focused training may increase appropriate documentation and cohesive clinical practice for primary care physicians. Clinically, overlooking other injuries and comorbidities may lead to prolonged recovery for the patient, particularly for patients with persistent or prolonged symptoms. Addressing these issues in a multidisciplinary approach using physical therapy, behavioral, and psychotherapy may help in decreasing the recovery time for certain patients. Retirement from sport in the pediatric population remains a controversial issue lacking evidenced-based studies and so must be done using a multidisciplinary approach that carefully weighs the individual athletes' medical history, clinical history, and cognitive function. Finally, there are currently no recommendations for the use of biomarkers for clinical diagnosis or management of concussions.

REFERENCES

1. Guskiewicz KM, Broglio SP. Acute sports-related traumatic brain injury and repetitive concussion. Handb Clin Neurol 2015;127:157.
2. McCrory P, Meeuwisse W, Aubry M, et al. Consensus statement on concussion in sport—the 4th international conference on concussion in sport held in Zurich, November 2012. Clin J Sport Med 2013;23(2):89.
3. McCrea MA, Nelson LD, Guskiewicz K. Diagnosis and management of acute concussion. Phys Med Rehabil Clin N Am 2017;28(2):271.
4. McCrory P, Meeuwisse W, Dvorak J, et al. Consensus statement on concussion in sport-the 5th international conference on concussion in sport held in Berlin, October 2016. Br J Sports Med 2017;51(11):838.
5. Centers for Disease Control and Prevention (CDC). Report to congress on traumatic brain injury in the United States: epidemiology and rehabilitation. Atlanta

(GA): National Center for Injury Prevention and Control; Division of Unintentional Injury Prevention; 2015.

6. Langlois JA, Rutland-Brown W, Wald MM. The epidemiology and impact of traumatic brain injury: a brief overview. J Head Trauma Rehabil 2006;21(5):375.

7. Schutzman S, Mannix R. Injury: head. In: Shaw K, Bachur R, editors. Fleisher and Ludwig's textbook of pediatric emergency medicine. 7th edition. Philadelphia: Wolters Kluwer; 2016. p. 247–53.

8. Mannix R, O'Brien MJ, Meehan IIIWP. The epidemiology of outpatient visits for minor head injury: 2005 to 2009. Neurosurgery 2013;73(1):129.

9. Bakhos LL, Lockhart GR, Myers R, et al. Emergency department visits for concussion in young child athletes. Pediatrics 2010;126(3):e550.

10. Taylor ME, Sanner JE. The relationship between concussion knowledge and the high school athlete's intention to report traumatic brain injury symptoms. J Sch Nurs 2017;33(1):73.

11. Cheng TA, Bell JM, Haileyesus T, et al. Nonfatal playground-related traumatic brain injuries among children, 2001-2013. Pediatrics 2016;137(6):e20152721.

12. McManemy J, Jea A. Neurotrauma. In: Shaw K, Bachur R, editors. Fleisher and Ludwig's textbook of pediatric emergency medicine. 7th edition. Philadelphia: Wolters Kluwer; 2016. p. 1280–7.

13. National Conference of State Legislatures: Injury Prevention Legislation Database/Opioid Abuse Prevention. Available at: http://www.ncsl.org/research/health/injury-prevention-legislation-database.aspx. Accessed October 27, 2017.

14. Arbogast KB, Curry AE, Metzger KB, et al. Improving primary care provider practices in youth concussion management. Clin Pediatr 2017;56(9):854.

15. Arbogast KB, Curry AE, Pfeiffer MR, et al. Point of health care entry for youth with concussion within a large pediatric care network. JAMA Pediatr 2016;170(7):e160294.

16. Centers for Disease Control and Prevention (CDC). National center for injury prevention and control. HEADS UP to health care providers: tools for providers. Available at; https://www.cdc.gov/headsup/providers/tools.html. Accessed October 27, 2017.

17. Kuppermann N, Holmes JF, Dayan PS, et al. Identification of children at very low risk of clinically-important brain injuries after head trauma: a prospective cohort study. Lancet 2009;374(9696):1160.

18. Zonfrillo MR, Topf S. Head trauma. In: Shaw K, Bachur R, editors. Fleisher and Ludwig's textbook of pediatric emergency medicine. 7th edition. Philadelphia: Wolters Kluwer; 2016. p. 595–7.

19. NCAA and Sport Science Institute Interassociation Consensus. Diagnosis and management of sport-related concussion best practices (2016). Available at: http://www.ncaa.org/sport-science-institute/concussion-diagnosis-and-management-best-practices. Accessed October 30, 2017.

20. Echemendia RJ, Meeuwisse W, McCrory P, et al. The sport concussion assessment tool 5th edition (SCAT5): background and rationale. Br J Sports Med 2017;51(11):848.

21. Davis GA, Purcell L, Schneider KJ, et al. The child sport concussion assessment tool 5th edition (child SCAT5): background and rationale. Br J Sports Med 2017;51(11):859.

22. Iverson GL, Gardner AJ, Terry DP, et al. Predictors of clinical recovery from concussion: a systematic review. Br J Sports Med 2017;51(12):941.

23. Patricios J, Fuller GW, Ellenbogen R, et al. What are the critical elements of sideline screening that can be used to establish the diagnosis of concussion? A

systematic review. Br J Sports Med 2017. https://doi.org/10.1136/bjsports-2016-097441.

24. Davis GA, Anderson V, Babl FE, et al. What is the difference in concussion management in children as compared with adults? A systematic review. Br J Sports Med 2017;51(12):949.

25. Alsalaheen B, Stockdale K, Pechumer D, et al. Validity of the immediate post concussion assessment and cognitive testing (ImPACT). Sports Med 2016; 46(10):1487.

26. Mucha A, Collins MW, Elbin RJ, et al. A brief vestibular/ocular motor screening (VOMS) assessment to evaluate concussions. Am J Sports Med 2014;42(10): 2479.

27. Schneider KJ, Leddy JJ, Guskiewicz KM, et al. Rest and treatment/rehabilitation following sport-related concussion: a systematic review. Br J Sports Med 2017; 51(12):930.

28. Solomon GS, Kuhn AW, Zuckerman SL. Depression as a modifying factor in sport-related concussion: a critical review of the literature. Phys Sportsmed 2016;44(1):14.

29. Kasamatsu T, Cleary M, Bennett J, et al. Examining academic support after concussion for the adolescent student-athlete: perspectives of the athletic trainer. J Athl Train 2016;51(2):153.

30. Olympia RP, Ritter JT, Brady J, et al. Return to learning after a concussion and compliance with recommendations for cognitive rest. Clin J Sport Med 2016; 26(2):115.

31. Wing R, Amanullah S, Jacobs E, et al. Heads up: communication is key in school nurses' preparedness for facilitating "return to learn" following concussion. Clin Pediatr 2016;55(3):228.

32. Dreer LE, Crowley MT, Cash A, et al. Examination of teacher knowledge, dissemination preferences, and classroom management of student concussions: implications for return-to-learn protocols. Health Promot Pract 2017;18(3):428.

33. Almeida A, Kutcher J. Sports and performance concussion. In: Daroff RB, Hitchen M, Chovan J, editors. Bradley's neurology in clinical practice. 7th edition. London: Elsevier; 2016. p. 860–6.

34. O'Neill JA, Cox MK, Clay OJ, et al. A review of the literature on pediatric concussions and return-to-learn (RTL): implications for RTL policy, research, and practice. Rehabil Psychol 2017;62(3):300–23.

35. Giza CC, Kutcher JS, Ashwal S, et al. Summary of evidence-based guideline update: evaluation and management of concussion in sports: report of the Guideline Development Subcommittee of the American Academy of Neurology. Neurology 2013;80(24):2250.

36. Guay JL, Lebretore BM, Main JM, et al. The era of sport concussion: evolution of knowledge, practice, and the role of psychology. Am Psychol 2016;71(9):875.

37. Guskiewicz KM, Bruce SL, Cantu RC, et al. Recommendations on management of sport-related concussion: summary of the national athletic trainers' association position statement. Neurosurgery 2004;55(4):891.

38. Harmon KG, Drezner J, Gammons M, et al. American medical society for sports medicine position statement: concussion in sport. Clin J Sport Med 2013;23(1):1.

39. Cantu RC. When to disqualify an athlete after a concussion. Curr Sports Med Rep 2009;8(1):6.

40. Concannon LG, Kaufman MS, Herring SA. The million dollar question: when should an athlete retire after concussion? Curr Sports Med Rep 2014;13(6):365.

41. McCrea M, Meier T, Huber D, et al. Role of advanced neuroimaging, fluid bio-markers and genetic testing in the assessment of sport-related concussion: a systematic review. Br J Sports Med 2017;51(12):919.

42. Roberts AH. Brain damage in boxers: a study of the prevalence of traumatic en-cephalopathy among ex-professional boxers. London: Pitman Medical & Scienti-fic Publishing Co., Ltd; 1969.

43. McKee AC, Stein TD, Kiernan PT, et al. The neuropathology of chronic traumatic encephalopathy. Brain Pathol 2015;25(3):350.

44. Manley GT, Gardner AJ, Schneider KJ, et al. A systematic review of potential long-term effects of sport-related concussion. Br J Sports Med 2017. https://doi.org/10.1136/bjsports-2017-097791.

45. Janssen PHH, Mandrekar J, Mielke MM, et al. High school football and late-life risk of neurodegenerative syndromes, 1956-1970. Mayo Clin Proc 2017; 92(1):66.

46. Deshpande SK, Hasegawa RB, Rabinowitz AR, et al. Association of playing high school football with cognition and mental health later in life. JAMA Neurol 2017; 74(8):909.

Management of Adult Patients in the Pediatric Emergency Department

Joy Ekezie, MB,BCh[a], Chad Garthe, MD[b],
Rachel Stanley, MD, MHSA[c],*

KEYWORDS

- Adults • Patient management • Pediatric emergency department
- Emergency medicine

KEY POINTS

- Increasing numbers of adult patients presenting to pediatric emergency departments.
- Description of stabilization and safe transfer of adult patients.
- Focus on the most common adult complaints presenting to the pediatric emergency department.

Adult patients often present to the pediatric emergency department (ED) for treatment of a wide variety of diseases. However, pediatric emergency medicine (PEM) physicians, like other pediatric specialists, are primarily trained to provide specialized care for children and adolescents and may lack experience in the evaluation and management of adult patients with acute illness or injury.

Studies have shown that the number of adult patients presenting to pediatric EDs has increased significantly since the introduction of the Emergency Medicine Transfer and Active Labor Act in 1986.[1,2] This law requires medical evaluation and stabilization of every patient who presents to an ED before transfer to another facility.[1] It is therefore important for physicians working in pediatric EDs to understand how best to triage, stabilize, and transfer adults presenting with emergency conditions.

Conflicts of Interest and Financial Disclosures: There are no commercial or financial conflicts of interest for any of the authors.
[a] Department of Pediatrics, Lagos University Teaching Hospital, PMB 12003, Lagos, Nigeria;
[b] Department of Emergency Medicine, The Ohio State University Medical Center, The Ohio State University, 1688 Canvasback Lane, Columbus, OH 43215, USA; [c] Division of Emergency Medicine, The Ohio State University, Nationwide Children's Hospital, 700 Children's Drive, Columbus, OH 43205, USA
* Corresponding author.
E-mail address: Rachel.stanley@nationwidechildrens.org

Pediatr Clin N Am 65 (2018) 1167–1190
https://doi.org/10.1016/j.pcl.2018.07.016
0031-3955/18/© 2018 Elsevier Inc. All rights reserved.

Adult patients presenting to the pediatric ED are either adults with chronic pediatric disorders or new adult patients who do not usually seek care in a pediatric ED. The complaints are wide and varied, including headache, syncope, chest pain, falls, respiratory distress, substance abuse, trauma, seizures, vomiting/dehydration, altered consciousness, strokelike symptoms, and manifestations of mental illness.[1,2] Examples of chronic pediatric disorders seen in adult patients in the pediatric ED include complex cyanotic congenital heart disease, severe global developmental delay, cystic fibrosis, and seizure disorder.[3] Management of these chronic pediatric disorders is not discussed here.

This article discusses the management of common complaints that adults present with to the pediatric ED. The focus is on triage/stabilization in the ED and transfer to an appropriate adult facility. The topics that are covered include:

1. Chest pain
2. Syncope
3. Seizures
4. Stroke
5. Shortness of breath (SOB)
6. Cardiac arrest/resuscitation

CHEST PAIN

Chest pain and symptoms consistent with myocardial ischemia (MI) account of 8% to 10% of the 119 million ED visits yearly.[4] Chest pain accounts for 11.9% to 14% of cases of adults presenting to pediatric EDs.[1,2] Acute MI (AMI) is one of the most critical diagnoses in an adult presenting with chest pain. AMI results in high mortalities and most deaths occur in the first 12 hours.[5] **Box 1** lists the common causes/differentials of chest pain. Management guidelines for adults with chest pain include resuscitation/stabilization (**Box 2**), history (**Box 3**), physical examination (**Box 4**), investigation, treatment, and transfer. **Fig. 1** shows a 12-lead electrocardiogram (ECG) showing

---

Box 1
Common causes of chest pain in adults

- Cardiovascular: acute coronary syndrome, angina, pericarditis/myocarditis, arrhythmias, cardiomyopathy, aortic dissection

- Respiratory: asthma, hypoxia, pneumonia, foreign body, cancer, pulmonary embolism

- Gastrointestinal: esophageal spasm, esophagitis, gastritis/peptic ulcer, gastroesophageal reflux disease, diverticular disease, gall bladder disease, pancreatitis

- Musculoskeletal: arthritis, costochondritis, muscular strain, trauma, fibromyalgia, rib fracture, fibrositis

- Psychogenic: somatoform disorder, anxiety/panic attacks, hyperventilation, depression

- Drug abuse: amphetamine, cocaine

- Miscellaneous: anemia (including sickle cell), herpes zoster, thyroid/adrenal problems, toxins

Data from Kontos MC, Roberts BD, Jesse RL, et al. Utility of the presenting electrocardiogram to predict mortality when troponin level is used to diagnose myocardial infarction. Acad Emerg Med 2006;13(5 Supplement 1):S37; and Agostini-Miranda A, Crown L. An approach to the initial care of patients with chest pain in an emergency department located in a non-cardiac center. Am J Med 2009;6:24–9.

Box 2
Resuscitation and stabilization for chest pain

- Airway: ensure patency of airway; suction if required
- Breathing: give supplemental oxygen if hypoxic
- Circulation: secure intravenous access; give bolus saline infusion if dehydrated
- Electrocardiogram

---

an ST-elevation myocardial infarction (STEMI). Elevation of the ST segment can be seen in some leads.[6]

Investigation (Electrocardiogram)

An initial ECG should be obtained as soon as possible to rule out MI. ECG is highly specific (77%–100%) in the first 12 hours depending on the criteria used but has poor sensitivity (28%–54%).[7] Ischemic changes are apparent at the time of presentation in only 20% to 30% of patients with acute MI, whereas 5% to 10% of patients with MI have normal findings on ECG at presentation.[8,9]

Treatment

Aspirin (325 mg) should be given immediately unless there is a major contraindication, such as active peptic ulceration, bleeding disorders, or severe allergy.[10] Aspirin acts as an inhibitor of cyclooxygenase-dependent platelet activity. Sublingual nitroglycerin

---

Box 3
History for chest pain

- Chest pain
  - Site, onset, nature/quality, severity, duration, aggravating and relieving factors, precipitating factor, radiation, and timing
  - The following features can be suggestive of MI:
    - Typical chest pain: (1) substernal, (2) provoked by exertion, (3) relieved by rest/nitroglycerin
    - Atypical chest pain: chest pain that does not satisfy all of the above typical chest pain criteria (note: there is no difference in the rate of MI in typical vs atypical chest pain)
    - Similar pain to previous MI
    - Other symptoms that may be associated with chest pain include diaphoresis, weakness, vomiting, nausea, palpitations, shortness of breath, and syncope
    - Atypical presentations are more likely in elderly persons, especially women in whom dyspnea may predominate over chest pain
  - Sudden-onset pleuritic chest pain with shortness of breath is suggestive of pulmonary embolism
  - Chest pain associated with cough, fever, and infiltrates on chest radiograph may suggest pneumonia
  - Sudden, severe tearing or sharp chest pain with syncope or other neurologic symptoms may suggest aortic dissection
- Significant past medical history includes previous history of AMI, hypertension, connective tissue disorders, hypercholesterolemia, and diabetes
- Family history of sudden death and coronary artery disease
- Other history such as smoking, obesity, and use of birth control pills or hormone replacement therapy may increase risk of thromboembolism

Data from Refs.[11,57–59]

> **Box 4**
> **Physical examination for chest pain**
>
> - Prominent murmurs (endocarditis)
> - Friction rub (pericarditis)
> - Fever with abnormal lung sounds (pneumonia)
> - Complete reproducible chest pain after palpation with no other suggestive findings (musculoskeletal)
> - Signs of significant heart failure with rales auscultated in the bilateral lung fields (not just including the bases) should be noted.
>
> *Data from* Kontos MC, Roberts BD, Jesse RL, et al. Utility of the presenting electrocardiogram to predict mortality when troponin level is used to diagnose myocardial infarction. Acad Emerg Med 2006;13(5 Supplement 1):S37; and Herren KR, Mackway-Jones K. Emergency management of cardiac chest pain: a review. Emerg Med J 2001;18(1):6–10.

(0.3 or 0.4 mg) should be given and repeated every 2 to 5 minutes if chest pain continues and if systolic BP is greater than 100 mm Hg, Discontinue sublingual nitroglycerin if BP deceases to less than 90 mm Hg.[11] Do not give sublingual nitroglycerin if there is evidence of inferior MI.[12] Intravenous (IV) morphine sulfate (2–4 mg IV) can be given every 5 to 30 minutes until pain improves or if there is hypotension or bradypnea.[13] **Fig. 2** shows the acute coronary syndromes algorithm from the American Heart Association (AHA).[14] After step 4 of this algorithm (ECG interpretation), rapid transportation to an appropriate adult facility should occur.

Transfer Promptly to an Appropriate Adult Facility, Preferably a Chest Pain Assessment Unit

Transfer should be completed as soon as possible so patients with MI can be identified rapidly and treated with percutaneous coronary revascularization, which is the

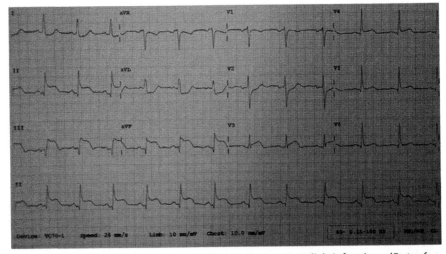

Fig. 1. Electrocardiogram showing an ST-elevation myocardial infarction. (*Data from* Heilman J. 12 lead ECG showing inferior and right ventricular infarct. 2014. Available at: https://commons.wikimedia.org/wiki/File:Inferior_and_RtV_MI_12_lead.jpg. Accessed December 4, 2017.)

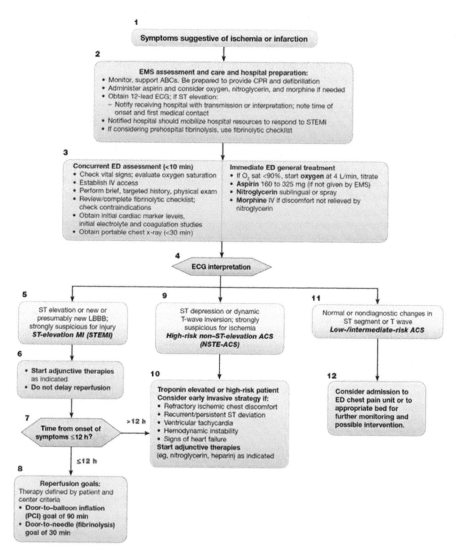

Fig. 2. Acute coronary syndromes algorithm from the American Heart Association. (*From* American Heart Association. Web-based integrated 2010 & 2015 American Heart Association guidelines for cardiopulmonary resuscitation and emergency cardiovascular care. Part 9: acute coronary syndromes. Available at: https://eccguidelines.heart.org/index.php/circulation/cpr-ecc-guidelines-2/part-9-acute-coronary-syndromes/. Accessed December 4, 2017.)

gold standard of treatment of STEMI. The goal for first medical contact to percutaneous coronary intervention is less than or equal to 90 minutes.[15] Most adult patients presenting to pediatric ED with chest pain benefit from a chest pain work up at an adult ED.

SYNCOPE

Syncope is defined as a sudden, transient loss of consciousness with loss of postural tone caused by cerebral hypoperfusion and spontaneous return to baseline function without intervention.[16,17] It is a symptom of an underlying illness, not a diagnosis. There is autonomic dysfunction with increased parasympathetic tone and inhibition of sympathetic activity leading to peripheral vasodilatation and bradycardia. This condition results in global cerebral hypoperfusion or focal hypoperfusion of the reticular activating system with loss of consciousness and postural tone.[16,17]

Syncope has a bimodal distribution with a peak in the second decade of life and also after age 70 years. It is mostly benign (vasovagal attack) in young people.[17] Syncope accounts for 6.7% to 22.6% of adult patients in pediatric EDs.[2,18]

The so-called rule of 15s states that approximately 15% of the following life-threatening conditions present with syncope: subarachnoid hemorrhage, acute coronary syndrome, aortic dissection, leaking aortic aneurysm, and ruptured ectopic pregnancy. Medications cause 5% to 15% of syncope.[19] **Box 5** lists the common causes of syncope.

Management guidelines for adults with syncope include resuscitation/stabilization (**Box 6**), history (**Box 7**), physical examination (**Box 8**), investigations, and transfer.

Investigations

ECG is recommended in the evaluation of most cases,[20] and may identify a cause in up to 7% of cases with evidence of cardiac ischemia or arrhythmia or MI.[19] ECG findings may include sinus bradycardia, atrioventricular block, prolonged QT interval, Brugada syndrome, and Wolff-Parkinson-White syndrome.[21] Normal ECG has a negative predictive value for MI as a cause for the syncope of greater than 99%.[22] Start continuous cardiac monitoring, and check blood glucose for hypoglycemia. Routine laboratory screening is not recommended because it seldom helps in evaluation and management of patients with syncope; in addition, laboratory screening in the pediatric ED is likely to delay transfer and definitive disposition of patients.[23,24]

Box 5
Common causes of syncope in adults

- Respiratory: pulmonary embolism, severe chronic obstructive pulmonary disease
- Cardiovascular: myocardial infarction, congestive heart failure, aortic dissection, cardiomyopathy, cardiac device, arrhythmias; these all cause hypoxia
- Neurologic: Parkinson disease, multiple sclerosis, other degenerative conditions
- Medications: diuretics, β-blockers, calcium channel blockers, angiotensin-converting enzyme (ACE) inhibitors, angiotensin receptor blockers, levodopa, α-blockers, nitrates, tricyclic antidepressants, antiarrhythmics, other medications that prolong QT interval (eg, antiemetics, antipsychotics, erythromycin, clarithromycin, hydroxychloroquine, quinine, loratidine, terfenadine, astemizole, methadone, domperidone, pentamidine)
- Psychiatric illnesses: major depressive disorder, anxiety
- Diabetes: hypoglycemia can cause syncope
- Substance abuse: narcotics, alcohol
- High altitude: causes hypoxia
- Hemorrhage: may lead to hypoxia/anoxia

Data from Patel PR, Quinn JV. Syncope: a review of emergency department management and disposition. Clin Exp Emerg Med 2015;2(2):67–74.

Box 6
Resuscitation and stabilization for syncope

- Airway: ensure patency of airway; suction if required
- Breathing: give supplemental oxygen if hypoxic
- Circulation: secure IV access; give bolus saline infusion if dehydrated
- Disability: give glucose if hypoglycemic
- Exposure: examine from head to toe for bruises, lacerations, bite marks, and so forth
- Most patients present after return to their normal baseline because syncopal attacks are usually brief (<1 minute). If longer lasting, rule out underlying illness such as seizures

Data from Welsh JT, Welsh T, Emerman C. Evaluation of syncope in the emergency department. Emergency Medicine Reports 2015;36(22):261–9.

Echocardiography is most useful in patients with a history of cardiac disease or abnormal ECG findings or clinical suspicion of aortic stenosis.[25] Certain risk factors present after a syncopal episode increases the likelihood of a more serious underlying cause of syncope and should prompt immediate referral to an adult emergency room.

Box 7
History for syncope

- Description of the episode (by the patient or someone who observed the event): onset, duration, precipitating factor, aura/prodrome, activity at time of onset, witnessed abnormal activity such as seizures, incontinence, tongue biting (suggestive of seizures)
- Triggers/precipitating factors: stress, fever, pain, micturition, defecation, coughing/sneezing, swallowing, diving, shaving, head turning, wearing a tight shirt collar or tie, exercise; these suggest a neurocardiogenic cause
- Exertional syncope is suggestive of a cardiac disorder (dysrhythmias, structural heart disease, cardiomyopathy)
- Onset: sudden onset with no prodrome (suggests a more serious cause, such as arrhythmia); gradual onset preceded by prodromal symptoms (usually suggests benign cause)
- Duration: brief (less than 1 to 2 minutes [true syncope]); more than a few minutes (may suggest a seizure)
- Posture: supine (arrhythmia); after prolonged standing (neurocardiogenic cause); standing up from a supine or seating position (orthostatic syncope, which is often benign)
- Associated symptoms: shakiness, sweating, hunger, dizziness (suggestive of hypoglycemia in a diabetic patient); blood loss (ruptured abdominal aortic aneurysm [AAA], ruptured ectopic pregnancy, rupture ovarian cyst, ruptured spleen); vaginal bleeding/menstrual irregularity (ectopic pregnancy); chest pain (acute coronary syndrome, pulmonary embolism); headache (subarachnoid hemorrhage or carbon monoxide poisoning); shortness of breath or leg pain (pulmonary embolism); specific weakness (neurologic cause); flank/abdominal pain (leaking abdominal aortic aneurysm)
- Medications (as listed earlier); substance abuse (alcohol, narcotics)
- Past medical history of any of the illnesses mentioned earlier
- Family history of sudden death, especially in relatives less than 45 to 50 years old may suggest cardiac syncope, such as Brugada syndrome
- Eating disorders, diuretic or laxative abuse, and inhalant abuse may be seen in adolescents

---

Box 8
Physical examination for syncope

- General examination: pallor (anemia from blood loss), cyanosis (from hypoxia), lateral tongue bite marks (in seizures), fever, dehydration, and evidence of trauma or fall.

- Cardiovascular: pulsus paradoxus (cardiac tamponade), systolic murmurs (hypertrophic cardiomyopathy or aortic stenosis; a murmur that gains intensity with Valsalva maneuvers and abolishes with squatting suggests hypertrophic cardiomyopathy), gallop rhythm/extra heart sound (S3 or S4) suggests congestive cardiac failure, and dysrhythmias.

- Neck: grade III/IV midsystolic murmur radiating to the neck with loss of S2 splitting (critical aortic stenosis), carotid stenosis, thyroid enlargement.

- Neurologic: usually normal. Any residual deficit suggests acute stroke, or a structural lesion, or a profound toxic or metabolic insult. Poor memory is a sign of concussion. Evidence of head injury could be from the fall caused by loss of muscle tone or an assault.

- Gastrointestinal: abdominal pain/tenderness, pulsatile abdominal mass (ruptured AAA), occult bleed seen on digital rectal examination.

Data from Patel PR, Quinn JV. Syncope: a review of emergency department management and disposition. Clin Exp Emerg Med 2015;2(2):67–74.

The San Francisco syncope rule is a rule for evaluating the risk of adverse outcomes in patients with syncope. The mnemonic for features of the rule is CHESS[26]:

C: history of congestive heart failure
H: hematocrit less than 30%
E: abnormal ECG
S: shortness of breath
S: a triage systolic BP of less than 90 mm Hg

These factors, in addition to age greater than 75 years, are all significant risk factors for serious outcome at 30 days. Serious outcome in this study is defined as "death, myocardial infarction, arrhythmia, pulmonary embolism, stroke, subarachnoid hemorrhage, significant hemorrhage, or any condition causing a return ED visit and hospitalization for a related event."[27]

Patients who satisfy any of the CHESS criteria cannot be considered low risk.[27,28]

Transfer

Patients should be transferred to an appropriate adult facility as soon as possible for further evaluation and treatment of the underlying cause.

SEIZURES

Seizures are a common presenting complaint in the ED, and status epilepticus complicates up to 7% of these seizures with a significant mortality.[29] Seizures account for about 2.4% of the complaints of adults presenting to the pediatric ED.[2]

Seizures may be provoked or unprovoked. Provoked seizures have been associated with a much higher mortality than unprovoked seizures.[30] Status epilepticus, defined as seizure activity lasting more than 5 minutes or more than 2 seizures without regaining baseline level of consciousness,[31] must be intervened in before transfer to an adult facility.

Common causes of provoked seizures are listed in **Box 9**.

> **Box 9**
> **Common causes of provoked seizures in adults**
>
> - Structural abnormalities: these can be caused by head injury, neurosurgical intervention, stroke, central nervous system (CNS) infections (such as neurocysticercosis, meningitis, encephalitis, neurosyphilis, human immunodeficiency virus, cat scratch, tuberculoma), brain abscess, CNS malignancy.
>
> - Metabolic/toxic disturbances: these include withdrawal from alcohol, benzodiazepines, barbiturates, or gamma hydroxybutyrate; organophosphate poisoning; sympathomimetic (cocaine, amphetamine) overdose; medications (such as isoniazid and tricyclic antidepressants); theophylline; hypoglycemia; extreme hyperglycemia; severe and rapidly developing hyponatremia or hypernatremia; severe hypocalcemia or hypercalcemia; severe hypomagnesemia; eclampsia (rarely, may present several weeks postpartum).
>
> *Data from* Garber BG, Glauser J. Evaluation and management of seizures in the emergency department. Emergency Medicine Reports 2017;38(12). Available at: https://www.reliasmedia.com/articles/140857-evaluation-and-management-of-seizures-in-the-emergency-department. Accessed December 12, 2018.

Management guidelines for adults with seizures include resuscitation/stabilization (**Box 10**) and aborting the seizures, history (**Box 11**), physical examination (**Box 12**), investigations, initiating treatment of underlying cause, and transfer.

Investigations

- Blood glucose[32]
- Serum sodium
- Pregnancy test (in any woman of child-bearing age to rule out eclampsia)

Treat Underlying Cause

Infection: if infection is suspected in a seizing, adult patient, consider giving broad-spectrum antibiotics such as ceftriaxone.

Ethanol withdrawal: in the case of ethanol withdrawal, administer IV Thiamine followed by a glucose infusion.

Eclampsia: for patients with eclampsia (>20 weeks pregnant or up to 3 weeks post-partum), give 2 to 6 g of IV magnesium every 5 to 10 minutes,[33] diazepam 5 mg IV every 5 minutes, and treat hypertension with 20 mg of IV labetalol or 5 to 10 mg of hydralazine. Transfer promptly to a facility with obstetric expertise because the definitive treatment is delivery and removal of the placenta.

Hypoglycemia: if hypoglycemia is suspected, administer 1 ampule of 50% dextrose every 5 minutes until euglycemic.

Hyponatremia: if hyponatremia is suspected (Na<120 mEq/L), give 3% normal saline (NS) at 100 mL of 3% NaCl infused intravenously over 10 minutes times 3 as needed.[34] In these conditions, the risks of the electrolyte disturbance exceed the risks of hypertonic saline therapy and fear of osmotic demyelination should not stop clinicians from giving aggressive treatment.[35]

Transfer

Patients should be transferred to an appropriate adult facility as soon as possible for further evaluation and treatment of the underlying cause.

STROKE

Stroke is an uncommon but important cause of presentation of adults to the pediatric ED, accounting for about 1% of the cases in one study.[2] The World Health

---

Box 10
Resuscitation and stabilization for seizures

- Airway: keep airway patent, suction if required, maintain airway with nasopharyngeal or oropharyngeal airway or intubation if necessary.
- Breathing: ensure that patient is breathing spontaneously, commence oxygen if necessary.
- Circulation: secure IV or intraosseous access.
- Disability: give IV thiamine 200 mg, then IV dextrose because vitamin B_1 deficiency induced by alcohol intoxication may be aggravated by glucose infusion. Also consider bicarbonate administration if a wide complex tachycardia is present and sodium channel blocker (eg, tricyclic antidepressant) overdose suspected.
- Exposure: check for signs of trauma or injury.

Abort the seizures (should be started during resuscitation)

- Benzodiazepines: used as first-line treatment. IV lorazepam 2 to 4 mg, or IV diazepam 5 to 10 mg, or intramuscular (IM) midazolam 10 mg (if there is a delay in establishing IV access). Doses can be repeated if the seizures continue.
- Second-line treatment: IV fosphenytoin (20–30 PE/kg at 150 PE/min IV), or IV valproic acid (20–40 mg/kg IV), or IV levetiracetam (20 mg/kg IV to maximum 60 mg/kg IV), or phenobarbital (20 mg/kg IV at 50–100 mg/min). Preferred second-line treatment is undergoing a multicenter clinical trial at the time of this writing.
- Give IV propofol if seizures refractory to the above (1–2 mg/kg induction dose; maintenance infusion: 30–200 µg/kg/min) Must intubate before giving IV propofol or give it during rapid sequence intubation.
- If intubated, patient must be transferred to hospital capable of continuous electroencephalogram (EEG) monitoring, whether medical intensive care unit (ICU) or neuro-ICU.
- Nonconvulsive status epilepticus is very difficult to diagnose in the ED without the aid of an EEG. In this clinical scenario, patients are likely to be intubated for airway protection and transferred to the nearest adult facility capable of continuous EEG monitoring.

Data from Refs.[28,31,32,60,61]

Box 11
History for seizure

- Patient's age
- Any previous provoked seizure
- Determine whether the first seizure was status epilepticus
- Time of day of first seizure occurrence
- Family history of seizures
- Associations such as postictal confusion, incontinence, and occurrence out of sleep
- Seek for a possible cause (as listed earlier)
- Consider other paroxysmal neurologic events and identify seizure mimics (discussed later in relation to differential diagnosis)

Data from AlEissa El. First adult seizure clinical presentation. 2017. Available at: https://emedicine.medscape.com/article/1186214-clinical. Accessed December 12, 2017.

Box 12
Physical examination for seizure

- Neurologic: look for signs of a focal brain lesion (lateralizing signs such as weakness of 1 side of the body or anisocoria)
- Cardiovascular: listen to heart sounds, identify murmurs if present
- Respiratory: breath sounds for underlying causes of hypoxemia
- Other systems: to identify comorbid conditions

Organization has identified stroke as the second leading cause of death in developed countries[36] and the most common cause of serious long-term disability in adults.[37]

Stroke can be broadly categorized into ischemic and hemorrhagic strokes. Hemorrhagic stroke is less common than ischemic stroke (15% and 85% respectively in most Western populations) but has a much higher mortality of about 50%.[38] Ischemia usually results from thromboembolic arterial occlusion with a progressive decrease in cerebral blood flow. Between the ischemic core and the normally perfused part of the brain at the periphery lies the ischemic penumbra, which is hypoxic and functionally inactive but still viable. This area is targeted by acute stroke therapies before necrosis occurs in hours to days.[38]

Hemorrhagic stroke is caused by rupture or leak of a cerebral blood vessel caused by uncontrolled hypertension, aneurysm, or overtreatment with anticoagulants. In hemorrhagic stroke, prompt hemostatic therapy is hypothesized to improve outcomes by reducing the volume of hematoma by cessation of bleeding or rebleeding.[39] Common causes of stroke are listed in **Box 13**.

The goal of acute management of adults with stroke in the pediatric ED is initial resuscitation/stabilization (**Box 14**), initial history (**Box 15**), and physical examination (**Box 16**). Strongly consider rapid transfer to a stroke unit in an adult facility as soon as possible. Laboratory testing and imaging are best left for the definitive care center.

Investigations

- Blood glucose; may be the only testing needed before transfer
- Electrolyte panel
- Complete blood count

Box 13
Common causes of stroke in adults

- Cardiac: atherosclerosis, arrhythmias, atrial fibrillation, defective heart valves, hypertension, aneurysm
- Diabetes mellitus
- Medications: oral contraceptives, hormone replacement therapy, anticoagulants
- Traumatic brain injury
- Others: smoking, obesity, sickle cell disease

Box 14
Resuscitation and stabilization for stroke

- Airway: ensure patency of airway, suction as required; intubate is Glasgow Coma Scale is less than 8
- Breathing: commence supplemental oxygen if necessary (oxygen saturation <94%)
- Circulation: secure IV access; hydration with normal saline
- Disability: Glasgow Coma Scale

- ECG
- Brain imaging (urgent computed tomography scan); best left for definitive care center

Transfer to Stroke Unit

Rapid transfer of patients to a stroke unit has been shown to reduce mortality by greater than or equal to 20%.[39,40] It has also been associated with improved functional outcomes.[41] The goal is to complete evaluation and administration of fibrinolytic therapy within 60 minutes of an arrival to an ED, which is best accomplished by dialing 911 for an Emergency Medical Services stroke team or using telestroke capabilities if available at the hospital.[42]

SHORTNESS OF BREATH

SOB is among the top 10 reasons for adult presentation to the ED.[43] The National Hospital Ambulatory Medical Care Survey in 2013 showed that SOB accounted for 3% of all adult ED presentations.[44] SOB accounts for about 9.5% of adult presentation to the pediatric ED.[2] SOB results from derangements in oxygenation and ventilation. Common causes are listed in **Box 17**. Management guidelines for adults with seizures include resuscitation/stabilization (**Box 18**), history (**Box 19**), physical examination (**Box 20**), investigations, and transfer.

Investigations

Chest radiograph and ECG are likely the most important investigations to obtain in the pediatric ED before transfer to an adult facility for definitive care.[45]

Box 15
History for stroke

- Find out onset of stroke because duration is the most important determinant of therapeutic options and should be determined as accurately as possible
- Ask about associated symptoms, such as seizures, fever, fall, to rule out infective cause and traumatic brain injury
- Previous history of stroke and neurologic deficits
- Past medical history of hypertension, diabetes, sickle cell anemia, hypercholesterolemia
- Tobacco use
- Family history of stroke
- Medications

Data from Davis S, Lees K, Donnan G. Treating the acute stroke patient as an emergency: current practices and future opportunities. Intern J Clin Pract 2006;60(4):399–407.

Box 16
Physical examination for stroke

- General examination: pallor (anemia/blood loss), fever
- Neurologic examination: level of consciousness, motor deficits, sensory deficits
- Cardiovascular examination: heart sounds
- Respiratory examination: breath sounds

- Chest radiograph:
  - Cardiomegaly, interstitial edema; for example, Kerley B lines, peribronchial cuffing, cephalization of blood vessels, vascular congestion: acute heart failure
  - Infiltrates: pneumonia
  - Hyperinflated lungs with flattened diaphragm: asthma or chronic obstructive pulmonary disease; if unilateral, think of foreign body
  - Pneumothorax: absence of normal lung markings to a portion of the lung field
  - Pleural effusion: white enhancement at the bilateral lung bases (pleural effusion has a very broad differential diagnosis)
- ECG:
  - ST segment changes: MI
  - Diffuse low-voltage electrical alternans: pericardial effusion
  - Right heart strain: pulmonary embolism

Transfer

Transfer patient as soon as the patient is stable to an appropriate facility for further evaluation and treatment of the underlying cause.

Box 17
Common causes of shortness of breath

- Respiratory: bronchial asthma exacerbations; chronic obstructive pulmonary disease; pulmonary embolism; pneumothorax; infections such as pneumonia, tuberculosis, epiglottitis, pertussis, severe tonsillitis, peritonsillar abscess, retropharyngeal abscess
- Cardiovascular: acute coronary syndrome, acute heart failure, arrhythmias, cardiac tamponade
- Neurologic: stroke may result in abnormal respiratory patterns (including apnea) and aspiration pneumonia; neuromuscular diseases (such as multiple sclerosis, Guillain-Barré syndrome, myasthenia gravis, amyotrophic lateral sclerosis) may result in weakness of respiratory muscles
- Trauma: blunt or penetrating injury to the neck or chest, facial burns, smoke inhalation
- Metabolic and toxic: poisoning (eg, organophosphates, salicylate, carbon monoxide), diabetic ketoacidosis, toxic inhalations (chlorine or anhydrous ammonia)
- Malignancy: lung cancer
- Others: sepsis, shock, complication of blood transfusion, drug overdose (cocaine, opioids, aspirin), anemia (from hemorrhage or hemolysis), peritonitis, massive obesity, anxiety/panic attacks

Data from Ahmed A, Graber MA. Evaluation of the adult with dyspnea in the emergency department. UpToDate: Waltham (MA); 2013.

Box 18
Resuscitation and stabilization for shortness of breath

- Airway: maintain patency of airway, suction if required, urgent intubation if necessary
- Breathing: oxygen supplementation
- Circulation: secure IV access; IV fluid may be required in anaphylaxis and asthma
- Disability: Glasgow Coma Scale
- Exposure: examine head to toe for signs of anaphylaxis or trauma
- Search for rapidly reversible causes:
  - Tension pneumothorax: immediate needle compression before radiograph
  - Pericardial tamponade: fluid boluses and emergent bedside pericardiocentesis
  - Upper airway foreign body: immediate consult to ear, nose, and throat for foreign body removal
  - Wheezing: nebulized beta-2 agonist (eg, salbutamol 5 mg), repeat as required; nebulized anticholinergic (eg, ipratropium bromide 0.5 mg, may be mixed with albuterol), repeat as required
  - Anaphylaxis: IM epinephrine (0.3 mg IM), antihistamines

Data from Ahmed A, Graber MA. Evaluation of the adult with dyspnea in the emergency department. UpToDate: Waltham (MA); 2013; and Woollard M, Greaves I. 4 Shortness of breath. Emerg Med J 2004;21(3):341–50.

Box 19
History for shortness of breath

- SOB: onset, course, severity, duration, triggers/precipitating factor, relieving factor, interventions so far
- Swelling of the lips, tongue, posterior pharynx, larynx, normal or erythematous skin (usually nonpruritic): angioedema caused by allergy, nonsteroidal antiinflammatory drug use, ACE inhibitor use
- Oropharyngeal swelling, hives, flushing, abdominal pain, vomiting, syncope, hypotension, tachycardia: anaphylaxis from insect bites, foods, medications
- Fever, sore throat, hoarseness, dysphagia: epiglottitis, pertussis
- Oropharyngeal swelling, pain, dysphagia, drooling, fever: Ludwig angina, severe tonsillitis, peritonsillar abscess, retropharyngeal abscess
- Dyspnea, wheezing, agitation, brief fragmented speech, depressed mental status in severe cases: asthma exacerbation
- Cough with hemoptysis: tuberculosis, pulmonary embolism, malignancy
- History of prolonged immobilization, recent trauma or surgery (particularly orthopedic), pregnancy oral contraceptive use and smoking, family history of hypercoagulability: pulmonary embolism
- Aspiration of dentures, food, medications, bones, coins (uncommon in adults)
- Blunt or penetrating injury to chest or neck or complications from medical procedures (such as central venous catheter placement): pneumothorax
- Previous history of SOB and severity (including requirement for advanced airway and ICU admission)
- Past medical history of asthma, chronic obstructive pulmonary disease (COPD), diabetes
- Medications and adherence; use of tobacco and drugs
- Psychogenic causes are diagnoses of exclusion in the ED

Data from Ahmed A, Graber MA. Evaluation of the adult with dyspnea in the emergency department. UpToDate: Waltham (MA); 2013.

Box 20
Physical examination for shortness of breath

- General examination: pallor (anemia), cyanosis (not common), clubbing (chronic hypoxemia), peripheral edema (heart failure), posture (sitting upright or tripod position)
- Signs of imminent respiratory arrest: depressed mental status, inability to maintain respiratory effort, cyanosis
- Signs of severe respiratory distress: retractions and use of accessory muscles, inability to lie supine, brief fragmented speech, profound sweating, agitation, dusky skin
- Respiratory:
  - Inspiratory stridor: obstruction above the vocal cords (eg, foreign body, epiglottitis, angioedema)
  - Expiratory stridor: obstruction below the vocal cords (eg, croup, foreign body, bacterial tracheitis)
  - Wheeze: asthma exacerbation, anaphylaxis, foreign body, acute heart failure, tumor
  - Crackles (rales): pneumonia, heart failure, pulmonary fibrosis
  - Decreased breath sounds: severe COPD, severe asthma, pneumothorax, pleural effusion
- Cardiovascular:
  - Extra heart sounds S3 or S4: heart failure, cardiomyopathy, MI
  - Muffled or distant heart sounds: cardiac tamponade
  - Murmurs: heart failure, compromised cardiac valves
  - Increased jugular venous pressure: heart failure, cardiac tamponade
  - Pulsus paradoxus: severe asthma, pulmonary embolism, cardiac tamponade

---

CARDIAC ARREST

Cardiac arrest is the sudden cessation of cardiac activity leading to unresponsiveness in patients with or without cardiac disease.[46] It accounts a small but important number of patients presenting to the adult ED,[47] and 15% to 20% of all deaths in the general population.[48] Presentation of adult patients with cardiac arrest is very rare in pediatric EDs, but it is essential for PEM physicians to rapidly institute corrective measures to improve outcomes.

Common causes of cardiac arrest are listed in **Box 21**.

The success of any resuscitation attempt depends on high-quality cardiopulmonary resuscitation (CPR) and defibrillation when indicated. While CPR is continued, there should be a search for reversible causes, which can be remembered with the mnemonic 5 Hs and 5 Ts:

Hs:
    Hypovolemia: 30 mL/kg NS boluses
    Hypoxia: secure airway with proper oxygenation
    Hydrogen ion (acidosis): bicarbonate (attempt to treat underlying cause of acidosis)
    Hypokalemia/hyperkalemia: hyperkalemia (calcium gluconate/calcium chloride, insulin/dextrose, albuterol, polystyrene sulfonate); hypokalemia (potassium chloride)
    Hypothermia: active rewarming
Ts:
    Tension pneumothorax: needle decompression/chest tube
    Tamponade (cardiac): pericardiocentesis
    Toxins: multiple treatments (antidotes)

Box 21
Common causes of cardiac arrest in adults

- Arrhythmias usually in a person with a preexisting heart condition such as:
  o Coronary artery disease
  o Valvular heart disease
  o Cardiomyopathy
  o Congenital heart disease
- Underlying rhythms associated with cardiac arrest are most commonly split into 2 different categories: shockable rhythms and nonshockable rhythms
- Pulseless ventricular tachycardia/ventricular fibrillation arrest constitute shockable rhythms
- Asystole/pulseless electrical activity arrest constitute nonshockable rhythms

Data from Sudden cardiac arrest. 2017. Available at: https://www.mayoclinic.org/diseases-conditions/sudden-cardiac-arrest/symptoms-causes/syc-20350634?p=1, 2017. Accessed December 12, 2017.

Thrombosis (pulmonary) (pulmonary embolism): tissue plasminogen activator (tPA)

Thrombosis (cardiac) (myocardial infarction): percutaneous coronary intervention or tPA

Resuscitation/Stabilization

Fig. 3 details the AHA adult cardiac arrest algorithm, including the 2015 update.[49]

Management

Tachycardia

Tachycardia has a wide differential diagnosis. Each rhythm has particular treatments. It is important when characterizing tachycardia to determine whether the patient is stable or unstable. A tachyarrhythmia (rhythm with a heart rate >100 beats/min) may be symptomatic or asymptomatic. The key to management of patients with tachycardia is to determine whether pulses are present. If pulses are present, then the clinician needs to determine whether the patient is stable or unstable and then provide treatment based on patient condition and rhythm. Drugs are generally not used to manage patients with unstable tachycardia. Immediate cardioversion is recommended.

Fig. 4 details the AHA adult tachycardia with a pulse algorithm.[50] Fig. 5A shows monomorphic ventricular tachycardia, and Fig. 5B shows polymorphic ventricular tachycardia.[51,52]

Management of pulseless ventricular tachycardia

Pulseless ventricular tachycardia is treated with CPR, epinephrine, and defibrillation from a high-energy shock. Biphasic defibrillation is 120 to 200 J. Monophasic defibrillation is 360 J. IV magnesium may terminate a polymorphic ventricular tachycardia such as torsades de pointes and can be given as 1 to 2 g IV/intraosseous (IO) in 10 mL of NS or 5% dextrose in water. Amiodarone can be considered if ventricular tachycardia is refractory to defibrillation or epinephrine. Consider giving during cardiac arrest as 300 mg IV/IO as the first dose. If a second dose is considered, give as 150 mg IV/IO. Lidocaine can also be considered. Lidocaine is given at a dose of 1 to 1.5 mg/kg IV/IO. This can be repeated to a maximum of 3 mg/kg. When using lidocaine, it should be noted that there has been no proven short-term or long-term efficacy in cardiac arrest.

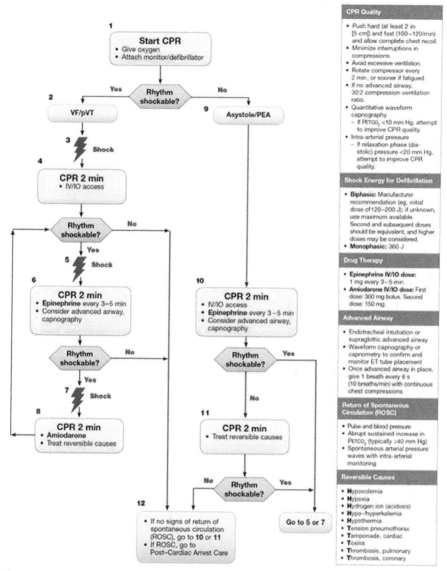

Fig. 3. AHA adult cardiac arrest algorithm including the 2015 update. (*Reprinted with permission Web-based Integrated 2010 & 2015 American Heart Association Guidelines for CPR & ECC. Part 7: Adult Advanced Cardiovascular Life Support ©2015 American Heart Association, Inc.*)

Management of ventricular tachycardia with a pulse

Ventricular tachycardia with a pulse is treated very similarly to pulseless ventricular tachycardia except IV magnesium has no role. The standard treatment of ventricular tachycardia is defibrillation. Consider sedation if the patient is conscious. Biphasic defibrillation is 120 to 200 J. Monophasic defibrillation is 360 J. Give epinephrine 1 mg every 3 to 5 minutes. Amiodarone can be given at a dose of 300 mg and a second

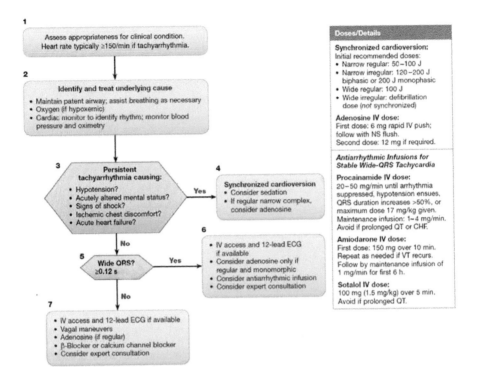

1

Assess appropriateness for clinical condition.
Heart rate typically ≥150/min if tachyarrhythmia.

2

Identify and treat underlying cause
- Maintain patent airway; assist breathing as necessary
- Oxygen (if hypoxemic)
- Cardiac monitor to identify rhythm; monitor blood pressure and oximetry

3

Persistent tachyarrhythmia causing:
- Hypotension?
- Acutely altered mental status?
- Signs of shock?
- Ischemic chest discomfort?
- Acute heart failure?

Yes →

4

Synchronized cardioversion
- Consider sedation
- If regular narrow complex, consider adenosine

No ↓

5

Wide QRS?
≥0.12 s

Yes →

6

- IV access and 12-lead ECG if available
- Consider adenosine only if regular and monomorphic
- Consider antiarrhythmic infusion
- Consider expert consultation

No ↓

7

- IV access and 12-lead ECG if available
- Vagal maneuvers
- Adenosine (if regular)
- β-Blocker or calcium channel blocker
- Consider expert consultation

Doses/Details

Synchronized cardioversion:
Initial recommended doses:
- Narrow regular: 50–100 J
- Narrow irregular: 120–200 J biphasic or 200 J monophasic
- Wide regular: 100 J
- Wide irregular: defibrillation dose (*not* synchronized)

Adenosine IV dose:
First dose: 6 mg rapid IV push; follow with NS flush.
Second dose: 12 mg if required.

Antiarrhythmic Infusions for Stable Wide-QRS Tachycardia

Procainamide IV dose:
20–50 mg/min until arrhythmia suppressed, hypotension ensues, QRS duration increases >50%, or maximum dose 17 mg/kg given. Maintenance infusion: 1–4 mg/min. Avoid if prolonged QT or CHF.

Amiodarone IV dose:
First dose: 150 mg over 10 min. Repeat as needed if VT recurs. Follow by maintenance infusion of 1 mg/min for first 6 h.

Sotalol IV dose:
100 mg (1.5 mg/kg) over 5 min. Avoid if prolonged QT.

Fig. 4. AHA adult tachycardia with a pulse algorithm. (*From* American Heart Association. Web-based integrated 2010 & 2015 American Heart Association guidelines for cardiopulmonary resuscitation and emergency cardiovascular care. Part 7: adult advanced cardiovascular life support. Available at: https://eccguidelines.heart.org/wp-content/themes/eccstaging/dompdf-master/pdffiles/part-7-adult-advanced-cardiovascular-life-support.pdf. Accessed December 4, 2017.)

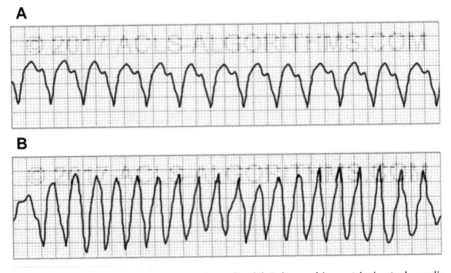

A

B

Fig. 5. (*A*) Monomorphic ventricular tachycardia. (*B*) Polymorphic ventricular tachycardia. (*From* Advanced cardiac life support. Other tachycardia rhythms. Available at: https://acls-algorithms.com/rhythms/other-tachycardias/. Accessed December 4, 2017.)

dose as warranted at 150 mg. If ventricular tachycardia is refractory to these measures, then lidocaine can be considered, given at the same dose as earlier at 1 to 1.5 mg/kg IV/IO with a maximum of 3 mg/kg.

Management of other forms of tachycardia

Fig. 6 shows examples of atrial fibrillation, atrial flutter, and supraventricular tachycardia.[53–55]

- Sinus tachycardia: treat underlying cause; for example, fluid resuscitation in sepsis
- Atrial fibrillation: stable, β-blocker (such as metoprolol 5 mg every 5 minutes), diltiazem bolus and infusion; unstable, synchronized cardioversion
- Atrial flutter: same as atrial fibrillation
- Superventricular tachycardia: stable, vagal maneuvers, adenosine 6 mg and 12 mg fast IV push; unstable,: synchronized cardioversion

Bradycardia

Bradyarrhythmia is any rhythm disorder with a pulse rate of less than 60 beats/min. Examples of this include sinus bradycardia or atrioventricular block. The adult

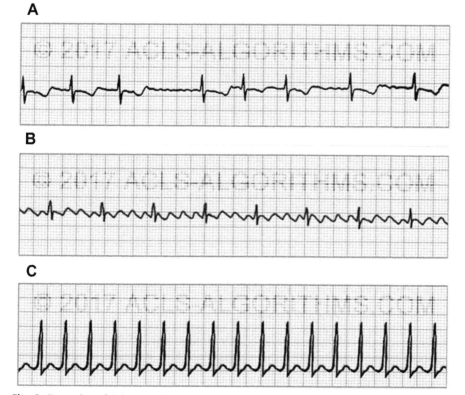

Fig. 6. Examples of (*A*) atrial fibrillation, (*B*) atrial flutter, and (*C*) supraventricular tachycardia. (*Data from* Advanced cardiac life support atrial fibrillation and supraventricular tachycardia. Available at: https://acls-algorithms.com/rhythms/atrial-fibrillation/, https://acls-algorithms.com/rhythms/supraventricular-tachycardia/. Accessed December 4, 2017.)

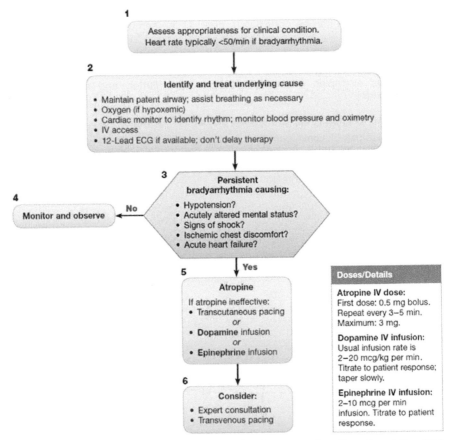

Fig. 7. AHA adult bradycardia with a pulse algorithm. (*From* American Heart Association. Web-based integrated 2010 & 2015 American Heart Association guidelines for cardiopulmonary resuscitation and emergency cardiovascular care. Part 7: adult advanced cardiovascular life support. Available at: https://eccguidelines.heart.org/wp-content/themes/eccstaging/dompdf-master/pdffiles/part-7-adult-advanced-cardiovascular-life-support.pdf. Accessed December 4, 2017.)

bradycardia with a pulse algorithm outlines the steps for assessment and management of patients presenting with symptomatic bradycardia with a pulse. A heart rate of less than 50 beats/min defines bradycardia.

Fig. 7 details the AHA adult bradycardia with a pulse algorithm.[50]

Pulseless electrical activity and asystole

Pulseless electrical activity is defined as any cardiac rhythm without the presence of a pulse. Asystole is an absent rhythm. These pulseless rhythms are treated with high-quality CPR and epinephrine. **Fig. 8** shows an example of asystole.[56]

Transfer

Once stabilized, patients should be transferred to an appropriate adult facility as soon as possible for further evaluation and treatment of the underlying cause.

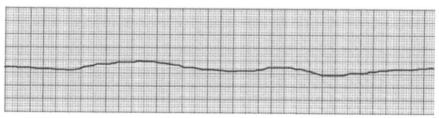

Fig. 8. Example of asystole. (*From* United Medical Education. Asystole. 2017. Available at: https://www.acls-pals-bls.com/algorithms/pals/. Accessed December 4, 2017.)

REFERENCES

1. Little WK, Hirsh DA. Adult patients in the pediatric emergency department: presentation and disposition. Pediatr Emerg Care 2014;30(11):808–11.
2. Baker MD, Schwartz GR, Ludwig S. The adult patient in the pediatric emergency department. Ann Emerg Med 1993;22(7):1136–9.
3. McDonnell WM, Kocolas I, Roosevelt GE, et al. Pediatric emergency department use by adults with chronic pediatric disorders. Arch Pediatr Adolesc Med 2010; 164(6):572–6.
4. Pitts SR, Niska RW, Xu J, et al. National Hospital Ambulatory Medical Care Survey: 2006 emergency department summary. Natl Health Stat Report 2008;(7): 1–38.
5. Norris RM. Fatality outside hospital from acute coronary events in three British health districts, 1994-5. United Kingdom Heart Attack Study Collaborative Group. BMJ 1998;316(7137):1065–70.
6. Heilman J. 12 lead ECG showing inferior and right ventricular infarct 2014. Available at: https://commons.wikimedia.org/wiki/File:Inferior_and_RtV_MI_12_lead. jpg. Accessed December 4, 2017.
7. Brush JE Jr, Brand DA, Acampora D, et al. Use of the initial electrocardiogram to predict in-hospital complications of acute myocardial infarction. N Engl J Med 1985;312(18):1137–41.
8. Forest RS, Shofer FS, Sease KL, et al. Assessment of the standardized reporting guidelines ECG classification system: the presenting ECG predicts 30-day outcomes. Ann Emerg Med 2004;44(3):206–12.
9. Kontos MC, Roberts BD, Jesse RL, et al. Utility of the presenting electrocardiogram to predict mortality when troponin level is used to diagnose myocardial infarction. Acad Emerg Med 2006;13(5 Supplement 1):S37.
10. Herren KR, Mackway-Jones K. Emergency management of cardiac chest pain: a review. Emerg Med J 2001;18(1):6–10.
11. Agostini-Miranda A, Crown L. An approach to the initial care of patients with chest pain in an emergency department located in a non-cardiac center. Am J Med 2009;6:24–9.
12. O'Gara PT, Kushner FG, Ascheim DD, et al. 2013 ACCF/AHA guideline for the management of ST-elevation myocardial infarction: executive summary: a report of the American College of Cardiology Foundation/American Heart Association Task Force on Practice Guidelines. J Am Coll Cardiol 2013;61(4):485–510.
13. Field JM, Hazinski MF, Gilmore D. Handbook of emergency cardiovascular care for healthcare providers from the American Heart Association. Dallas (TX): American Heart Association; 2006.

14. American Heart Association. Web-based integrated 2010 & 2015 American Heart Association guidelines for cardiopulmonary resuscitation and emergency cardiovascular care. Part 9: acute coronary syndromes. Available at: https://eccguidelines.heart.org/index.php/circulation/cpr-ecc-guidelines-2/part-9-acute-coronary-syndromes/. Accessed December 4, 2017.

15. Jneid H, Addison D, Bhatt DL, et al. 2017 AHA/ACC clinical performance and quality measures for adults with ST-elevation and non-ST-elevation myocardial infarction: a report of the American College of Cardiology/American Heart Association Task Force on Performance Measures. Circ Cardiovasc Qual Outcomes 2017;10(10) [pii:e000032].

16. Patel PR, Quinn JV. Syncope: a review of emergency department management and disposition. Clin Exp Emerg Med 2015;2(2):67–74.

17. Welsh JT, Welsh T, Emerman C. Evaluation of syncope in the emergency department. Emerg Med Rep 2015;36(22):261–9.

18. Bourgeois FT, Shannon MW. Adult patient visits to children's hospital emergency departments. Pediatrics 2003;111(6 Pt 1):1268–72.

19. Lemonick DM. Evaluation of syncope in the emergency department. Am J Clin Med 2010;7(1):11–9.

20. Huff JS, Decker WW, Quinn JV, et al. Clinical policy: critical issues in the evaluation and management of adult patients presenting to the emergency department with syncope. Ann Emerg Med 2007;49(4):431–44.

21. Iwai S. Syncope: an evidence-based approach. Evidence-based cardiology consult. London: Springer; 2014. p. 553–63.

22. Kapoor WN, Karpf M, Wieand S, et al. A prospective evaluation and follow-up of patients with syncope. N Engl J Med 1983;309(4):197–204.

23. Martin GJ, Adams SL, Martin HG, et al. Prospective evaluation of syncope. Ann Emerg Med 1984;13(7):499–504.

24. Eagle KA, Black HR. The impact of diagnostic tests in evaluating patients with syncope. Yale J Biol Med 1983;56(1):1–8.

25. Sarasin FP, Junod AF, Carballo D, et al. Role of echocardiography in the evaluation of syncope: a prospective study. Heart 2002;88(4):363–7.

26. Quinn JV, Stiell IG, McDermott DA, et al. Derivation of the San Francisco Syncope Rule to predict patients with short-term serious outcomes. Ann Emerg Med 2004;43(2):224–32.

27. Quinn J, McDermott D, Stiell I, et al. Prospective validation of the San Francisco Syncope Rule to predict patients with serious outcomes. Ann Emerg Med 2006;47(5):448–54.

28. Birnbaum A, Esses D, Bijur P, et al. Failure to validate the San Francisco Syncope Rule in an independent emergency department population. Ann Emerg Med 2008;52(2):151–9.

29. Huff JS, Melnick ER, Tomaszewski CA, et al. Clinical policy: critical issues in the evaluation and management of adult patients presenting to the emergency department with seizures. Ann Emerg Med 2014;63(4):437–47.e5.

30. Lapalme-Remis S, Cascino GD. Imaging for adults with seizures and epilepsy. Continuum (Minneap Minn) 2016;22(5, Neuroimaging):1451–79.

31. Trinka E, Cock H, Hesdorffer D, et al. A definition and classification of status epilepticus–Report of the ILAE task force on classification of status epilepticus. Epilepsia 2015;56(10):1515–23.

32. Garber BG, Glauser J. Evaluation and management of seizures in the emergency department. Emerg Med Rep 2017;38(12). Available at: https://www.reliasmedia.

com/articles/140857-evaluation-and-management-of-seizures-in-the-emergency-department. Accessed December 12, 2018.

33. Sibai BM. Magnesium sulfate prophylaxis in preeclampsia: lessons learned from recent trials. Am J Obstet Gynecol 2004;190(6):1520–6.

34. Verbalis JG, Goldsmith SR, Greenberg A, et al. Diagnosis, evaluation, and treatment of hyponatremia: expert panel recommendations. Am J Med 2013;126(10):S1–42.

35. Sterns RH, Nigwekar SU, Hix JK. The treatment of hyponatremia. Seminars in nephrology 2009;29(3):282–99.

36. The top 10 causes of death 2017:3. Available at: http://www.who.int/mediacentre/factsheets/fs310/en/. Accessed December 12, 2017.

37. Zweifler RM. Management of acute stroke. South Med J 2003;96(4):380–5.

38. Davis S, Lees K, Donnan G. Treating the acute stroke patient as an emergency: current practices and future opportunities. Int J Clin Pract 2006;60(4):399–407.

39. Mayer SA. Ultra-early hemostatic therapy for intracerebral hemorrhage. Stroke 2003;34(1):224–9.

40. Collaborative systematic review of the randomised trials of organised inpatient (stroke unit) care after stroke. Stroke Unit Trialists' Collaboration. BMJ 1997;314(7088):1151–9.

41. How do stroke units improve patient outcomes? A collaborative systematic review of the randomized trials. Stroke Unit Trialists Collaboration. Stroke 1997;28(11):2139–44.

42. Jauch EC, Saver JL, Adams HP Jr, et al. Guidelines for the early management of patients with acute ischemic stroke: a guideline for healthcare professionals from the American Heart Association/American Stroke Association. Stroke 2013;44(3):870–947.

43. Niska R, Bhuiya F, Xu J. National hospital ambulatory medical care survey: 2007 emergency department summary. Natl Health Stat Report 2010;26(26):1–31.

44. Centers for Disease Control and Prevention. National hospital ambulatory medical care survey: 2010 emergency department summary tables 2013. Available at: https://www.cdc.gov/nchs/data/ahcd/nhamcs_emergency/2010_ed_web_tables.pdf. Accessed December 12, 2017.

45. Ahmed A, Graber MA. Evaluation of the adult with dyspnea in the emergency department. Waltham (MA): UpToDate; 2013.

46. Pandian GR, Thampi SM, Chakraborty N, et al. Profile and outcome of sudden cardiac arrests in the emergency department of a tertiary care hospital in South India. J Emerg Trauma Shock 2016;9(4):139–45.

47. Johnson NJ, Salhi RA, Abella BS, et al. Emergency department factors associated with survival after sudden cardiac arrest. Resuscitation 2013;84(3):292–7.

48. Deo R, Albert CM. Epidemiology and genetics of sudden cardiac death. Circulation 2012;125(4):620–37.

49. Link MS, Berkow LC, Kudenchuk PJ, et al. Part 7: adult advanced cardiovascular life support: 2015 American Heart Association guidelines update for cardiopulmonary resuscitation and emergency cardiovascular care. Circulation 2015;132(18 Suppl 2):S444–64.

50. American Heart Association. Web-based integrated 2010 & 2015 American Heart Association guidelines for cardiopulmonary resuscitation and emergency cardiovascular care. Part 7: adult advanced cardiovascular life support. Available at: https://eccguidelines.heart.org/wp-content/themes/eccstaging/dompdf-master/pdffiles/part-7-adult-advanced-cardiovascular-life-support.pdf. Accessed December 4, 2017.

51. ACLS Algorithms. Monomorphic ventricular tachycardia 2017. Available at: https://acls-algorithms.com/rhythms/other-tachycardias. Accessed December 12, 2017.
52. ACLS Algorithms. Polymorphic ventricular tachycardia 2017. Available at: https://acls-algorithms.com/rhythms/other-tachycardias. Accessed December 12, 2017.
53. ACLS Algorithms. Atrial fibrillation 2017. Available at: https://acls-algorithms.com/rhythms/atrial-fibrillation. Accessed December 12, 2017.
54. ACLS Algorithms. Atrial flutter 2017. Available at: https://acls-algorithms.com/rhythms/atrial-flutter. Accessed December 12, 2017.
55. ACLS Algorithms. Supraventricular tachycardia 2017. Available at: https://acls-algorithms.com/rhythms/supraventricular-tachycardia. Accessed December 12, 2017.
56. United Medical Education. Asystole 2017. Available at: https://www.acls-pals-bls.com/algorithms/pals/. Accessed December 4, 2017.
57. Bayer AJ, Chadha JS, Farag RR, et al. Changing presentation of myocardial infarction with increasing old age. J Am Geriatr Soc 1986;34(4):263–6.
58. Hermann LK, Weingart SD, Yoon YM, et al. Comparison of frequency of inducible myocardial ischemia in patients presenting to emergency department with typical versus atypical or nonanginal chest pain. Am J Cardiol 2010;105(11):1561–4.
59. Kannel WB, Abbott RD. Incidence and prognosis of unrecognized myocardial infarction. An update on the Framingham study. N Engl J Med 1984;311(18):1144–7.
60. ESETT - The Established Status Epilepticus Treatment Trial. 2017. Available at: https://nett.umich.edu/clinical-trials/esett. Accessed December 12, 2017.
61. Misra UK, Kalita J. Management of provoked seizure. Ann Indian Acad Neurol 2011;14(1):2–8.

Indications and Interpretation of Common Laboratory Assays in the Emergency Department

Andrea T. Cruz, MD, MPH

KEYWORDS

- False negative • False positive • Laboratory abnormalities • Pediatric
- Reference ranges

KEY POINTS

- No single component of the complete blood cell count or inflammatory marker can reliably exclude bacteremia or meningitis in a febrile child.
- Laboratory results may well be normal for a child presenting to the emergency department (ED) shortly after the onset of symptoms, given the natural history of when laboratory tests are thought to increase in response to a given stimulus.
- Not all abnormal laboratory tests require follow-up while a child is in the ED.
- Specimen handling and processing can have an impact on laboratory results in predictable ways.

INTRODUCTION

Laboratory evaluation is commonly performed to allow clinicians to increase or decrease their index of suspicion for a child having a certain disease process. It is estimated that each patient who presents to an emergency department (ED) has at least 7 laboratory or other studies obtained.[1] One modified Delphi study found little consensus in diagnostic approaches in emergency medicine.[2] Although laboratory tests provide the opportunity to alter the post-test probability of different disease processes, the more laboratory tests are obtained, the greater the probability that at least one of those tests falls outside the normal range. In addition, the turn-around time of laboratory tests has a direct impact on ED length of stay.[1] Most physicians are unaware of the costs of laboratory tests, with one study in family physicians noting that only one-quarter of cost estimates were accurate to within 25% of the actual

Disclosures: The author has no disclosures or conflicts of interest.
Department of Pediatrics, Sections of Emergency Medicine and Infectious Diseases, Baylor College of Medicine, 6621 Fannin Street, Suite A2210, Houston, TX 77030, USA
E-mail address: atcruz@texaschildrens.org

Pediatr Clin N Am 65 (2018) 1191–1204
https://doi.org/10.1016/j.pcl.2018.07.005
0031-3955/18/© 2018 Elsevier Inc. All rights reserved.

costs of the test, with physicians routinely underestimating test cost.[3] Even when physicians were presented with Medicare allowable fees, ordering patterns did not change.[4]

It is also important for clinicians to recognize how reference ranges are established. In most cases, normal ranges represent 2 SDs above and below the mean. Laboratories should report the ranges considered normal based on a child's age. This is particularly important for providers practicing at facilities that predominantly care for adults, in which normal ranges may be those for adult patients. Certain laboratory tests are often higher in neonates and young children than older children and adults (and may thus appear falsely elevated using adult norms); these include alkaline phosphatase, ammonia, aspartate aminotransferase (AST), bilirubin, γ-glutamyl transferase (GGT), creatine kinase, potassium, thyroid-stimulating hormone, and thyroxine. Conversely, some tests have lower norms for children than for adults. These include amylase, creatinine, and haptoglobin.

Given the increased resource utilization and transmission of cost to patients and their families, the first question a clinician should be asking is how a given laboratory test would alter clinical management. This article reviews some of the most commonly obtained laboratory and other tests in the pediatric ED, discusses common patterns of laboratory abnormalities seen in certain conditions, and reviews some spurious conditions that can have an impact on test interpretation.

TESTS
Complete Blood Cell Counts and Acute-phase Reactants

Fever is one of the most common reasons children present to EDs, and a complete blood cell count (CBC) is often obtained in febrile children, despite the known low sensitivity and positive predictive value of elevated absolute neutrophil count (ANC) and white blood cell count (WBC) in identifying children with bacteremia and meningitis.[5] Even the presence of extreme leukocytosis, defined as a WBC count of greater than or equal to 25,000 cells/mm^3, has a sensitivity of only 25% to 40% for bacterial etiologies.[6-8] The presence of profound neutropenia in association with fever in a child without other reasons for neutropenia, however, should increase the index of suspicion for overwhelming bacterial infection. There are fewer data on how other CBC parameters (eg, bandemia and toxic granulation) allow for risk stratification. **Table 1** describes hematologic and other reasons for abnormalities in the CBC.

Given the limitations in CBC parameters in differentiating viral from bacterial etiologies, use of acute-phase reactants, including erythrocyte sedimentation rate (ESR), C-reactive protein (CRP), and procalcitonin (PCT), have been used to attempt to identify children at risk for serious bacterial infections (SBIs), which include bacteremia, acute bacterial meningitis, and urinary tract infection (UTI). A limitation in the ESR is that it takes longer to increase and decrease than other inflammatory markers. CRP and PCT are more temporally increased with fever, but CRP is commonly elevated with bacterial and nonbacterial pathogens. PCT, in contrast, is more likely to be increased in bacterial infections.[9] In part, this is because elevations in PCT require disruptions in several components of the cytokine pathway, to a far greater degree than do elevations in ESR or CRP. Therefore, PCT may be superior to other inflammatory markers not only in terms of differentiating bacterial from other pathogens but also in identifying the severity of disease. For example, some studies have used PCT to differentiate between cystitis and pyelonephritis.[10] Cutoffs for optimal PCT have varied, however, with some studies using a cutoff of greater than or equal to 0.5 ng/mL[9] and others using a threshold of greater than or equal to 2 ng/mL to

Table 1
Interpretation of complete blood cell count and acute-phase reactant parameters

Parameter	Hematologic Causes for Elevation	Nonhematologic Causes for Elevation	Hematologic Causes for Depression	Nonhematologic Causes for Depression
WBC	Infection, malignancy	Demargination after seizures; systemic corticosteroids	Overwhelming infection	Clumped WBCs
Bandemia		Bacteremia, *Clostridium difficile*, *Shigella*, adenovirus; variation in classification of bands vs neutrophils by the laboratory	N/A	N/A
Toxic granulation	Autophagocytosis	Severe infection, rheumatologic disease	N/A	N/A
Atypical lymphocytes	Malignancy	CMV, EBV, hepatitis C, streptococcal infection, syphilis, rheumatologic disease, Addison, drugs (eg, phenytoin)	N/A	N/A
Hemoglobin	Polycythemia in children with cyanotic heart disease	Hemoconcentration	Anemias; marrow disorders (including malignancy); hemolysis	Hemodilution
Schistocytes	Hemolytic uremic syndrome; hemolytic anemia; DIC; TTP	Hemolysis from prosthetic valves	N/A	N/A

(continued on next page)

Table 1
(continued)

Parameter	Hematologic Causes for Elevation	Nonhematologic Causes for Elevation	Hematologic Causes for Depression	Nonhematologic Causes for Depression
MCV	Macrocytic anemia (vitamin B_{12}, folate deficiency); marrow disorders	Hypothyroidism; drugs (hydroxyurea, MTX, antiretrovirals)	Iron deficiency anemia; thalassemia; sideroblastic anemia	Lead toxicity; micronutrient (copper, zinc) deficiency
Platelets	Recovery from anemia and ITP; post-splenectomy	Infection; nephrotic syndrome; vasculitides; rheumatologic conditions; drug reaction (eg, enoxaparin)	ITP; DIC; marrow disorders; anemia (iron deficiency, vitamin B_{12}, folate); Wiskott-Aldrich syndrome; thrombocytopenia with absent radii syndrome	Clumped platelets; lupus; drug-induced; ECMO; hemangiomas; splenomegaly; cyanotic congenital heart disease
ESR	Anemia	Receipt of IVIG; infection; rheumatologic	Can be falsely depressed with polycythemia, sickle cell	N/A
CRP	N/A	Infection; rheumatologic; drug reaction; malignancy	N/A	Can be falsely depressed in hepatic failure
PCT	N/A	Infection; receipt of chemotherapeutic agents; GVHD; rheumatologic; cardiac surgery; severe burns; multiorgan system failure	N/A	N/A
D-dimer	DIC	Thrombotic disease; high levels of rheumatoid factor; malignancy; recent surgery; sickle cell disease	N/A	N/A

Abbreviations: DIC, disseminated intravascular coagulation; ECMO, extracorporeal membrane oxygenation; GVHD, graft versus host disease; ITP, immune thrombocytopenia (formerly idiopathic thrombocytopenic purpura); IVIG, intravenous immunoglobulin; MCV, mean corpuscular volume; MTX, methotrexate; TTP, thrombotic thrombocytopenic.

2.5 ng/mL.[11] PCT increases within 2 hours to 4 hours of the inciting event and peaks by 12 hours to 24 hours.

A common scenario is when a child with unexplained fever has slightly elevated (<2 times the upper limit of normal [ULN]) inflammatory markers. For the ED provider, who often is seeing the child for the first time, it is often unclear if these markers are trending upward or downward. One option is close follow-up with the child's pediatrician after the ED stay to trend inflammatory markers. It is also important to realize that no inflammatory marker is sufficiently sensitive in the child with fever of short duration.[9]

It is likely that a combination of CBC parameters and inflammatory markers results in a better decision tool for the evaluation of febrile children than a single parameter used in isolation. For example, one study of febrile children found that absolute band count and PCT were the 2 screening tests most associated with SBIs.[12] Other studies have found that the ANC is the WBC parameter most correlated with bacteremia and meningitis.[5] Thus, combining ANC with inflammatory markers may be promising and offer increased accuracy over use of any single parameter.

Although CBC parameters and inflammatory markers may be more nonspecific for many forms of SBIs, leukocytosis and elevated inflammatory markers are associated with community-acquired pneumonia (CAP). Many fever algorithms recommend obtaining chest radiography for a WBC greater than or equal to 20,000/mm^3 even in the absence of auscultory findings. A study conducted after the widespread introduction of the pneumococcal conjugate vaccine found that 15% of children with leukocytosis greater than or equal to 20,000/mm^3 had occult pneumonia.[13] Given that the national guidelines for pediatric CAP recommend against antibiotic treatment in otherwise healthy preschool-aged children,[14] use of PCT may be a way of decreasing antibiotic utilization. One study found that no child with CAP had typical bacterial pathogens detected if the PCT was less than 0.1 mg/mL.[15]

A common reason children are evaluated in the ED is for prolonged fever. The extent of ED evaluation that should be conducted in a well-appearing, previously healthy child with a nonfocal examination is not well established. A tiered approach, of obtaining laboratory tests for common infectious etiologies, followed by outpatient follow-up with the child's primary care provider, is reasonable. The ED evaluation may consist of the following tests, based on known pathogens causing prolonged fever: CBC and blood culture; urinalysis and urine culture; chest radiograph; inflammatory markers; and serologies for Epstein-Barr virus (EBV), cytomegalovirus (CMV), and *Bartonella*. A monospot assay for EBV can also be considered for older children; sensitivity in the preschool-aged population is poor. Although not all these test results return during a child's ED visit, the results may benefit providers who see the child in follow-up.

One critical disease to identify in a child with prolonged fever is Kawasaki disease (KD). Providers should ask about KD symptoms, which may have occurred at any time during the febrile illness, even if not present at the time of the ED visit. Laboratory findings consistent with KD include anemia, thrombocytopenia, hepatic transaminitis, hypoalbuminemia, elevation in inflammatory markers, and sterile pyuria.

Metabolic Panels

Electrolytes, renal function testing, and hepatic panels are obtained for several reasons in the ED, including for children with abdominal pain and abdominal trauma. Laboratory tests are not useful in ruling acute appendicitis in or out in the child with undifferentiated abdominal pain.[16] Another common reason chemistry panels are ordered is in children with dehydration. Although serum bicarbonate is correlated with clinical dehydration scores,[17] ED providers should avoid hospitalizing well-appearing children who have

Table 2
Patterns of liver injury

Pattern	Causes	Aspartate Aminotransferase	Alanine Aminotransferase	Aspartate Aminotransferase/Alanine Aminotransferase	Alkaline Phosphatase	γ-Glutamyl Transferase	Direct Bilirubin	Indirect Bilirubin	Albumin	Prothrombin Time
Acute viral hepatitis	Hepatitis A–E, CMV, EBV	↑↑	↑↑	↓	↑↔	↑↔	↑	↔	↓↔	↑↔
Drug-induced	Acetaminophen, isoniazid	↑↑	↑↑	↔	↑↔	↑↔	↑	↔	↓↔	↑↔
Shock liver (ischemic hepatitis)	Hypoxemia, sepsis, heart failure	↑↑↑	↑↑↑	↑	↑↔	↑↔	↑	↑	↓	↑↑
Cholestasis, extrahepatic	Choledochal cysts; choledocholithiasis; biliary strictures; parasitic infections	↑	↑	↔	↑↑	↑↑	↑↔	↑↔	↓↔	↑↔
Cholestasis, intrahepatic	Cholangitis; sickle cell; drug toxicity; hepatic allograft rejection; infiltrative disease; TPN	↑	↑	↔	↑↑	↑↑	↑	↔	↓↔	↑↔
Isolated GGT elevation	Pancreatic disease; MI; AKI; drugs (phenytoin, barbiturates)	↔	↔	↔	↔	↑	↔	↔	↔	↔
Isolated hyperbilirubinemia (direct)	Dubin–Johnson syndrome; Rotor syndrome	↔	↔	↔	↔	↔	↑	↔	↔	↔

Condition	Cause								
Isolated hyperbilirubinemia (indirect)	Hemolysis; Gilbert syndrome; Crigler-Najjar syndrome; drug toxicity	↔	↔	↔	↑	↔	↔	↔	↔
Rhabdomyolysis or heat stroke	Heat injury; drugs	↑↑	↑	↑↔	↑	↑↔	↑	↔	↑↔
Vitamin K deficiency or malabsorption	Hemorrhagic disease of the newborn, drugs (coumadin, phenytoin), fat malabsorption	↔	↔	↑↔	↑↔	↑↔	↔	↑	↑
NAFLD	Obesity	↑	↑	↑↔	↑↔	↑	↔	↔	↔
Alcoholic liver disease	Alcohol abuse	↑	↑↔	↑	↑↔	↑↔	→	↑↔	
Disorders of bone turnover	Osteoporosis, Paget disease, bony metastases	↔	↑	↔	↔	↔	↔	↔	

Abbreviations: ↑, increased; ↓, decreased; ↔, normal; AKI, acute kidney injury; MI, myocardial infarction; TPN, total parenteral nutrition.

successfully orally rehydrated only because they have a low serum bicarbonate. The American College of Emergency Physicians states that no single laboratory variable can accurately predict the degree of dehydration in a child, and laboratory evaluation should be targeted to specific concerns rather than obtained indiscriminantly.[18] The single most useful test in a dehydrated child may be a serum glucose rather than bicarbonate.

AST and alanine aminotransferase (ALT) often are obtained to evaluate for medical or traumatic liver injury. There is no single widely accepted threshold value that should prompt imaging to evaluate for hepatic injury. One recent pediatric study found that AST less than 200 IU/L, combined with a reassuring examination and normal pancreatic enzymes, had a negative predictive value of 99% for abdominal trauma.[19] Lower cutoffs may be considered, however, if the mechanism of injury is unclear, as is the case for suspected nonaccidental trauma. Laboratory parameters consistent with different forms of liver pathology are reviewed in **Table 2**. One common reason for transaminase elevation is nonalcoholic fatty liver disease (NAFLD), estimated to occur in more than 10% of American children.[20] Although some patients with NAFLD progress to end-stage liver disease in the long term, in childhood, isolated elevations in aminotransferases may be the only finding.

Table 3
Interpretation of blood gases

Disorder	pH	P_{CO_2}	HCO_3	Base Excess	Compensation[a]
Metabolic acidosis	↓	↔	↓	↓	Begins within 30 min; failure to compensate indicates substantial respiratory or neurologic disease
Respiratory acidosis	↓	↑	↔	↔	Renal compensation can require up to 3–5 d
Metabolic alkalosis	↑	↔	↑	↑	Begins within 30 min; failure to compensate indicates substantial respiratory or neurologic disease
Respiratory alkalosis	↑	↓	↔	↔	Renal compensation can require up to 3–5 d
Primary metabolic acidosis with respiratory compensation	↓	↓	↓	↓	P_{CO_2} decreases by 1.2 mm Hg for every 1 mEq/L reduction in HCO_3 [a]Aspirin toxicity can cause metabolic acidosis and a respiratory alkalosis
Primary respiratory acidosis with renal compensation	↓	↑	↑	↑	HCO_3 increases by 1 mEq/L for every 10 mm Hg increase in P_{CO_2}
Mixed respiratory and metabolic acidosis	↓	↑	↓	↓	Often seen in patients with multiorgan system dysfunction receiving multiple treatments
Primary metabolic alkalosis with respiratory compensation	↑	↓	↑	↑	P_{CO_2} increases by 0.7 mm Hg for each 1 mEq/L increase in HCO_3
Primary respiratory alkalosis with renal compensation	↑	↓	↓	↓	HCO_3 decreases by 2 mEq/L for every 10 mm Hg decrease in P_{CO_2}
Mixed respiratory and metabolic alkalosis	↑	↓	↑	↑	Often seen in patients with multiorgan system dysfunction receiving multiple treatments

[a] Compensation values listed are for acute expected compensation; generally, compensation does not result in full normalization of pH.

When a liver panel is obtained, physicians may note abnormal findings in parameters not initially of interest, such as elevations in alkaline phosphatase or in GGT. Although both parameters may be elevated in hepatobiliary disease, a normal GGT in the presence of an elevated alkaline phosphatase is more indicative of bone disease (eg, bony metastases and renal osteodystrophy). An isolated elevated GGT should not prompt evaluation for other pathology nor should an alkaline phosphatase less than 2 times the ULN. Alkaline phosphatase greater than or equal to 2 times the ULN should prompt evaluation of the biliary tree and hepatic parenchyma with a hepatic ultrasound.

Table 4
Interpretation of urine drug screens

Drug	How Soon Test Becomes Positive After Use	Time Remains Positive in Urine (d)	False-Positive Results Due to
Amphetamines	4–6 h	1–3 (up to 10 d in chronic usage)	Pseudoephedrine, ephedrine, β-blockers, bupropion, fluoroquinolones, labetalol, metformin, promethazine, trazodone, tricyclic antidepressants, Vicks (camphor-based metholated eucalyptus oil) inhaler
Barbiturates	2–4 h	4–6	Nonsteroidal anti-inflammatory drugs
Benzodiazepines	2–7 h	1–7	Nonsteroidal anti-inflammatory drugs, efavirenz, sertraline
Cocaine	2–6 h	1–4	[b]
Lysergic acid diethylamide	0–3 h	1–5	Amitriptyline, bupropion, diltiazem, fentanyl, fluoxetine, haloperidol, labetalol, metoclopramide, risperidone, sertraline, trazodone, verapamil
Marijuana	1–3 h	Days–months[a]	Marinol, nonsteroidal anti-inflammatory drugs, efavirenz
3,4-methylenedioxy methamphetamine (Ecstasy)	2–7 h	2–4 d	Bupropion, trazodone
Opiates	1–6 h	1–3	Poppy seeds, antibiotics (fluoroquinolones, rifampin, rifapentine), diphenhydramine, naloxone, quetiapine (Seroquel), tramadol, verapamil
Tricyclic antidepressants	8–12 h	2–7	Quetiapine (Seroquel)
Phencyclidine	4–6 h	1–14	Bath salts, cough/cold medications (including dextromethorphan), diphenhydramine, ketamine, lamotrigine, tramadol

[a] Chronic users can have positive urine drug tests for cannabinoids months after cessation of usage.
[b] Previous reports that amoxicillin can cause falsely positive cocaine assays on UDSs have been refuted.

Blood Gases

Blood gases are useful in helping differentiate among causes of acid-base imbalances or to monitor response to therapy (such as in an intubated patient). The common blood gas findings associated with various conditions are summarized in **Table 3**. Physicians should be cautious about obtaining blood gases in children with respiratory distress who are protecting their airways. Many of these children have hypercarbia, but this is not a stand-alone reason for intubation. Pediatric acute lung injury experts achieved strong consensus on accepting permissive hypercapnia in children with respiratory distress.[21] In addition, many children with chronic pulmonary parenchymal disease have baseline hypercarbia. Correction of hypercarbia should not be the goal in these patients, lest they lose their respiratory drive.

Urine Drug Screens

Urine drug screens (UDSs) are commonly obtained in patients with altered mentation or as part of medical clearance for psychiatric patients (discussed later). The utility of the UDS is controversial, because the presence of a substance in the urine does not mean that it is contributing to the patient's presentation. One study found that fewer than 5% of cases in which UDS was obtained was management altered by the results (all were in young children exposed to drugs in the home).[22] In one study of approximately 900 pediatric psychiatry patients, the UDS results did not alter management or the ED-based intervention.[23] Moreover, falsely positive UDS results are common (**Table 4**).[24,25] One possible role for the UDS is to evaluate for cocaine in a child or adolescent with suspected myocardial infarction, to avoid using β-blockers.

Evaluation of the Patient with Psychiatric Disease

Many children present to the ED for medical clearance before transfer to psychiatric facilities. There is substantial controversy over the utility of routine laboratory evaluation in the medical clearance process, given that most pathology may be evident based on historical features and examination findings. This is particularly the case in a patient with preexisting psychiatric diagnoses. The American Association for

Table 5
Recommendations for medical clearance of psychiatric patients in the emergency department

Evaluation	Examples
Identify medical mimics	Encephalopathy, intoxication or substance withdrawal, diabetes, hypothyroidism
Identify potential conditions that require care that may be more than can be handled by a psychiatric facility	Autism, impairments in activities of daily living
Recommend additional evaluation if:	Cognitive deficits or delirium Positive review of systems (eg, fever) Focal neurologic findings (including head injury) Substance intoxication or withdrawal Decreased level of consciousness Abnormal vital signs

Data from Wilson MP, Nordstrom K, Anderson EL, et al. American Association for Emergency Psychiatry Task Force on medical clearance of adult psychiatric patients. Part II: controversies over medical assessment, and consensus recommendations. West J Emerg Med 2017;18:640–6; with variables pertinent to the pediatric population.

Emergency Psychiatry Task Force on Medical Clearance of Adult Psychiatric Patients has published screening recommendations, summarized in **Table 5**.[26] There is no standard combination of laboratory tests that is used for medical clearance across EDs. Rather, practice variation often is driven by the admission requirements of local inpatient psychiatric facilities.

Although most data on medical clearance stems from the adult literature, one study evaluating more than 1000 pediatric psychiatric ED visits demonstrated that in fewer than 1% of cases did laboratory evaluation change disposition decisions, and findings changed management decisions in fewer than 6% of cases. The most common abnormal laboratory findings were abnormal urinalyses and iron-deficiency anemia in menstruating adolescents.[27] Although the UDS was positive in approximately 7% of pediatric patients, this did not alter disposition.

Table 6
Interpretation of urinalysis values

Parameter	Normal Range[a]	False-Positive Results	False-Negative Results
pH	4.5–8.0	Alkali urine seen with: vegetarian diet, medications (amphotericin, acetazolamide, salicylates), urine stored at room temperature prior to processing	Acidic urine seen with: high protein diet, cranberry consumption, diarrhea, phenylketonuria, alkaptonuria
Urine specific gravity	1.005–1.035	Falsely high urine specific gravity seen with glycosuria, proteinuria, receipt of colloids, intravenous contrast	Falsely low urine specific gravity seen with alkaline urine
Urobilinogen	0.2–1 mg/dL	Chlorpromazine, sulfa drugs, para-aminosalicylic acid	High nitrite concentrations
Ketones	Negative	Dehydration, glucocorticoids, valproate	Severe ketoacidosis
Glucose	Negative	Cystitis	Vitamin C
Protein	Negative	Concentrated or alkaline urine, drugs (acetazolamide, cephalosporins)	Dilute or acidic urine, multiple myeloma
Blood	Negative	Myoglobin, menstrual blood	Vitamin C, high nitrites and protein, urine dipsticks with prolonged air exposure
Leukocyte esterase	Negative	Antibiotics (imipenem, meropenem, clavulanate), *Trichomonas*, eosinophils in urine	Acidosis, hyperglycemia, high ketones, vitamin C
Nitrites	Negative	Urine stored at room temperature before processing	Urine not in bladder long enough for bacteria to reduce nitrate to nitrite, malnutrition, UTI caused by organisms that cannot convert nitrate to nitrite (yeast, Gram-positive organisms)

[a] Assuming normal renal function.

Urinalysis

Urinalysis is one of the most commonly obtained tests in the ED. Optimally, the urine would be transported to a laboratory promptly for evaluation, rather than left at room temperature before processing. Leaving urine at room temperature for hours can result in an alkaline pH, darker color, increased turbidity, decreased glucose and ketones, increased nitrites (due to bacterial overgrowth), and decreased urinary WBC and red blood cell (due to the alkaline pH). Thus, most laboratories recommend that urinalysis be performed within 2 hours of specimen collection. Aside from specimen handling, other causes of falsely positive or falsely negative components of the urinalysis are summarized in **Table 6**.

Although in most cases in the pediatric ED, urinalyses are obtained to evaluate for UTI or hematuria, other components of the urinalyses may be abnormal and warrant additional evaluation. Elevated urine bilirubin can be seen with hemolytic processes, hepatic disease, or biliary obstruction. Urine urobilinogen, in contrast, is elevated in hemolytic disease and hepatic disease but is low in biliary obstruction, because bilirubin cannot enter circulation and undergo renal excretion.

SUMMARY

The ease of ordering laboratory tests in the ED can lead to complacency about ordering and a false sense of reassurance for the risk-averse provider. It is important for providers to be cognizant that the more tests are ordered, the higher the risk that one of these tests is falsely abnormal. Evaluation of these falsely abnormal tests entails additional laboratory evaluation. Prior to ordering a test, providers should consider how a test result will alter management for that patient. Recognition of falsely positive and falsely negative tests may then help guide additional evaluation.

REFERENCES

1. Li L, Georgiou A, Vecellio E, et al. The effect of laboratory testing on emergency department length of stay: a multihospital longitudinal study applying a cross-classified random-effect modeling approach. Acad Emerg Med 2015; 22:38–46.
2. Schuur JD, Carney DP, Lyn ET, et al. A top-five list for emergency medicine: a pilot project to improve the value of emergency care. JAMA Intern Med 2014;174: 509–15.
3. Sá L, Costa-Santos C, Teixeira A, et al. Portuguese family physicians' awareness of diagnostic and laboratory tests costs: a cross-sectional study. PLoS One 2015; 10:e0137025.
4. Sedrak MS, Myers JS, Small DS, et al. Effect of a price transparency intervention in the electronic health record on clinician ordering of inpatient laboratory tests: the PRICE randomized clinical trial. JAMA Intern Med 2017;177:939–45.
5. Cruz AT, Mahajan P, Bonsu BK, et al. Accuracy of complete blood cell counts to identify febrile infants 60 days or younger with invasive bacterial infection. JAMA Pediatr 2017;171:e172927.
6. Shah SS, Shofer FS, Seidel JS, et al. Significance of extreme leukocytosis in the evaluation of febrile children. Pediatr Infect Dis J 2005;24:627–30.
7. Danino D, Rimon A, Scolnik D, et al. Does extreme leukocytosis predict serious bacterial infections in infants in the post-pneumococcal conjugate vaccine era? The experience of a large, tertiary care pediatric hospital. Pediatr Emerg Care 2015;31:391–4.

8. Brauner M, Goldman M, Kozer E. Extreme leukocytosis and the risk of serious bacterial infections in febrile children. Arch Dis Child 2010;95:209–12.

9. Gomez B, Mintegi S, Bressan S, et al. Validation of the "Step-by-Step" approach in the management of young febrile infants. Pediatrics 2016;138:e20154381.

10. Shaik N, Borrell JL, Evron J, et al. Procalcitonin, C-reactive protein, and erythrocyte sedimentation rate for the diagnosis of acute pyelonephritis in children. Cochrane Database Syst Rev 2015;(1):CD009185.

11. Pontrelli G, De Crescenzo F, Buzzetti R, et al. Accuracy of serum procalcitonin for the diagnosis of sepsis in neonates an children with systemic inflammatory response syndrome: a meta-analysis. BMC Infect Dis 2017;17:302.

12. Mahajan P, Grzybowski M, Chen X, et al. Procalcitonin as a marker of serious bacterial infections in febrile children younger than 3 years old. Acad Emerg Med 2014;21:171–9.

13. Rutman MS, Bachur R, Harper MB. Radiographic pneumonia in young, highly febrile children with leukocytosis before and after pneumococcal conjugate vaccination. Pediatr Emerg Care 2009;25:1–7.

14. Bradley JS, Byington CL, Shah SS, et al. The management of community-acquired pneumonia in infants and children older than 3 months of age: clinical practice guidelines by the Pediatric Infectious Diseases Society and the Infectious Diseases Society of America. Clin Infect Dis 2011;53:e25–76.

15. Stockmann C, Ampofo K, Killpack J, et al. Procalcitonin accurately identifies hospitalized children with low risk of bacterial community-acquired pneumonia. J Pediatric Infect Dis Soc 2018;7(1):46–53.

16. Benabbas R, Hanna M, Shah J, et al. Diagnostic accuracy of history, physical examination, laboratory tests, and point-of-care ultrasound for pediatric acute appendicitis in the emergency department: a systematic review and meta-analysis. Acad Emerg Med 2017;24:523–51.

17. Kinlin LM, Freedman SB. Evaluation of a clinical dehydration scale in children requiring intravenous rehydration. Pediatrics 2012;129:e1211–9.

18. Colletti JE, Brown KM, Sharieff GQ, et al. The management of children with gastroenteritis and dehydration in the emergency department. J Emerg Med 2010;38:686–98.

19. Streck CJ, Vogel AM, Zhang J, et al. Identifying children at very low risk for blunt intra-abdominal injury in whom CT of the abdomen can be safely avoided. J Am Coll Surg 2017;224:449–58.

20. Goyal NP, Schwimmer JB. The progression and natural history of pediatric nonalcoholic fatty liver disease. Clin Liver Dis 2016;20:325–38.

21. Rimensberger PC, Cheifetz IM, Pediatric Acute Lung Injury Consensus Conference Group. Ventilatory support in children with pediatric acute respiratory distress syndrome: proceedings from the pediatric acute lung injury consensus conference. Pediatr Crit Care Med 2015;16(5 Suppl 1):S51–60.

22. Christian MR, Lowry JA, Algren DA, et al. Do rapid comprehensive urine drug screens change clinical management in children? Clin Toxicol (Phila) 2017;55:977–80.

23. Shihabuddin BS, Hack CM, Sivitz AB. Role of urine drug screening in the medical clearance of pediatric psychiatric patients: is there one? Pediatr Emerg Care 2013;29:903–6.

24. Saitman A, Park H-D, Fitzgerald RL. False-positive interferences of common urine drug screen immunoassays: a review. J Anal Toxicol 2014;38:387–96.

25. Food and Drug Administration. Drugs of abuse tests. Available at: https://www.fda.gov/MedicalDevices/ProductsandMedicalProcedures/InVitroDiagnostics/DrugsofAbuseTests/ucm125722.htm. Accessed September 20, 2017.

26. Wilson MP, Nordstrom K, Anderson EL, et al. American Association for Emergency Psychiatry Task Force on medical clearance of adult psychiatric patients. Part II: controversies over medical assessment, and consensus recommendations. West J Emerg Med 2017;18:640–6.

27. Donofrio JJ, Santillanes G, McCammack BD, et al. Clinical utility of screening laboratory tests in pediatric psychiatric patients presenting to the emergency department for medical clearance. Ann Emerg Med 2014;63:666–75.

Pediatric Disaster Preparedness

Marie M. Lozon, MD*, Stuart Bradin, DO

KEYWORDS

- Pediatric • Disaster • Triage • Mass casualty • Incident command • Preparedness

KEY POINTS

- Disasters can involve child victims and only recently were the special needs of children considered in planning.
- Children's body size and physiology impacts how they are affected by disaster scenarios, such as blast injuries and biologic or chemical weapons.
- The differences between adults and children must be considered during triage of victims in a mass casualty to maximize lives saved.
- Pediatric and emergency providers must recognize early signs of potential biologic or chemical weapon release to protect both the patient, health care workers and facilities.
- Physicians in emergency or urgent care settings should have familiarity with their own facility's disaster plans and the universal methods of management of disasters in health care settings.

INTRODUCTION

Providers who practice pediatric emergency medicine (PEM), general emergency medicine (EM), or hospital pediatrics, or who staff pediatric urgent care clinics must be aware of and be prepared to manage manmade or natural events that involve a large number of people, including children, that is, disaster planning. The definition of "disaster" varies depending on the context. In the United States, The Federal Emergency Management Agency, the body tasked with responding to disasters, uses a simple definition: "an occurrence that has resulted in property damage, death(s) or injuries to the community." The Stafford Act is the legislation under which disasters are declared and the federal government begins to work with state and local governments to mitigate the damage.[1]

Disclosure Statement: The authors have no commercial relationships with any entities or subject matter discussed in this article.
Department of Emergency Medicine, University of Michigan Health System, 1500 East Medical Center Drive, Ann Arbor, MI 48109, USA
* Corresponding author.
E-mail address: Mlozon@umich.edu

pediatric.theclinics.com

As the United States became more invested in preparation for both manmade and natural disasters in the wake of 9/11 and Hurricane Katrina, advocates for children recognized that much of the previous disaster planning did not consider children's needs. The aftermath of such catastrophes includes obvious material losses, but also serious psychological effects, the loss of a child's medical home, and disruption of schooling. The National Commission on Children and Disasters was charged by the president and congress to undertake a comprehensive review of disaster laws, programs, and policies to assess the gaps in plans for children.[2] The commission's report, published in 2010, made pointed recommendations to improve planning for recovery, address children's mental health needs, pediatric focused training for responders, pediatric-specific countermeasures for biologic, chemical, radiologic, and many other threats.

Although there has been progress, in 2015 Save the Children issued the National Report Card on Protecting Children in Disasters and found that 79% of the National Commission's recommendations remained unfulfilled (although 21% were met, 54% of those were only partially met).[3]

A recent review in the *American Journal of Public Health* highlights the progress that has been made, with pediatric disaster expertise being developed by the American Academy of Pediatrics, Emergency Medical Services for Children, along with legislation and federal agencies focused on the needs of children. The creation of the National Advisory Committee on Children and Disasters in 2014 helped to inform federal efforts and spur progress.[4]

The Office of the Assistant Secretary for Preparedness and Response (ASPR), has specified the need for regional health care organizations to be able to respond to pediatric surge and provide some initial, stabilizing care in the event of a mass casualty or illness.[5]

In an emergency department (ED), urgent care setting, or hospital, the first evidence of a disaster may be the arrival of very sick or injured patients that outstrips the capability of the organization, either owing to the complexity of the injuries or the numbers of victims. Hospitals, to comply with regulatory rules, have developed internal disaster definitions, thresholds, and response plans.[6] For providers who could be called on to care for children in a disaster, this article provides an overview of likely pediatric disaster scenarios facing PEM/EM/urgent care pediatricians.

Many PEM physicians receive preparedness training during residency or fellowship, such as exercise participation, often while completing emergency medical services rotations; however, in some training programs, there is limited focus on the needs of children.

Studies of the aftereffects of hurricanes and manmade catastrophes (Hurricane Katrina, school shootings) led PEM leaders to push for disaster planning and to consider the special needs of children because it is well-recognized that most children with illness and injury present to community EDs not staffed by providers with specific training in the evaluation and management of pediatric conditions. Advocates for improvements in the emergency care for children have long provided guidelines, resources, and metrics to push for a higher standard of care.[7,8]

The National Incident Management System defines and provides a comprehensive approach to management of untoward events and guides all levels of government, nongovernmental organizations, and the private sector to be able to work together with a shared taxonomy and processes to successfully leverage the capabilities that our national systems provide, including the incident command system, emergency operations center structures, and multiagency coordination groups. These systems are scalable and can work for one hospital or the whole country.[9] Residents training in EM or PEM are often required or encouraged by their programs to take Federal Emergency Management Agency training courses, found online, to introduce the concepts of incident command (the basic organizing principle of disaster management). These courses are available at the Federal Emergency Management Agency website and useful for those charged with providing emergency care in any setting.[10]

CHILDREN'S UNIQUE NEEDS IN DISASTER PREPARATION

Pediatric focused providers know that children are not little adults. They have unique needs and are more vulnerable to the effects of certain mass casualty events. Children with special health care needs, such chronic illness or technological dependency, must also be considered in any disaster planning.[11] In some events, children may be disproportionately impacted, such as in the 2009 to 2010 H1N1 influenza pandemic, or present with atypical signs and symptoms or earlier in the course of the illness than adults.

Physical Characteristics

Children have an increased baseline respiratory rates, which increases the risk for absorbing larger amounts of aerosolized agents (eg, sarin, anthrax). High vapor density agents are heavier than air and concentrate closer to the ground, within the breathing zone of children. Thus, even small doses of a toxin may be dangerous because the same amount of agent ingested, absorbed, or inhaled by a child will mean a higher dose/body weight than an adult. Children have thinner, less keratinized, more permeable skin, with a proportionally larger surface area/volume ration, which allows for greater transdermal absorption of toxins, greater injury from vesicants/corrosive chemicals, and faster absorption of nerve agents. This higher body surface area promotes rapid heat loss when a child is exposed or wet and increases the risk for hypothermia. This issue is especially important in the context of the need for decontamination.

Children have less fluid reserves than adults and are particularly at risk for dehydration and shock, especially if diarrhea, vomiting, poor appetite, or fever arises from illness induced by a biological agent or there are fluid losses from chemical/vesicant exposure or radiation sickness.

An immature immune system makes children more likely to get ill from an exposure and, once infected, more likely to develop severe disease. Immature blood–brain barriers increase risk for central nervous toxicity from nerve agents[12] and increases susceptibility to effects of even low levels of radiation.[13]

Smaller size and stature make children more prone to polytrauma, especially in a blast event. Head injury is common given their proportionally larger heads. Intrathoracic and abdominal injuries owing to blunt trauma are also high because children have more compliant chest walls and less developed abdominal musculature.[11,12,14–19]

Development and Psychological Characteristics

Children are more vulnerable to disasters by virtue of their reliance on their caregivers for assistance and the potential for getting separated from their families.[20] Infants and younger children may not be ambulatory and able to flee or seek shelter independently. They may unable to verbally express complaints or symptoms.[21] In a biological or chemical event, health care providers will be in personal protective equipment, which could be frightening for a young child.

The risk for posttraumatic stress disorder is magnified in the child witnessing an injury to or death of a parent/family member or who becomes separated from family. Teens are at high risk for unrecognized psychological trauma.[19,21] The following link (https://www.luriechildrens.org/globalassets/documents/emsc/disaster/planning-and-care guidelines/pedsneodisastersurgepocketguidejune20173.pdf) outlines many of the vulnerabilities of children.

PRINCIPLES OF EVALUATION AND MANAGEMENT OF PEDIATRIC DISASTERS

The ED management of mass injury or illness that could be considered a disaster will follow generally accepted principles of setting up an incident command and gathering available resources, but when the victims are children, providers will have to be mindful of not only the special characteristics already discussed, but also other nuances that could impact pediatric disaster care. Examples include the following: (a) differences in triage, because many recommended antibiotics for biological agents are not used routinely in children (tetracycline or quinolones),[22] (b) the currently available vaccines for biological agents used for mass terror are not approved for children (eg, anthrax, plague) and those that are available may be more dangerous in children or restricted in their use (eg, smallpox), (c) antidote dosing and administration may be difficult for responders unfamiliar with pediatric weight-based dosing, and (d) autoinjectors (eg, used in nerve gas release) are not widely available in pediatric sizes.

Child-safe sheltering and reunification of children with their caregivers (in addition to the provision of appropriate disaster medical care) are critical components of pediatric disaster planning. Young children may not be able to identify themselves or caretakers and may be too scared or stressed to provide accurate information. Currently, planning for family reunification is fragmented and a unified all-hazards family reunification tool does not exist in the United States. Delayed reunification can result in increased health care costs and further cause harm. An updated emergency information form should be maintained that includes emergency contacts and medical information; it is especially important for children with special health care needs. When managing a disaster in the ED or hospital setting, there may be unaccompanied children who must be reunited with their families. Many pediatric specialty centers may have child life or social work staff to assist with managing support and reunification; those facilities that do not specialize in pediatrics, but that could receive victims, should have a plan. According to the World Health Organization, the goal of family reunification is to ensure children's protection by prioritizing the identification, registering, and documenting of unaccompanied children as quickly as possible. This process is quite complex and must include a knowledge of pediatric vulnerabilities and responses to a disaster, multilayered planning and communication between local, regional, national, and governmental agencies as well as a plan for the appropriate use of resources, tracking, and coordination of services.[23]

TRIAGE IN DISASTER VERSUS STANDARD TRIAGE

PEM and EM physicians, by virtue of emergency training, are familiar with the care of the injured child, but in a mass casualty incident involving children with blunt or penetrating trauma (explosion, building collapse, active shooter) or special injuries, such as severe burns, their practice site may have to stand up their disaster plan and manage until assistance arrives or transfer can be made to a higher level of care. Routine triage, the norm in EDs, is the process to identify the sickest patients and initiate care, notwithstanding the possibility of poor outcome or death. This strategy differs from disaster triage, where resources can be limited and the same intensity of care may not be provided to all.[16] Triage goals change and the priority becomes maximizing the number of lives saved[24]; that is, doing the greatest good for the greatest number of victims. Care is directed toward those who may be salvageable and for whom immediate intervention can improve chances for survival.[16,24,25]

Mass casualty triage is intended to distinguish those requiring immediate life-saving care from those for whom care could be delayed.[24] Many use color-coding systems to identify priority. Red/immediate denotes those with life-threatening injuries but potentially salvageable with immediate medical attention. Yellow/delayed indicates potentially serious injuries that require urgent but not immediate intervention for survival. Green/minor category, often termed the walking wounded, have minimal injuries that require care but can wait longer periods for treatment. Black/expectant are those victims who have died or are likely to die even with immediate intervention. Disaster plans must include for the provision of palliative care for these victims.[14,16,26]

Most existing triage systems are adult focused; there is a need for a reliable pediatric mass casualty triage tool.[24] Several pediatric triage systems exist, but none have been validated.[14] No one perfect system exists because each has strengths and weaknesses, especially outside a simulated setting.[25,27–29]

The Simple Triage and Rapid Treatment (START) triage system was designed for first responders to easily categorize both adult and pediatric victims by severity of injury. Rapid assessment of airway patency, neurologic function, and the ability to walk are the basis of this system. However, the appropriateness of this system in children may be limited. JumpSTART, developed in 1995, is the most commonly used pediatric mass casualty triage system, especially under 8 years of age (although useful until patient has obvious signs of pubertal development). It accounts for age-dependent physiologic differences in respiratory rate, circulation, and mentation between adults and children. For instance, an important distinction is that assessment of adequacy of circulation is based on presence of pulse, not capillary refill. This system recognizes that the ability to follow commands is not reliable in the pediatric patient[16,24,30] (**Fig. 1**).

The Sort, Assess, Life-saving interventions, Treatment/Transport (SALT) triage system was developed to simplify and standardize disaster triage for victims of all ages; however, it is not a pediatric-specific triage tool. This method emphasizes continual reassessment and incorporates the most effective components of existing systems. Lifesaving interventions such as hemorrhage control, opening the airway, 2 rescue breaths in children, needle decompression of tension pneumothorax, and use of auto-injector antidotes are implemented before the designation of a triage category if supplies are available and the responder is competent in their use. If performed in a timely fashion, survival can be dramatically increased (**Fig. 2**).[16,31]

DECONTAMINATION OF THE PEDIATRIC PATIENT

Decontamination is not generally the role of the PEM provider, but is most often done at the scene of the contaminant release (primary decontamination) and the detailed methodology is beyond the scope of this article. When victims self-present or are not fully decontaminated, then ED personnel trained in hazardous material decontamination, often ED paramedics or technicians, or specially trained nurses, will perform the decontamination in a designated room near the entrance to the department or in external structures. Decontamination can be frightening for small children and can contribute to hypothermia if done improperly. Thankfully, removal of the child from the area of contamination, removal of clothes, and simple soap and water rinsing removes most harmful substances.

JumpSTART Pediatric MCI Triage

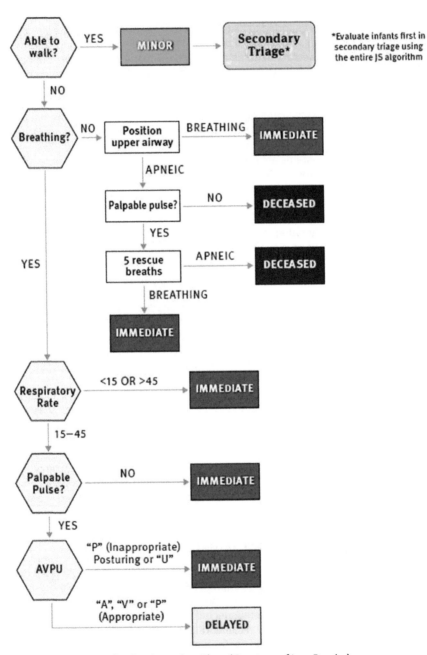

Fig. 1. JumpSTART pediatric triage algorithm. (*Courtesy of* Lou Romig.)

SALT Mass Casualty Triage Algorithm (Sort, Assess, Lifesaving Interventions, Treatment/Transport)

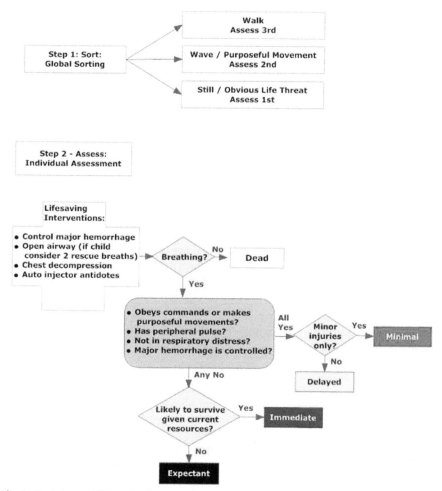

Fig. 2. Sort, Assess, Life-saving interventions, Treatment/Transport (SALT) triage. AVPU, alert, verbal, painful, unresponsive; MCI, mass casualty incident. (*Adapted from* Lerner EB, Cone DC, Weinstein ES, et al. Mass casualty triage: an evaluation of the science and refinement of a national guideline. Disaster Med Public Health Prep 2011;5(2):129–37.)

BIOLOGICAL AGENTS IN DISASTER

Many properties of bioagents make them useful weapons of war and terror. Inexpensive and easily produced, some are ubiquitous in soil, such as, *Clostridium botulinum*, which can be readily grown in a culture medium by a trained person. Biological agents are substantially deadlier and cheaper than other weapons. They provide brand name recognition with accompanying fear and chaos. When deployed, the agent is largely silent, and the incubation period can vary from hours to weeks, which increases the risk for delayed diagnosis and enhances the potential for a greater number of victims and the possibility to overwhelm the system. Biological agents also have a potential for dissemination over large geographic areas. Morbidity and mortality can be high because person-to-person transmission is possible for many agents and diagnosis and treatment may be difficult. Dissemination can be airborne or through food and water supplies. Presenting symptoms are often vague and flulike, such as fever, chills, respiratory symptoms, myalgias, or headache and only a short window of opportunity exists between the identification of the initial cases and a second wave of the population becoming ill. ED and primary care providers are often at the front line of recognition and treatment. Knowledge of presenting signs and symptoms and appropriate management are crucial for prompt recognition of a biological agent release and rapid response.[12,21,32]

The US Centers for Disease Control and Prevention has identified 35 biological agents that can potentially cause harm and overwhelm the current medical system. These are classified into categories based on (a) ease of transmission and dissemination, (b) potential for major public health impact, (c) potential public panic and social disruption, and (d) requirements for public health preparedness. Biologic agents are prioritized by the Centers for Disease Control and Prevention based on the impact to public health, with level A being most concerning owing to ease of dissemination and transmission and mortality risks (level C are still of great concern but not as highly prioritized). Level A agents include anthrax, smallpox, plague, botulism, tularemia, and viral hemorrhagic fevers. These agents pose the greatest risk for mortality and threat to public health, and are discussed elsewhere in this article.[11–13,33–35]

Providers must maintain a high index of suspicion if a biologic attack is to be recognized and appropriate management initiated. There are several clues that suggest a bioagent event:

- Any single case of an uncommon agent
- An unusually large number of patients with the same disease or symptoms
- Many unexplained deaths
- Dead animals
- More severe disease than expected
- Disease unusual for season or geographic region
- Failure to respond to standard therapy for a specific pathogen
- Disease transmitted by a vector unusual for the region
- Unusual route of exposure for the disease
- Disease in an unusual population or age group

ANTHRAX

The most problematic biologic threat is believed to be inhalational anthrax,[12,36] Not transmitted person to person, it has an incubation person of 1 to 6 days, beginning with a flulike illness characterized by fever, headache, cough, and chest tightness. A 1- to 2-day period of improvement is followed by rapid deterioration resulting in shock, cyanosis, and sepsis. Hemorrhagic meningitis is seen in up to 50% of patients. Chest radiographs may show a widened mediastinum. The prognosis is grave with mortality rates approaching 95% if therapy is started later than 48 hours from the onset of symptoms. No widespread vaccination distribution is currently available[12,35–37] (**Fig. 3**).

PLAGUE

Plague occurs naturally in septicemic, bubonic, and pneumonic forms, caused by the gram-negative rod *Yersinia pestis*. Pneumonic plague, with easy dissemination via aerosolization, is the most likely form to be seen in a terror attack. Unlike naturally occurring plague, a biological attack would present with respiratory symptoms without

Anthrax

Biological Agent
The bacteria *Bacillus anthracis*

Indications of Terrorist Release
The sudden appearance in a region of a large number of patients with flulike illness (particularly off flu season), respiratory symptoms, and a high fatality rate, with nearly ½ of all deaths occurring w/in 24-48 hrs from time that symptoms begin, would suggest a release of inhalation anthrax as a biological weapon.

Possible Means of Exposure
Inhalation, ingestion, and cutaneous

Incubation
Cutaneous: 1–12 d
Gastrointestinal: 3–7 d
Inhalational (most likely in bioterror attack): 1–60 d

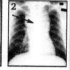

(1) Cutaneous anthrax lesion on hand, about 5 days after exposure. (2) Inhalational anthrax; arrows point to the widened mediastinum.

Primary Symptoms of Inhalational Anthrax
Flulike symptoms (e.g., fever, malaise, myalgias, headache, abdominal pain, vomiting, coughing, chest pain) but no nasal congestion; increasingly severe respiratory symptoms, including dyspnea, stridor, and cyanosis, and expansion of the mediastinum seen on chest X-ray.

Diagnostic Tool of Choice
Tissue/blood culture

Treatment
Immediate initiation of IV antibiotics:
(1st choice = ciprofloxacin or doxycycline)

Post-Exposure Prophylaxis
Antibiotic therapy P.O.
(1st choice = ciprofloxacin)

Vaccine
Available

Infection Control
• Use standard precautions.
• Isolation of patient not indicated.
• Note that anthrax spores are resistant in the environment and decontamination efforts will be difficult.

Fig. 3. Anthrax. PO, per os.

the development of buboes. It results in a multilobar, hemorrhagic, necrotizing pneumonia. Symptoms start within 6 days of exposure, rapidly progressing to severe pneumonia with hemoptysis. Untreated, pneumonic plague is highly lethal, resulting in nearly 100% mortality. Antibiotics, including doxycycline and aminoglycosides, are effective if begun within 24 hours of the onset of symptoms. It is highly contagious[11,12,34,37] **(Fig. 4).**

SMALL POX

Smallpox is a viral infection with prominent skin findings, associated systemic toxicity, and a historical 30% mortality rate.[33] Any identified case of small pox would be considered an act of terrorism. Smallpox was declared eradicated by the World Health Organization and no child has been routinely vaccinated against small pox since 1971.[37] More than 80% of adults and 100% of children are susceptible to variola.[11] There is an incubation period of 7 to 19 days after exposure. Initial symptoms are

Plague

Biological Agent
The bacteria *Yersinia pestis*

Indications of Terrorist Release
In a bioterrorism attack, *Y. pestis* would likely be released as an aerosol and inhaled; a large number of previously healthy persons rapidly progressing from flulike symptoms to cough, dyspnea, chest pain, to severe pneumonia and death suggestive of attack; most natural cases in the U.S. occur in southwestern states.

Possible Means of Exposure
Inhalation; person-to-person

Incubation
Bubonic: 2–8 d
Pneumonic (most likely in bioterror attack): 1–8 d

Bubonic plague patient with swollen, ruptured inguinal lymph node ("bubo").

Right hand of a plague patient displaying acral gangrene.

Primary Symptoms of Pneumonic Plague
Fulminant onset w/ high fever, chills, headache, extreme malaise, and myalgias; cough and hemoptysis w/in 24 hrs; nausea, vomiting, and abdominal pain may also occur; rapidly progresses to dyspnea, stridor, cyanosis, respiratory failure, and circulatory collapse.

Diagnostic Tool of Choice
Culture, serology, Gram/Wright stain, chest x-ray

Treatment
When plague is suspected and diagnosed early, a health care provider can prescribe specific antibiotics (generally streptomycin or gentamycin). Certain other antibiotics are also effective.

Post-Exposure Prophylaxis
Doxycycline or ciprofloxacin

Vaccine
No longer available (discontinued by its manufacturers in 1999)

Infection Control
• Use standard precautions.
• Mask suspected pneumonic plague patients in ER/transport; isolate confirmed patients, using strict droplet precautions.
• Decontaminate surfaces, clothing, and bedding thoroughly.

Fig. 4. Plague. ER, emergency room.

nonspecific: fever, malaise, vomiting, headache, and myalgias. Two or 3 days later, a red, macular rash develops, progressing to papules, and then pustules. The rash spreads centrifugally. Lesions are synchronous, not in different stages as seen in varicella. Death occurs from multisystem organ failure from overwhelming viremia. The diagnosis is clinical because no widely available assays exist; suspicion for exposure must be reported immediately to the health department because patients need to monitored for a minimum of 17 days and in proper isolation precautions. Management is supportive. No antivirals that have been approved by the US Food and Drug Administration are recommended at present, although cidofovir has been shown to be useful in animal models. Vaccine within 96 hours of exposure offers good protection against developing disease and limiting the severity of illness. All close contacts require isolation and vaccination.[12,33,37] Vaccination is not without risk: side effects include vaccinia to encephalitis. Contraindications include pregnancy, eczema, and immunocompromise[34] (**Fig. 5**).

BOTULINUM TOXIN

Botulinum toxin, produced by *C botulinum*, is the most lethal toxin known to humankind. It causes the inhibition of the release of acetylcholine resulting in paralysis. Death is due to respiratory failure. Even with intensive supportive care, recovery is prolonged, taking months. Although it can be spread via food or wound infection, inhalational botulism would be the most likely form of a bioterrorism attack. Symptoms present within 24 hours of exposure: cranial nerve palsies initially, followed by descending paralysis, and progression to respiratory failure. Patients are lucid with no altered mentation. Supportive care and ventilatory support are the mainstays of therapy. Treatment of secondary infections is vital, but aminoglycosides and clindamycin must be avoided because they worsen neuromuscular blockade. Antitoxin is available and should be administered upon onset of symptoms. This agent may be in short supply if a large-scale attack occurs. It does not reverse current paralysis, but may limit progression and prevent nerve damage if administered early.[33–35,37]

Smallpox

Biological Agent
The Variola major virus

Indications of Terrorist Release
Since smallpox has been eradicated in the world since 1977, even one confirmed case would indicate a probable terrorist attack.

Possible Means of Exposure
Inhalation of airborne droplets; contact with skin sores, secretions, or clothing or bedding

Incubation
7–17 d

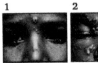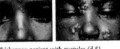

1) Chickenpox patient with pustules (d 5), 2) Smallpox patient with pustules (d 5).

Primary Symptoms
Initial symptoms are flulike, including fever, vomiting, myalgias, physical exhaustion; rash appears ~ d 12 post-exposure, at which point patient becomes highly contagious; then formation of macular rash → papules → vesicles → pustules → scabs, most densely on face and limbs, including palms and soles of feet (ie, centrifugal distribution, unlike chickenpox, in which lesions are distributed evenly over the body, beginning on the trunk); lesions go through stages at the same time (unlike chickenpox, in which new lesions form and scab over at different times).

Diagnostic Tool of Choice
Culture followed by PCR and RFLP (by BSL-4 laboratory(, electron microscopy

Treatment
Vaccination up to 4 d after exposure

Post-Exposure Prophylaxis
Vaccination

Vaccine
Currently available to high-risk groups (First responders, etc.)

Infection Control
- Use standard, contact, droplet, and airborne precautions.
- Patients and contacts should wear N95 mask or better.
- Consider bedding and clothing of patients potentially infectious.
- Quarantine/respiratory isolation/vaccination program for patients and secondary contacts will be necessary in the event of an outbreak.

Fig. 5. Smallpox. PCR, polymerase chain reaction; RFLP, restriction fragment length polymorphism.

VIRAL HEMORRHAGIC FEVERS

Viral hemorrhagic fevers include Ebola, Marburg, and Lassa viruses. Highly infectious, these RNA viruses cause high fever, flulike symptoms, and bleeding from multiple sites. Spread by aerosolized particles, a 2- to 21-day incubation period is followed by the onset of high fever, headache, myalgias, malaise, abdominal pain, and mucous membrane bleeding. As symptoms evolve and progress, death is due to hypotension and shock. Care is supportive and requires vigorous fluid resuscitation, vasoactive agents to support circulation, and infusion of blood products. Parenteral ribavirin has been used to treat some cases of Lassa fever; vaccines are under development at present. During the most recent outbreak in Liberia, West Africa, health care workers were at extreme risk for acquiring the disease. Mortality can be quite high—the Zaire subtype approaches 90%. Owing to the highly contagious nature of these illnesses, great care should be taken handling body fluids and use/donning/doffing of appropriate personal protective equipment . Owing to their highly infectious nature, any case of a viral hemorrhagic fever in the United States should be considered a public health emergency.[34,37,38]

The US Army Medical Research Institute on Infectious Diseases has excellent public resources on all important biologic agents and can be found at http://www.usamriid. army.mil/education/docs/Quick_Bio-Agents_Giude.pdf.

CHEMICAL AGENTS

Exposure to toxic gases with deliberate intent to inflict harm has claimed countless lives throughout recent history. Examples include phosgene, chlorine, and mustard gas releases in World War I; Zyklon B gas in World War 2; Agent Orange during the Vietnam War and the Iraq–Iran War in the 1980s; the release of Sarin gas in Tokyo in 1995; and, most recently, the civilian attacks with nerve gas in the current Syrian war that included many pediatric victims. Chemical agents pose great risk to unprepared health care workers who must recognize the signs and symptoms of a release (toxidrome), identify the need for rapid decontamination, and provide appropriate medical management. Agents typically exist as liquids and are disseminated as vapors or aerosols with both inhalation and dermal threats. Direct and systemic toxicity is possible via either route.[12,15,39]

General treatment begins with getting the victim out of danger, triage, and decontamination. Decontamination is typically with soap/water and prevents secondary exposure of health care workers/facilities and minimizes continued absorption by the patient. Care must be taken to avoid hypothermia both before and after decontamination.[14,15,33] Nerve agents are the most toxic chemical warfare agents, similar to, but much more potent than, organophosphate pesticides; 1 drop to the skin can cause death within 20 minutes. Cholinergic symptoms are caused by the inhibition of acetylcholinesterase, producing a toxidrome—salivation, bronchospasm, altered mentation, autonomic instability, and pinpoint pupils. Paralysis, fasciculation and respiratory arrest follow nicotinic hyperstimulation. Central nervous system effects include seizures and coma. Death, typically owing to respiratory failure, can occur within 5 to 10 minutes without appropriate management. Treatment consists of antidotes for both muscarinic (atropine) and nicotinic (2-PAM) toxicity. Atropine is indicated for any patient exhibiting signs or symptoms of a nerve agent exposure. Benzodiazepines are used to treat and prevent seizures. Children may present atypically with tachyarrythmias, pronounced hypotonia, weakness, and respiratory insufficiency, plus seizures more commonly than in adults (**Fig. 6**).[12,15,37]

Chemical Agents Overview

Examples of Chemical Agents
Nerve Agents; Blister Agents (also known as "vesicants" or "mustard agents"); Chemical Asphyxiants (also known as "blood agents"); Pulmonary Irritants (also known as "choking agents")

Indications of Terrorist Release
Most chemical agents work relatively fast, hence the presence of one would initially primarily be detected by the symptom pattern victims were experiencing.

PRIMARY CHARACTERISTICS
Nerve Agents
See next panel of this brochure.

Blister Agents
Examples: Lewisite (military code name L),

mustards (HD, HN, HT), phosgene oxime (CX); **Common odors:** Odorless, garlic, mustard, onion, geraniums, pepper; **Onset of symptoms:** Immediate (L, CX) to 2–48 hrs (HD); **Symptoms:** Erythema, pruritus, burning of the skin, large blister formation, eye and airway irritation, sore throat, cough, chest pain, profuse rhinorrhea, copious pulmonary secretions, nausea and vomiting can also occur; **Rx:** Iodophors for skin; dimercaprol for L

Chemical Asphyxiants
Examples: Hydrogen cyanide (AC), cyanogen chloride (CK), arsine (SA); **Common odors:** Bitter almonds, garlic; **Onset of symptoms:** Most immediate, SA may be delayed by hrs; **Symptoms:** AC/CK—Irritation to eyes, nose, and airways; dyspnea, agitation, weakness,

nausea, vomiting, muscular trembling; SA—Conjunctival redness, garlic breath odor, headache, thirst, shivering, weakness, abdominal pain; **Rx:** Sodium nitrite/sodium thiosulfate for AC and CK; supportive

Pulmonary Irritants
Examples: Phosgene (CG), chlorine (CL), diphosgene (DP), chloropicrin (PS), and ammonia; **Common odors:** Green corn, newly mown hay; **Onset of symptoms:** Usually rapid, effects of CL may be delayed; **Symptoms:** Burning eyes, nose, and throat; conjunctival injection, lacrimation, rhinorrhea, laryngeal spasm, chest pain and tightness, dyspnea; after 3 hrs to days, respiratory symptoms may progress to pulmonary edema and respiratory failure; **Rx:** Supportive

Nerve Agents

Examples of Nerve Agents
Sarin (military code name GB), tabun (GA), soman (GD), cyclosarin (GF), VX, VE, VG, VM

Indications of Terrorist Release
Since nerve agents in their pure form are odorless and colorless, an attack would initially primarily be identified by the symptoms victims were experiencing.

Possible Means of Exposure
Inhalation, absorption through mucous membranes; dermal absorption upon contact with the liquid form (particular danger for VX, which is most commonly an oily, amber-colored liquid)

Time from Exposure to Illness
Inhalation: Seconds to minutes
Dermal absorption: 1 min to 18 h

Primary Symptoms of Inhalational Exposure
Miosis (13% will have dilated pupils); dimmed or blurred vision; lacrimation; rhinorrhea; sudden excess oral, nasal, and respiratory secretions; headache; dyspnea/wheezing; sweating; sneezing; urinary and fecal incontinence; vomiting; sudden loss of consciousness; muscle fasciculations; seizure; flaccid paralysis.

Primary Symptoms of Dermal Exposure
May include localized sweating, fasciculations, nausea, vomiting, diarrhea, generalized diaphoresis, generalized weakness, miosis; large exposure will resemble inhalational exposure.

Diagnostic Tool of Choice
Clinical syndrome + percent reduction of RBC-cholinesterase

Treatment
Atropine and pralidoxime

Prophylaxis
The Army has awarded a $156.6 million contract to the DynPort division of Computer Sciences Corp. for development of an anti-nerve gas agent that protects against a wide range of nerve gases for up to 60 d.

Decontamination
Thorough decontamination of patient is important as risk of secondary contamination is high.

Nerve agent antidote kits (NAAK), also known as Mark-1 kits, contain 1 dosage of the antidotes atropine and pralidoxime.

Fig. 6. Overview of chemical and nerve agents.

PANDEMIC INFLUENZA

Influenza remains a significant threat for mass illness. 2018 marks the 100th anniversary of the 1918 Influenza Pandemic, which killed 2% of the world's population.[40] The ability of the virus to undergo genetic reassortment allows for the rapid development of new influenza strains to which a population has little or no previous immunity. Influenza remains a significant cause of morbidity and mortality; each year, more than 30,000 deaths result from influenza in the United States.[41] Influenza is one of the most common pediatric infectious diseases, occurring annually in up to 20% of children worldwide. The rate in preschool children can exceed 40% during an epidemic.[42] The ability to contain regional outbreaks of the disease, and thereby slow the progression of an emerging pandemic, is constrained, given the relative ease in worldwide travel. Influenza infections are associated with a range of symptoms and presentations that vary by age, making clinical diagnosis challenging.[41]

Clinical symptoms of illness reported with novel influenza A (H1N1) were similar to those seen with seasonal influenza: fever, cough, sore throat, malaise, headache, myalgia, arthralgia, and fatigue. Children also presented with gastrointestinal symptoms, more frequently than seen with previous influenza strains. The most commonly reported complication of H1N1 infection was pneumonia, which at times was accompanied by a necrotizing disease or empyema. Other described complications were dehydration, encephalopathy, and exacerbation of underlying chronic disease, as also seen with seasonal influenza. Although pandemic H1N1 influenza seemed to disproportionately affect older children and those with chronic medical conditions, particularly neurodevelopmental disorders and asthma, the relative severity of the illnesses seen in hospitalized children seemed to be unchanged from previous influenza seasons.[42]

Influenza is classified into types, subtypes, and strains. The 3 types of influenza viruses are A, B, and C. Influenza A is the most common form of the virus affecting children and the one that leads to epidemics. Influenza B occurs less frequently, but has the potential to cause epidemics. Influenza C is uncommon in humans. Influenza A viruses are further divided into subtypes based on 2 surface proteins: hemagglutinin (H) and neuraminidase (N). A change from natural mutations that occur in influenza virus strains is termed antigenic drift, a process that occurs continuously. With influenza A infection, a new subtype may be formed from the reassortment of 2 or more influenza virus strains (often combining animal and human strains), a process that is termed antigenic shift. This phenomenon can cause a pandemic, as occurred in 2009 with the novel influenza A (H1N1) virus.[42] Today, the use of the term pandemic by the World Health Organization is reserved for the occurrence of worldwide events and not for the emergence of a new strain. Declaration of a pandemic by the World Health Organization raises global awareness of a disease outbreak and allows for aggressive preparedness and response planning. Such a declaration does not necessarily imply a more virulent disease course; it simply signals worldwide spread of the disease. The year 2009 will be remembered as the year of the influenza pandemic owing to novel virus with a swine origin A (H1N1). After the first wave appeared in late spring and summer, some experts predicted that the subsequent wave would infect 30% to 50% of the population, lead to 1.8 million hospitalizations, and cause 90,000 deaths. Although this virus did prove to be unusually virulent for children and young adults compared with seasonal influenza, it was quite mild in its effect on older adults, and the overall attack rate was substantially lower than predicted with the number of infections, hospitalizations, and deaths was far below early estimates, and the strain on our health care system was far less than was initially feared.[43]

The American Academy of Pediatrics publishes policies on the prevention and treatment of influenza that may change based on circulating strains. For patients with evidence of mild to moderate disease and no underlying high-risk conditions, treatment with supportive therapy alone is reasonable. Antiviral therapy is best indicated for those with a more severe disease or in whom a high-risk condition predicts increased morbidity and mortality resulting from an influenza infection.[41] Invasive pneumococcal disease and community-acquired methicillin-resistant *Staphylococcus aureus* can complicate pediatric influenza.[42]

SUMMARY: PREPARING FOR DISASTER

Recognition of the need for attention to the vulnerabilities of children in the planning for disaster response has advanced in recent decades, especially with respect to inclusion in shelter planning, need for attention to mental health, countermeasures appropriate for children, special care for the technology dependent child, and potentially better triage systems. A positive outcome of these efforts are better preparation for the disaster of one.

The National Pediatric Readiness Project, sponsored by the federally funded Emergency Medicine Services for Children in a coalition with the American Academy of Pediatrics, the American College of Emergency Physicians, and the Emergency Nurses Association, has pushed for the adoption of guidelines around equipment needs and training required for the proper care of children in the ED.[7] PEM, EM, and other pediatric providers wishing to gain improved knowledge of activities around disaster preparedness in their communities can join pediatric committees of the regional health care coalitions, which can be found through state health and human services departments or through federal resources at ASPR Technical Resources, Assistance Center, and Information Exchange (TRACIE). Resources and training in disaster life support, mass event preparedness and specific all-hazards preparedness for your region can be found through the ASPR TRACIE program or your regional health care coalition. One of the most important community contributions of the pediatric provider can be the education of prehospital personnel, EM, and primary care providers, nurses, and other colleagues who do not routinely care for large numbers of children and advocating for pediatric preparedness in your care facility and your community.

REFERENCES

1. Robert T. Stafford disaster relief and emergency assistance act. 1988.
2. National Commission on Children and Disasters. 2010 Report to the President and Congress. 2010.
3. Children Still at risk: U.S. children 10 years after Hurricane Katrina; 2015 National Report Card on Protecting Children in Disasters. 2015.
4. Dziuban EJ, Peacock G, Frogel M. A child's health is the public's health: progress and gaps in addressing pediatric needs in public health emergencies. Am J Public Health 2017;107(S2):S134–7.
5. 2017-2022 Health care preparedness and response capabilities. In: response OotASfPa, ed.
6. Centers for Medicare and Medicaid Services emergency preparedness rules. ed. 2016.
7. Gausche-Hill M, Ely M, Schmuhl P, et al. A national assessment of pediatric readiness of emergency departments. JAMA Pediatr 2015;169(6):527–34.
8. Emergency medical services for children improvement and innovation center. 2018. Available at: https://emscimprovement.center/.
9. National incident management system. 2017.
10. Introduction to the Incident Command System (ICS 100) for Healthcare/Hospitals. 2017. Available at: https://training.fema.gov/is/courseoverview.aspx?code=IS-100.HCb.
11. Redlener I, Markenson D. Disaster and terrorism preparedness: what pediatricians need to know. Dis Mon 2004;50:1–40.
12. Henretig FM, CT. Chemical and biologic terrorism. In: SM S, editor. Pediatric emergency medicine secrets. 3rd edition. Philadelphia: Elsevier Saunders; 2015. p. 555–66.
13. David M. Pediatrics and terrorism. In: Shapira SC, HJ, Cole LA, editors. Essentials of terror medicine. New York: Springer; 2009. p. 365–90.
14. Kim K. Disaster planning in the pediatric emergency department. Pediatr Emerg Med Rep 2013;18(5).
15. Seeyave D, Bradin SA. Pediatric mass casualty events: toxic exposures. Critical decisions in emergency medicine. 29(5):13–21.
16. Seeyave D, Bradin, SA. Disaster preparedness for the pediatric population. Crit Decisions Emerg Med 28(12):2–13.
17. Burke RV, Iverson E, Goodhue CJ, et al. Disaster and mass casualty events in the pediatric population. Semin Pediatr Surg 2010;19:265–70.

18. Bartenfeld MT, Peacock G, Griese SE. Public health emergency planning for children in chemical, biological, radiological, and nuclear (CBRN) disasters. Biosecur Bioterror 2014;12(4):201–7.

19. White SR, Henretig FM, Dukes RG. Medical management of vulnerable populations and co-morbid conditions of victims of bioterrorism. Emerg Med Clin North Am 2002;20:365–92.

20. Phillips BD, SL. Populations with functional or access needs. Koegnig and Schultz's disaster medicine comprehensive principles and practices. 2nd edition. New York: Cambridge University Press; 2016. p. 137–62.

21. Chung S, AT. Disaster preparedness. In: Tenenbein M, SR, editors. Strange and Schafermeyer's pediatric emergency medicine. New York: McGraw Hill; 2015. p. 805–9.

22. Scarfone RJ, HF, et al. Emergency department recognition and management of victims of biological and chemical terrorism. Pediatric emergency medicine. Lippincott Williams & Wilkins; p. 125–52.

23. AL N. Family reunification- concepts and challenges. Clin Pediatr Emerg Med 2009;10(3):195–207.

24. Lyle K, TT, Graham J. Pediatric mass casualty: triage and planning for the prehospital provider. Clin Pediatr Emerg Med 2009;10(3):173–85.

25. Lerner EB, Cone DC, Weinstein ES, et al. Mass casualty triage: an evaluation of the science and refinement of a national guideline. Disaster Med Public Health Prep 2011;5(2):129–37.

26. Bradin S, Lozon M, et al. Planning for children in disasters: a hospital toolkit. 2015.

27. Cross KP, Cicero MX. Head-to-head comparison of disaster triage methods in pediatric, adult, and geriatric patients. Ann Emerg Med 2013;61(6):668–76.e7.

28. Jones N, White ML, Tofil N, et al. Randomized trial comparing two mass casualty triage systems (JumpSTART versus SALT) in a pediatric simulated mass casualty event. Prehosp Emerg Care 2014;18(3):417–23.

29. Nadeau NL, Cicero MX. Pediatric disaster triage system utilization across the United States. Pediatr Emerg Care 2017;33(3):152–5.

30. Lou R. 2002. Available at: https://chemm.nlm.nih.gov/StartPediatricTriage Algorithm.pdf.

31. SALT mass casualty triage: concept endorsed by the American College of Emergency Physicians, American College of Surgeons Committee on Trauma, American Trauma Society, National Association of EMS Physicians, National disaster life support education consortium, and state and territorial injury prevention directors association. Disaster Med Public Health Prep 2008;2(4):245–6.

32. Kienstra AJ, EE. Bioterrorism and its impact on the emergency department. Clin Pediatr Emerg Med 2002;3(4):231–8.

33. FM H. Preparation for terrorist threats: biologic and chemical agents. Clin Pediatr Emerg Med 2009;10(3):130–5.

34. Darling RG, Catlett CL, Huebner KD, et al. Threats in bioterrorism. 1: CDC category A agents. Emerg Med Clin North Am 2002;20:273–309.

35. A. Biological, chemical, & nuclear emergencies: a physician's resource manual. In: Technologies TMSotSoNYaE, ed.

36. Inglesby TV, O'Toole T, Henderson DA, et al. Anthrax as a biological weapon, 2002: updated recommendations for management. JAMA 2002;287(17):2236–52.

37. Hamele M, Poss WB, Sweney J. Disaster preparedness, pediatric considerations in primary blast injury, chemical, and biological terrorism. World J Crit Care Med 2014;4(3):15–23.

38. McNutt S, Darling, RG. Bioterrorism and the emergency physician: on the front lines. Emergency medicine practice: an evidence-based approach to emergency medicine. Vol 42002.

39. RS. Chemical warfare agents. Clin Pediatr Emerg Med 2002;3(4):239–47.

40. Simonsen L, Chowell G, Andreasen V, et al. A review of the 1918 herald pandemic wave: importance for contemporary pandemic response strategies. Ann Epidemiol 2018;28(5):281–8.

41. CG M. Challenges in diagnosis and management in the emergency department. Emerg Med Pract An Evidenced Based Approach Emerg Med 2009;11(11).

42. R G. Pediatric influenza in the emergency department setting. Pediatr Emerg Med Pract 2010;7(11).

43. JA W. A(H1N1) 'Swine Flu' 2009/2010: where we've been, what we now know, where we may be heading. Pediatr Emerg Med Rep 2010;15(3).

Advances in Medical Education and Implications for the Pediatric Emergency Department

Sarah Tomlinson, MD[a],*, Michele M. Carney, MD[b],
Margaret Wolff, MD[b]

KEYWORDS

- Medical education • Clinical teaching • Learning environment • Entrustment
- Pediatrics • Emergency medicine

KEY POINTS

- The learning environment encompasses both the learner's written curriculum and the "hidden" curriculum, which refers to the social factors of the practice of medicine, including relationships, values, and behaviors encountered in clinical practice.
- Spending a few minutes at the beginning of a shift talking with the learner to gauge skill set and knowledge base can provide the opportunity to tailor teaching on shift to the learner's priorities or desired goals.
- Entrustment is a critical part of a trainee's education in becoming an autonomous physician. Building on each patient encounter in a shift creates graduated autonomy in a short amount of time.
- Creating opportunities for faculty development aimed at improving clinical teaching or encouraging interest in medical education is paramount in improving the efforts of physician educators.
- Teaching techniques, such as the one-minute preceptor, can be used effectively in the busy environment of the pediatric emergency department.

INTRODUCTION

The learning environment plays a fundamental role in medical education.[1] The Accreditation Council for Graduate Medical Education (ACGME) recently brought the clinical

Disclosure Statement: The authors have no financial disclosures to make.
[a] Departments of Emergency Medicine and Pediatrics, University of Michigan, 1540 East Hospital Drive, CW 2-737, Ann Arbor, MI 48109-4260, USA; [b] Departments of Emergency Medicine and Pediatrics, University of Michigan, 1500 East Medical Center Drive, SPC 5303, Taubman Center, B1 - 354, Ann Arbor, MI 48109-5303, USA
* Corresponding author. 1540 East Hospital Drive, CW 2-737, Ann Arbor, MI 48109-4260.
E-mail address: shamilt@med.umich.edu

Pediatr Clin N Am 65 (2018) 1221–1227
https://doi.org/10.1016/j.pcl.2018.07.008
0031-3955/18/© 2018 Elsevier Inc. All rights reserved.

learning environment into the spotlight by implementing the Clinical Learning Environment Review for all ACGME-accredited training programs.[2] This focus is fueled by research demonstrating the profound impact the educational environment has on performance, learning, satisfaction, and well-being.[1] Given the magnitude of this, it is important to understand the scope of this concept and how supervising physicians and learners can positively influence the clinical learning environment. This article defines the clinical learning environment, followed by a comprehensive review of the current state of research, and culminated by advocating for best practices that positively influence it.

THE LEARNING ENVIRONMENT

The learning environment is vast and complex and encompasses all aspects of a learner's education, including both the written and "hidden" curriculum. The written curriculum refers to subjects and systems that need to be taught to all learners as outlined by a medical school or residency program. In contrast, the hidden curriculum refers to the social factors of the practice of medicine, such as the values and behaviors of physicians and other health care providers that a learner is exposed to.[3] The hidden curriculum is also influenced by how the learner perceives the environment, rather than the environment itself. Thus, the terms, *environment* and *climate*, are often used interchangeably.[4] Miller[5] created a framework to describe the complexity of the learning environment and the interactions between the components. The levels described are the individual learner, the group, the organization, the community, and the society. This framework is used as the basis for this discussion of the different components of the learning environment, and how these components can be targeted to improve education in the pediatric emergency department (ED) is examined. The multitude of factors that contributes to the complexity of the learning environment provides an opportunity for intervention at various levels to customize the learning environment for individual learners to help them succeed.

The Learner

The learner is at the center of this framework, underpinning the notion that the learning environment is different for every individual. A variety of factors, such as individual preferences and motivations, affect learners' ability to succeed and influence how they experience the educational environment. There is increasing diversity in terms of age, gender, ethnic background, and socioeconomic status of medical students. All these factors affect the way in which an individual is most successful in acquiring an education. Recognizing the different needs of these individuals can lead to improvements in the educational environment and make it more appealing to a broader audience.[6]

Another important consideration at the learner level for medical trainees is adult learning theory. Adult learners want to be actively involved in their learning and require relevance to their practice to maximize information retention.[7] Adult learners also desire clear goals and feedback on their performance.[8] Many of these characteristics can be the focus for educational intervention when approaching a learner in the clinical environment.

Implementation Strategies: The Learner

As a supervisor in the ED, it is unfeasible to anticipate the needs of every learner. One approach is to take a few minutes at the start of a shift to provide introductions. This immediately establishes the relationship between the learner and the teacher and welcomes learners into the learning environment. In addition to basics, such as name, stage of training, and current training program, other considerations might include prior experience in pediatrics and emergency medicine. These questions can provide vital information for their expected knowledge base and skill set. Asking questions, such as "What are you looking to learn this shift?" and "What type of patients would you like to see today?" can allow assessing what their goals are for the shift. If information is able to be put into context for learners based on their goals, it becomes more meaningful for them. For example, if a resident is about to embark on a career as a general pediatrician at a community practice, a case discussion might be framed by asking, "If you saw this patient in the office, what characteristics would prompt you to transfer this patient to the ED?" Framing teaching within these types of statements allows learners to see the relevance in what they are doing, even if they are not planning to pursue a career in pediatric emergency medicine. Additionally, providing learners with expectations for a shift creates a clear set of goals for them and creates a standard by which to provide assessment and feedback.

The Group

The group level consists of the social interactions that play a role in the learning environment, such as the interactions between supervising physicians and learners. Physicians are all expected to be teachers to residents and students at some point in their careers, whether in the classroom or at the bedside. Despite this, physicians are not given formal training in education unless those who desire it actively seek it out. Most teaching habits stem from personal experiences, both positive and negative, as students and trainees. Physicians seek to model those behaviors from positive experiences, and to cast out negative behaviors of others that they have encountered. Irby and Papadakis[9] reviewed several studies that showed excellent teachers not only demonstrate clinical competence but also are able to target their teaching to the learner's level of knowledge through a varied catalog of teaching scripts. These excellent teachers not only provide direction and feedback but also solicit feedback from learners on their performance and engage in self-reflection themselves.[9] Identifying these characteristics is essential because effective clinical teachers have a positive outcome on students' learning and experiences.[9] These characteristics can be the impetus for creating a faculty development curriculum aimed at fostering these qualities and improving the skills of clinician teachers.

Making entrustment decisions in the pediatric ED is a difficult process but paramount to a trainee's education in becoming an autonomous physician. Stakes are high in the pediatric ED because patients are small and easily harmed by medical errors. According to Ten Cate and colleagues,[10] there are 5 categories that affect the ability to entrust: trainee factors, supervisor factors, situation, task, and the relationship between the trainee and supervisor. Trainee factors and the relationship to the supervisor are difficult in an ED setting because trainees come and go frequently. It is difficult to build a relationship with trainees in the short time they are rotating in the department. The supervisor must be able to quickly assess competence to gauge entrustment. Other factors at play are trainees' abilities to be trustworthy and honest and know when they are beyond their abilities. If trainees are found untrustworthy, it is hard to entrust them with complex tasks. Trainees must be aware that entrustment is not given but earned. The supervisor factors are primarily related to teaching style and personality. If physician educators are open to alternative options, they may grant autonomy more readily. Comfort level and confidence of the faculty in their ability also play key roles. The environment of the ED and of the institution as a whole also plays large roles in the ability to entrust and provide autonomy. If there are complex situations happening simultaneously, the physician educator may compensate by doling out orders instead of allowing trainees to make independent decisions. In addition, if the institution mandates its faculty to provide in-depth patient contact, this may also hinder autonomy. Risk-averse physicians may find it more difficult to trust others for fear of retribution. The final category is task. Complex tasks are more difficult to entrust to a trainee without supervision because there are high stakes if a mistake is made. There is a fine balance between entrustment/autonomy and supervision. If too much autonomy is given, the student may become overwhelmed; if too little, the student does not learn independent thinking.

Implementation Strategies: The Group

Creating opportunities for professional development in the field of medical education is paramount in improving the skills of clinician teachers. This can be achieved in several ways. Creation of a faculty development curriculum with workshops to focus on specific teaching techniques, providing feedback, and promoting autonomy encourages clinicians to incorporate these techniques into their current practice. Peer mentoring can be helpful to clinicians to navigate the particular challenges to effective teaching that they experience in their work environment. Encouraging and supporting interested clinicians to pursue additional training in medical education in the form of a course, conference, or fellowship can generate educational leadership within a group.

When it comes to the challenges of entrustment, there are several unique ways in which pediatric emergency medicine physicians can entrust and provide autonomy in the department. At the beginning of a shift, set expectation and goals for the shift, especially if a trainee is new to the department. As the shift advances, and trainees have fulfilled their duties well, more autonomy should be granted and trainees should take ownership of the patients. In this model, if ownership is shared between faculty and trainee, with the trainee as the primary clinician and the faculty in the supporting role, the trainee will incur the responsibility and want to provide good care. If faculty are dictating management and not allowing trainees to practice medicine, trainees feels like note writers and not active players in the management of the patient.[11] If the trainees have a different management plan or style, they should be allowed to execute it as long as it is within standard of care. To help facilitate ownership of the patient, it is important to step back and be a silent observer until a trainee needs help. In this way, the patient care team knows the trainee is in charge and will initiate care without faculty input. If it becomes necessary for the attending physician to take over and direct care, as in a critical resuscitation, then after the situation has been stabilized, pertinent teaching points of the case should be reviewed. It is imperative for trainees to create treatment plans independent of faculty input; otherwise, they will simply tailor the plan to faculty preference, thereby hindering learning.

The Organization

The organization level of the learning environment focuses on the physical features and cultural characteristics of the pediatric ED. Often it is these features and characteristics that can create many challenges in executing effective clinical teaching. The ED is a busy clinical setting full of uncertainty with competing demands for both learners' and teachers' attention.[12] Managing many patients can decrease the amount of time available for teaching.[12] Learning and service are often performed simultaneously, and, in times of high patient acuity or emergent situations, education can become secondary to the delivery of patient care. Interactions with a given learner may be brief; often in the ED, supervisors are working with a trainee for one shift or even a partial shift. Lastly, there is no way to control what types of encounters learners are exposed to, so if learners have identified a gap in their knowledge or training (eg, respiratory distress in the neonate), there is no guarantee that this type of patient encounter will be available during his shift.

Emergency medicine is a team-based practice with many members on the patient care team, leaving students struggling to find their place within the ED as a learner. Students may feel isolated from the rest of the patient care team or may not feel welcomed in the department. The ED if often staffed by residents and trainees of varying levels of training/education. It can be challenging to tailor teaching to trainees of different residency backgrounds and different levels of training and to constantly switch focus when working with multiple learners.

Teaching within pediatrics is also challenging in that parents may be more reluctant to incorporate students or trainees into their child's care, particularly in the realm of procedural teaching.[13] Because children are not always willing participants in their own care, sometimes there is only one opportunity to solicit a particular physical examination finding or to perform patient care functions. Balancing this with the needs of multiple learners can be challenging; for example, both emergency medicine and pediatrics residents need to learn how to reduce a radial head subluxation as part of their training, but there is only one opportunity to do so in a single patient. Additionally, certain illnesses are rare in children, and events, such as resuscitations, cardiac arrest, respiratory failure, and advanced airway control, are less commonly seen in the pediatric population. As such, the possibility exists that not all educational needs of learners are met during their clinical experience.

Implementation Strategies: The Organization

Teaching in a busy clinical environment like the ED can be daunting, but there are strategies to make it a successful learning environment for students and trainees. Teaching is most readily accomplished during a trainee's case presentation and at the bedside. As discussed previously, taking a few minutes to orient to learners, their stage of training, and their goals for the shift can provide a great foundation on which to build during the course of the shift together. This can be performed by directly questioning a learner and can be augmented by observing the learner's performance during a patient encounter. Taking these steps allow the teacher to focus on what steps the learner should accomplish next based on what the learner already knows. One specific technique that exists for teaching in a busy clinical environment is called the one-minute preceptor and mirrors, at least in part, what most clinicians do as part of their staffing model with trainees. This is a 5-step model whereby the teacher (1) gets a commitment from the learner about what the learner thinks is going on with the patient, (2) asks for rationale or explanation for this commitment, (3) teaches a general principle, (4) provides positive feedback to the learner, and (5) corrects errors and makes suggestions for improvement.[14] This technique can be adapted to trainees of all levels and not only provides the context to teach a focused principle or idea but also provides real-time feedback to learners on their performance.

Another way to incorporate teaching in the ED is through the use of bedside teaching techniques. Aldeen and Gisondi[12] discuss the importance of bedside teaching in the ED, even in times of high patient volumes or high patient acuity. They offer specific strategies for how to execute bedside teaching in the ED. One such strategy is to "choose the right time to teach," knowing which forms of teaching work best in a given scenario.[12] For example, a resuscitation may be the appropriate time for observational learning, such as having a medical student observe airway assessment and how the decision is made to place an advanced airway. A calm and cooperative infant presenting for evaluation of respiratory symptoms may be an ideal opportunity to discuss with a junior resident the physical examination findings differentiating an upper respiratory tract infection from a lower respiratory tract infection. Bedside teaching can be interspersed throughout the shift and does not have to be performed on every patient. Instead, bedside teaching may focus on 2 to 3 common chief complaints that present to an ED or on a patient with interesting examination findings. Lastly, if a culture of education is created in a department, senior residents can also lead short bedside teaching sessions with junior residents or medical students.

Other opportunities exist for enriching the learning environment of the ED. Orienting the new members of a patient care team (ie, the resident or the student) to the "usual players" (nurses, paramedics, and technicians) and promoting their inclusion in patient care activities can make learners feel like they are part of the patient care team. Building a work environment in which all members of the care team are acknowledged and respected also allows learners to feel comfortable asking questions identifying their own gaps in knowledge, creating targets for teaching. Learners will also seek to model these behaviors in their own future practice. Lastly, informing patients and their families of the role of the learner in the patient care team minimizes their reluctance in allowing trainees to participate in their care and can encourage patients to identify the resident as "their doctor" while the teacher takes a supervising doctor role.

SUMMARY

The pediatric ED is rich with educational opportunities. By exploring individual levels of the learning environment in the pediatric ED, potential barriers to providing meaningful educational experiences for learners are identified. Recognizing these barriers allows physician educators to execute strategies in their unique environment to balance service requirements in a busy clinical setting with the needs of a variety of learners. Improving the educational environment for learners contributes not only to their growth into autonomous physicians but also to their overall well-being and satisfaction in their education and training.

REFERENCES

1. Schonrock-Adema J, Bouwkamp-Timmer T, van Hell EA, et al. Key elements in assessing the educational environment: where is the theory? Adv Health Sci Educ Theory Pract 2012;17(5):727–42.
2. Long TR, Doherty JA, Frimannsdottir KR, et al. An early assessment of the ACGME CLER program: a national survey of designated institutional officials. J Grad Med Educ 2017;9(3):330–5.
3. Harden RM. The learning environment and the curriculum. Med Teach 2001; 23(4):335–6.
4. Soemantri D, Herrera C, Riquelme A. Measuring the educational environment in health professions studies: a systematic review. Med Teach 2010;32(12):947–52.
5. Miller JG. Living systems. New York: McGraw-Hill; 1978.
6. Roff S, McAleer S. What is educational climate? Med Teach 2001;23(4):333–4.
7. Knowles MS. The modern practice of adult education: from pedagogy to andragogy. New York: Cambridge; 1980.
8. Ramani S, Leinster S. AMEE guide no. 34: teaching in the clinical environment. Med Teach 2008;30(4):347–64.
9. Irby DM, Papadakis M. Does good clinical teaching really make a difference? Am J Med 2001;110(3):231–2.
10. Ten Cate O, Hart D, Ankel F, et al. Entrustment decision making in clinical training. Acad Med 2016;91(2):191–8.

11. Saxon K, Juneja N. Establishing entrustment of residents and autonomy. Acad Emerg Med 2013;20(9):947–9.
12. Aldeen AZ, Gisondi MA. Bedside teaching in the emergency department. Acad Emerg Med 2006;13(8):860–6.
13. McCarthy ML, Chaudoin LT, Mercurio MR, et al. Parents' perspective on trainees performing invasive procedures: a qualitative evaluation. Pediatr Emerg Care 2017. [Epub ahead of print].
14. Irby DM, Wilkerson L. Teaching when time is limited. BMJ 2008;336(7640):384–7.

Recent Advances in Technology and Its Applications to Pediatric Emergency Care

Marisa C. Louie, MD[a,b,*], Todd P. Chang, MD, MAcM[c],
Robert W. Grundmeier, MD[d]

KEYWORDS

- Pediatric emergency medicine • Ultrasonography • Electronic health records
- Clinical decision support • Simulation-based training • Clinical competence
- Free open access medical education

KEY POINTS

- Technology offers opportunities to provide better care for patients through point-of-care ultrasound examination, innovative devices to facilitate procedures and examinations, and electronic health record tools, such as timely clinical decision-making support and patient tracking.
- Technology also offer opportunities to provide better training and education for pediatric emergency medicine providers through the use of mannequin, virtual, and augmented reality-based simulations and online/electronic resources.
- Although new technology is often appealing, its effectiveness should be critically evaluated before its adoption.

INTRODUCTION

Technology can provide tools, information, and education in settings it was previously unavailable or difficult to attain. This is particularly true for pediatric emergency

Disclosure: The authors have no commercial or financial conflicts of interest to declare.
[a] Department of Emergency Medicine, University of Michigan Medical School, Mott Children's Hospital, 1540 East Hospital Drive, CW 2-737, Ann Arbor, MI 48109, USA; [b] Department of Pediatrics, University of Michigan Medical School, Mott Children's Hospital, 1540 East Hospital Drive, CW 2-737, Ann Arbor, MI 48109, USA; [c] Pediatric Emergency Medicine, Keck School of Medicine at University of Southern California, Children's Hospital Los Angeles, 4650 Sunset Boulevard Mailstop 113, Los Angeles, CA 90027, USA; [d] Department of Biomedical and Health Informatics, Perelman School of Medicine at the University of Pennsylvania, Children's Hospital of Philadelphia, Roberts Center, 2716 South Street, 15th Floor, Philadelphia, PA 19146, USA
* Corresponding author. Department of Pediatrics, University of Michigan Medical School, Mott Children's Hospital, 1540 East Hospital Drive, CW 2-737, Ann Arbor, MI 48109.
E-mail address: mclouie@med.umich.edu

Pediatr Clin N Am 65 (2018) 1229–1246
https://doi.org/10.1016/j.pcl.2018.07.013
0031-3955/18/© 2018 Published by Elsevier Inc.

medicine (PEM), where patients seek care at any time or day with needs that are encountered infrequently and in places where pediatric specialty expertise is not readily available. For example, a child might present with concerns for appendicitis to an emergency department (ED) that does not have radiology capability in the overnight hours. Another child might require a cricothyrotomy, a procedure that is infrequently encountered and thus rarely practiced. A third patient with complex congenital heart disease might present in extremis to a community ED that is unfamiliar with their care needs. Advances in technology create potential solutions for all these and many other similar scenarios.

This article seeks to discuss key advances in technology that are transforming PEM. Technological advances affect all aspects of patient care, from before the visit to well after discharge. We have organized major advances into those that occur at the bedside, at the desktop, and beyond.

AT THE BEDSIDE CLINICAL CARE
Point-of-Care Ultrasound Examination

Perhaps one of the most widely adopted technologies in PEM is the expansion of point-of-care ultrasound (POCUS) examination. Although POCUS has been a longstanding feature of adult emergency care, its use in children is particularly valuable given the increased concern for radiation exposure. Mechanical advances allowing good quality images to be obtained using small, portable devices also makes ultrasound accessible in low-resource settings. **Table 1** lists some common POCUS examinations in PEM.

In addition to the uses listed in **Table 1**, there are many other possible uses for PEM POCUS, such as biliary system assessments, scrotal examinations, and optic nerve diameter measurements, which are better described in the adult literature. However, many questions have yet to be answered and may be depend on local practice patterns. For example, is performing POCUS judicious time management in a setting where radiology-based ultrasound examination is readily available? Conversely, should POCUS be used to rule-in diagnoses to conserve radiology resources? What are the training requirements and competency criteria? Should images be stored in the patient's medical chart as radiology-acquired images would be? Will there be a lag in its acceptance among the clinicians who provide definitive management for POCUS-identified problems? In health care, as in daily life, opportunities to integrate new technologies into daily practice poses new questions and potential for regulation and rules.

Videolaryngoscopy

Videolaryngoscopy (VL) is increasingly used as an alternative to direct laryngoscopy (DL) for intubation.[33] The camera, located at the end of the blade, can provide an improved view by obviating the need to optically align the mouth, pharynx, and larynx. It also allows visualization for supervising providers in settings where trainees or additional staff are present. To date, studies in pediatric ED patients are scarce. In a retrospective study, Eisenberg and colleagues[34] found that VL and DL had similar success and complication rates, even though patients were more likely to have difficult airway characteristics in the VL group. A recent metaanalysis examined outcomes comparing the 2 techniques as performed by anesthesiologists and also found no significant difference in first-pass success rates. However, they demonstrated a lower overall success rate and longer time to intubation (mean difference, 5.49 seconds; 95% confidence interval, 1.37–9.60 seconds) with VL. Airway trauma, an oft-cited VL

Table 1 Common POCUS examinations encountered in PEM		
Examination Type	**Indication(s)**	**Comments**
FAST	Rapid identification of abdominal, pericardial and pleural fluid and pneumothorax	• Difficult to rule out abdominal free fluid with sensitivities of 27%–66%[1–3] • May allow avoidance of computed tomography scanning in patients with a low risk of intraabdominal injury[4]
Right lower quadrant	Diagnosis of appendicitis	• Metaanalysis with sensitivity 86% (95% CI, 79%–90%) and specificity 91% (95% CI, 87%–94%)[5] • Excellent agreement between PEM and Radiology performed examinations[6]
Soft tissue	Differentiation between cellulitis and abscess	Increased sensitivity relative to clinical abscess examinations,[7–9] or at least in cases of clinical uncertainty[10]
Chest (outside of FAST)	Diagnosis of pneumonia	Per metaanalysis[11]: • Sensitivity, 96% (95% CI, 94%–97%) • Specificity, 93% (95% CI, 90%–96%) • Positive likelihood ratio, 15.3 (95% CI, 6.6–35.3) • Negative likelihood ratio, 0.06 (95% CI, 0.03–0.11)
Bone	Fracture diagnosis	• Sensitivity $\geq$83%, specificity $\geq$85%, generally higher in long bones of the extremities[12–22] • Potential poorer sensitivity for fractures in small bones and near joints[12,15,22] • Equally or less painful than radiographs[13,19,21,22]
Procedural guidance	Dynamic guidance for central venous access	Increased success rate of central venous cannulation per metaanalysis (RR, 1.32; 95% CI, 1.10–1.58)[23]
	Dynamic guidance for peripheral and venous access	• High overall (80%–91% in 2 studies) first attempt (68%) success rates for peripheral venous access[24,25] • May reduce procedure time and total number of attempts[24]
	Landmark identification for lumbar puncture	• Higher success rate[26,27] • Fewer traumatic taps[26]

(continued on next page)

Table 1 (continued)		
Examination Type	**Indication(s)**	**Comments**
IVC measurements with or without aortic measurements	Identification of intravascular fluid status	Conflicting evidence: • May correlate with volume status[28,29] • May not sensitively detect dehydration[30,31] • May not correlate with central venous pressure measurements[32] • Unclear optimal measurement (IVC:aortic diameter vs IVC:aortic cross-sectional area)[28]

Abbreviations: CI, confidence interval; FAST, Focused assessment with sonography for trauma; IVS, inferior vena cava; PEM, pediatric emergency medicine; POCUS, point-of-care ultrasound; RR, relative risk.

concern, occurred in no VL subjects. However, the authors cite lower quality evidence as a significant limitation of their conclusions.[35]

Both previous studies included patients with and without difficult airways. However, patients with a difficult airway may benefit the most from VL. One retrospective study of a pediatric difficult intubation registry compared GlideScope (Verathon Inc, Bothell, WA) VL with DL. GlideScope use had a significantly higher rate of initial success compared with DL (odds ratio, 7.9; 95% confidence interval, 4.2–14.7) with no increased risk of airway trauma.[36]

One concern regarding VL is that increasing use will result in reduced comfort with DL, because the fundamental hand–eye coordination skills differ. Because VL may not be available in low-resource settings and depends on an airway relatively clean of secretions and debris, expertise with DL is key for PEM physicians. Tools such as the C-MAC (Karl Storz, Tuttlingen, Germany) can circumvent this issue by allowing both forms of laryngoscopy with the same tool.

Cardiopulmonary Resuscitation Assistive and Feedback Devices

As evidence for high-quality chest compressions for cardiopulmonary resuscitation (CPR) has emerged, so too have technologies to help achieve the compressions. The American Heart Association and the Canadian Heart & Stroke Foundation both recognize the need for compressions of a precise depth, between 5 and 6 cm for adult patients.[37,38] Providers without technological assistance are prone to poor quality CPR, leading to poorer outcomes.[39,40] Any delay in CPR or defibrillation is also associated with poorer outcomes. These needs have led to further technological adjuncts to improve the quality and timing of CPR during resuscitation, particularly in out-of-hospital resuscitation.[41] Most devices are meant for adult CPR, although some case reports for pediatric resuscitation do exist.

Mechanical CPR devices, such as the LUCAS 3 device (Lund University Cardiopulmonary Assist System, Lund University, Lund, Sweden), have existed for quite some time. From a purely physics point of view, mechanical devices for adult CPR tend to provide superior compression quality than manual CPR,[42] although the clinical evidence for patient outcomes has been mixed and possibly harmful.[43,44] To date, there is no out-of-the-box solution for pediatric chest compressions, although there is a case report that used towels under an 11-year-old patient to overcome the chest height gap.[45]

For manual CPR, feedback devices have been shown to improve compression quality. Devices include portable versions placed under the compressors' hands to measure depth, rate, and recoil, as well as measurements provided by defibrillator pads that sense similar movement. These include the Laerdal CPRmeter (Laerdal, Stavanger Norway), the Philips Q-CPR "puck" (Philips, Amsterdam, Netherlands). and the sensing defibrillator pads from Zoll (Chelmsford MA). The use of any feedback device—whether visual feedback or computerized feedback—has been associated with improved quality of CPR.[46–48] It should be noted that human feedback—when other providers provide feedback on CPR quality based on their own eyes—is inferior to mechanical feedback.[49]

Finally, early bystander CPR and defibrillation have been associated with improved outcomes in out-of-hospital cardiac arrest for all ages. To improve bystander CPR, particularly in remote areas away from emergency services, delivery drones with both automated external defibrillators and communication devices to help assist remotely have been trialed, with improved response times in rural areas when compared with actual emergency medical services personnel.[50] The same network resources could be vital for pediatric resuscitations, although pediatric data have yet to be gathered.

System-Targeted Apps and Tools

The development of apps and tools for system-specific purposes can assist with diagnosis and be valuable teaching adjuncts in PEM, especially when patient cooperation is limited. For example, the iExaminer (Welch Allyn, Skaneateles Falls, NY) is an adaptor system that attaches a smart phone to the Welch Allyn PanOptic and uses an app to capture an image. Day and colleagues[51] demonstrated that images could be obtained with the iExaminer system in patients in the pediatric ED. Among a study population presenting for nonocular complaints, clinically adequate images were captured in 91% of children aged 2 to 18 years and 16% of children under the age of 2 years. Furthermore, mean examination time was only 3 minutes 24 seconds.

Similarly, the CellScope Oto (CellScope, Inc., San Diego, CA) can be used to capture views of the tympanic membrane. Richards and colleagues[52] demonstrated that physicians in a pediatric ED found the CellScope easy to use even without training, with enhanced visualization of the tympanic membrane; it was also a good teaching tool. After performing an examination with a traditional otoscope, a subsequent CellScope examination resulted in diagnostic changes that would be likely to affect management in 6% of attending examinations.

AT-THE-DESKTOP CLINICAL CARE

Health information technology available at the bedside—especially in the form of electronic health record (EHR) systems, clinical decision support (CDS), and telemedicine—offers tremendous opportunities to improve the quality, efficiency, and effectiveness of clinical care. Meaningful use incentive programs have expedited implementation efforts in many US health systems.[53] Unfortunately, these incentive programs have had less benefit for the delivery pediatric health care, largely because many EHRs lack features that are essential for pediatrics.[54] Nevertheless, research efforts in the last decade involving EHRs and related health information technology in PEM settings have yielded promising results in the domains of diagnostic accuracy, management of specific clinical problems, medication safety, documentation quality, family engagement, patient flow, and telemedicine applications.

Clinical Decision-Making Tools

More than one-half of the articles (n = 12) we reviewed described clinical decision tools that were either derived or implemented using EHR systems. All but one addressed specific clinical problems. The remaining article addressed a diagnostic decision support system that was not focused on any single clinical problem. Six articles described process or patient outcomes as part of an implementation effort. The remaining articles described system development and validation efforts.

One team decreased abdominal computed tomography (CT) use by developing a clinical practice guideline for the management of abdominal pain and implementing an electronic CDS tool that included a web-based risk stratification tool, a standardized order set, and an alert that appeared when an ultrasound examination or CT scan was ordered. In an interrupted time-series trial, a 20-percentage point decrease in CT use was observed with no increases in appendiceal perforations, return visits within 30 days, or ED duration of stay.[55]

In a sepsis clinical pathway implementation effort that included a paper-based decision tool combined with an electronic order set, the authors observed a decrease in time to intravenous access (from 37 to 24 minutes) and first dose of antibiotics (from 92 to 55 minutes).[56] The project cooccurred with EHR implementation and the authors' cautioned that without care EHR implementation may hinder ongoing quality improvement efforts.

Four articles described the implementation of a decision rule addressing pediatric blunt head trauma and the related use of CT scans. One study team reported the results of a usability evaluation to design a decision tool that better supports clinical workflow.[57] Another team identified chief complaints that should trigger additional data capture related to blunt injury[58] and proposed the use of web service technologies to rapidly implement the decision tool.[59] The results of an implementation project were highly variable by site, but the intervention resulted in modest decreases in the rate of CT imaging among children at very low risk of clinically important traumatic brain injury.[60]

In a randomized, clinical trial studying paper versus electronic implementation of a clinical practice guideline for asthma care, the authors found no difference in their primary outcome (time to disposition decision) between the study arms. For both study arms, the authors used a Bayesian network that accurately and automatically identified children experiencing an asthma flare based on information collected at triage to initiate asthma care (before physician involvement). At a prespecified sensitivity level of 85%, the Bayesian network identified children experiencing an asthma flare with a positive predictive value of 69.9%.[61]

In a multisite retrospective study, the investigators found no impact of clinical decision tools for acute gastroenteritis (either paper based or electronic) on hospitalization rate and ED return visits within 72 hours. However, they did find that initiation of oral rehydration therapy at triage did reduce ED return visits, suggesting this may be a promising target for future implementation efforts.[62]

Using machine learning approaches, a team of authors developed a Bayesian network to estimate the probability of pyloric stenosis before imaging. Based on the performance of the network, if it were implemented, clinicians would have ordered 22% fewer imaging tests without missing any cases of pyloric stenosis.[63]

In a natural language processing experiment, 1 article described the development and validation of an algorithm to screen EHR narrative documentation with the goal of identifying children with Kawasaki disease. At the 2 study sites, the algorithm had a sensitivity of 93.6% and a specificity of 77.5%. The authors suggested that the algorithm could be implemented as a real-time reminder system to identify children in whom further evaluation for Kawasaki disease should be considered.[64]

A team of authors described the development of a tool to improve the documentation of information related to cerebrospinal fluid shunts. The authors described how this documentation tool, available across the continuum of care, could support future decision support, quality improvement, and research efforts.[65]

One group of authors evaluated a web-based diagnosis decision support system designed to increase the number of clinically relevant diagnoses considered during pediatric acute health care encounters. The primary outcome was the frequency of "unsafe workups," defined as a failure to consider all medically important conditions. Although the system was only used for a minority of acute visits, there was a 12.5 percentage point decrease in unsafe workups after the use of the system.[66]

Medication Safety

Medication safety has been identified as an important issue in the pediatric emergency care setting.[67] Our review identified 2 articles specifically addressing medication safety issues in PEM settings related to medication allergy documentation and prescribing errors.

A team of investigators compared the accuracy of allergy information recorded as part of routine ED care (in either paper or electronic form) with information collected by the study team through a structured verbal interview. In this study, triage personnel identified children allergic to medication with a sensitivity of 74% and a specificity of 93%.[68]

In a pre–post study design, investigators evaluated the impact of CDS that addressed prescription errors related to allergies, drug–drug interactions, dose range errors, and dose frequency errors. The absolute reduction in errors was 3.1 percentage points (from 10.4% of prescriptions before implementation to 7.3% after implementation). Drug dosage errors were most common and decreased by 2.6 percentage points after implementation (from 8.0% to 5.4% of prescriptions).[69]

Family Engagement

Health information technology provides new mechanisms for capturing information electronically directly from patients and their parents. Two articles included in our review addressed methods of engaging families in PEM settings; one focused on system design and one on describing implementation results.

One investigator described the design of an idealized system using technology to support collaborative management of pediatric asthma that incorporates the expertise of patients and their parents alongside that of clinicians.[70]

In a study with alternating intervention and control periods at 2 pediatric EDs, the study team evaluated the impact of electronically collecting information directly from parents on documentation completeness and errors (either omission or commission). The system demonstrated the feasibility of collecting information electronically directly from parents to support "parent-driven decision support" and increased the completeness of pain medication documentation by 13 percentage points.[71]

Patient Flow

The EHR can have significant impact on patient flow in any clinical setting, and these effects may be exaggerated in the pediatric ED owing to patient volumes that are often unpredictable, the variable acuity of illness, and the complexity of patient flow. Although the EHR can provide many tools such as tracking boards, template documentation, and order sets that plausibly improve the efficiency of clinical care, these benefits are not always realized. Three articles in our review specifically examined specific EHR features and their impact on aspects of patient flow.

In a natural experiment, a team of researchers evaluated the effect of EHR implementation on patient flow measures in the pediatric ED, such as time to be placed in a room, time to be seen by a physician, and ED duration of stay. They noted a negative impact on patient flow (longer wait times and duration of stay) despite increased staffing during EHR implementation and increased numbers of children leaving the ED before being seen. However, these impacts were temporary and patient flow measures returned to baseline 3 months after implementation.[72]

A team of authors used Lean development design principles to rapidly implement and refine an electronic documentation tool and assessed its impact on duration of stay in the pediatric ED. The electronic tool was designed to improve the quality of discharge summaries provided to referring physicians. They observed a temporary increase in duration of stay by 15 minutes for patients who were discharged home from the ED during the first 6 weeks after implementation, with a subsequent return to a new baseline duration of stay that was 7 minutes longer than before implementation.[73]

One article described the process of adapting a vendor-supplied ED tracking board for use in a pediatric ED setting to address common problems with patient flow. In a case study, the investigators described the impact of the tracking board on rates of pain reassessment after an intervention. Although statistical significance was not reported, they found that reassessment rates increased from a baseline of 50% to 65% to more than 85% after adding a pain reassessment reminder feature to the tracking board.[74]

Clinical Image Capture

With the widespread adoption of EHRs, the ability to capture patient photographs and other nonradiologic images and store them electronically in the chart has become widely available. These images can facilitate discussion with off-site consultants, follow disease processes over time, and enable clinical education, whether in the context of visual diagnoses or in providing feedback, such as with laceration repairs. Unfortunately, there are no reports in the literature around the usefulness of these images in PEM. An analysis of photographs uploaded into the EHR at Brigham and Women's Hospital over the course of a year indicated dermatology, ophthalmology, and surgery as the major users.[75] However, anecdotally, PEM providers find use of photographs helpful, especially in the context of skin wounds and infections. The report of an iOS image capture application included emergency medicine among the residents who tested the device, the overwhelming majority of whom found it useful or very useful for clinical practice.[76] Furthermore, a small dermatology study suggested clinical images alter management, with fewer changes in management observed after in-person evaluation when phone consultation was accompanied by digital images than when the consultation relied exclusively on a verbal report.[77]

Telemedicine

Telemedicine in the form of a teleconsult offers specialty expertise to community and rural EDs, the benefits of which are exemplified with telestroke care among adults[78] The teleconsult literature in PEM has primarily focused on pediatric critical care consultation for ED patients and has demonstrated increased provision of optimal care before transfer[79–81] and improved resource use.[82–84]

Telemedicine in the form of e-visits for acute illnesses is an emerging practice that can in theory expand the availability of PEM expertise and can potentially replace low-acuity ED visits with less costly e-visits.[85] There are multiple commercial providers of acute care telemedicine visits, such as HealthTap and Teladoc. However, 2 studies of commercial acute care telemedicine providers found poor adherence to established guidelines for common conditions.[86,87] Furthermore, treating physicians may not have knowledge of local resources for additional testing and follow-up, if needed. Health systems that provide primary, subspecialty, and emergency care are now also launching acute care e-visits.[88] This advance has the potential to provide improved transitions of care and communication with the patient's primary care provider as recommended by the American Academy of Pediatrics.[89] However, it remains to be seen whether offering e-visits in lieu of in-person visits within a patient's existing health system will result in good quality of care.

BEYOND DIRECT CLINICAL CARE

Technology for PEM is frequently applied for learning, education, and skills training purposes. Although today's learners are technologically adept,[90] a blind worship of technological mesmerism is not recommended. Rather, we propose a judicious and purposeful use of technology for PEM education, particularly when the technological platform allows for learning or assessing skills that are more difficult to do so under traditional methods.[91]

Simulation-Based Training

Simulation, particularly for high-stakes, low-frequency events, has been used in PEM for a variety of resuscitative scenarios and for procedural skills. Techniques for simulation may include mannequin-based training, serious games (eg, screen-based) training, and virtual reality (VR; head-mounted display VR) training (**Figs. 1** and **2**).

Although a high-fidelity mannequin is not always needed for every learning objective,[92] the technology to simulate the various states of patient disease or injury without facilitator input adds to the realism and fidelity of the ultimate scenario. Companies such as Laerdal, Gaumard Scientific (Miami, FL), and CAE Inc (Montreal, Canada) have various simulators that promote resuscitation training. These mannequin-based scenarios for resuscitation are universally beloved, with typical immediate gains in knowledge and performance.[93–95] However, appropriate learning transfer occurs with well-conducted debriefing to promote reflection.[96,97]

Procedures requiring psychomotor skills in PEM, such as intubation, umbilical line placement, and lumbar puncture, are often taught using task training mannequins. These mannequins allow learners to practice the hand–eye coordination and movements required to complete their procedures.[98] The evidence typically shows improved confidence and performance for most tasks, although studies that demonstrate clinical outcomes are relatively rare.[99] As an example, Barsuk and colleagues[100,101] have shown decreased catheter-related infections after task training for catheter insertions.

Screen-based simulations tend to be more portable than the mannequin-based ones and are often done asynchronously.[102,103] This advantage allows trainees and practitioners to practice or test at their own time. The term "serious game" falls under the umbrella of screen-based simulations: a video game with the primary intent of education and the secondary intent of entertainment is classified as a serious game (as opposed to Angry Birds, which incidentally teaches physics).[102,103] Time management exercises for PEM are often used on a screen-based simulator or in a serious games format.[104] Screen-based simulations are particularly costly to produce, because all costs are upfront, but thereafter can be distributed ad infinitum. These types of simulations have some levels of evidence, but are less frequently

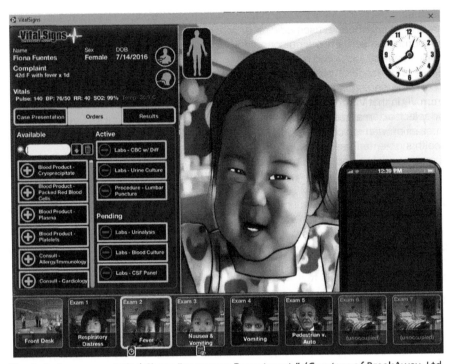

Fig. 1. Serious game: "Vital Signs: Emergency Department." (*Courtesy of* BreakAway, Ltd., Hunt Valley, MD.)

studied than mannequin-based simulations based on the cost prohibitions as mentioned.[105–107]

Finally, the newest form of simulation is head-mounted display VR. This system is in contrast with the older (and now outdated) definition of VR, which was the use of 3-dimensional avatars on a computer screen, such as in Second Life.[108] Current VR devices completely occlude visual and auditory stimuli from the outside and can detect user positioning. Devices as of this writing include the HTC Vive (HTC, New Taipei City, Taiwan) and Oculus Rift (Oculus CR, Menlo Park, CA). These devised are technically part of screen-based simulations because they include a screen system within the

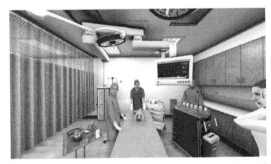

Fig. 2. Virtual reality training module for pediatric emergency medicine. (*Courtesy of* Todd P. Chang, MD, MAcMc, Los Angeles, CA.)

headset, but have potential for geospatial simulations, such as navigating a disaster arena or a crowded resuscitation room.

Augmented reality is the practice of a holographic image or text superimposed on reality, currently achieved by a special set of glasses. At the time of this writing, Google Glass is no longer in production, but Microsoft HoloLens (Microsoft Inc, Redmond, WA) is the predominant augmented reality device. Augmented reality is differentiated from VR in that VR attempts to occlude all external stimuli (except for the user's hands or select externalized items), whereas augmented reality is primarily meant to allow interaction with the outside world with the holography being a secondary component. Most augmented reality present menus, text-based information, and simple holography over a real object; Pokémon Go, along with similar app-based programs, are the beginnings of augmented reality.

Augmented reality in PEM education is still nascent as of this writing, but its potential use is with real patient education or even software-based recognition of signs and symptoms on real patients. Disaster medicine is the most likely use of augmented reality in the actual health care setting. A new term called mixed reality has also emerged with the developers in this sphere; mixed reality provides about a 50-50 mix of superimposed holography that is particularly reactive to changes in real surroundings. The technology will continue to improve for mixed reality as an asset in the near future.

Online Networks, Free Open Access Meducation

Emergency medicine has led the way in online and other electronic reference resources as well as simple platforms to collaborate and discuss PEM topics. Social media resources that spur collaborations[109] and other methods of e-learning such as blogs, wikis, podcasts, and other web resources are particularly prevalent.[110] Specific to PEM, the PEMNetwork emerged as a collaborative through the American Academy of Pediatrics, which currently has a simple blog format as part of the Free Open Access Meducation.[111] Because of the explosion of various online materials, there is current concern over the quality of many of these items; a simple gestalt assessment method seems to be insufficient.[112] Because most online content is ranked by popularity rather than content accuracy, curation methods have also popped up.[109,113] Over time, we will see further levels of hierarchy in the Free Open Access Meducation movement for expectations of quality educational materials.

SUMMARY

We have highlighted promising results demonstrating the capabilities of current bedside technology to avoid radiation-based studies, improve health care outcomes, and enhance education in PEM. Desktop technology has already offered improvements for a number of clinical problems through CDS, and tremendous opportunities remain. The potential for health information technology to improve care collaboration by directly engaging patients and their families is particularly appealing. Simultaneously, the use of technology beyond the bedside in the form of simulation-based training and online learning allows PEM providers to better prepare for the delivery of bedside care. As with all advances in care, research to better define the best tools, identify appropriate indications, and measure quality will ensure we continuously advance care for our patients.

REFERENCES

1. Fox JC, Boysen M, Gharahbaghian L, et al. Test characteristics of focused assessment of sonography for trauma for clinically significant abdominal

free fluid in pediatric blunt abdominal trauma. Acad Emerg Med 2011;18(5): 477–82.

2. Holmes JF, Gladman A, Chang CH. Performance of abdominal ultrasonography in pediatric blunt trauma patients: a meta-analysis. J Pediatr Surg 2007;42(9): 1588–94.

3. Calder BW, Vogel AM, Zhang J, et al. Focused assessment with sonography for trauma in children after blunt abdominal trauma: a multi-institutional analysis. J Trauma Acute Care Surg 2017;83(2):218–24.

4. Menaker J, Blumberg S, Wisner DH, et al. Use of the focused assessment with sonography for trauma (FAST) examination and its impact on abdominal computed tomography use in hemodynamically stable children with blunt torso trauma. J Trauma Acute Care Surg 2014;77(3):427–32.

5. Benabbas R, Hanna M, Shah J, et al. Diagnostic accuracy of history, physical examination, laboratory tests, and point-of-care ultrasound for pediatric acute appendicitis in the emergency department: a systematic review and meta-analysis. Acad Emerg Med 2017;24(5):523–51.

6. Doniger SJ, Kornblith A. Point-of-care ultrasound integrated into a staged diagnostic algorithm for pediatric appendicitis. Pediatr Emerg Care 2018;34(2): 109–15.

7. Adams CM, Neuman MI, Levy JA. Point-of-care ultrasonography for the diagnosis of pediatric soft tissue infection. J Pediatr 2016;169:122–7.e1.

8. Iverson K, Haritos D, Thomas R, et al. The effect of bedside ultrasound on diagnosis and management of soft tissue infections in a pediatric ED. Am J Emerg Med 2012;30(8):1347–51.

9. Sivitz AB, Lam SH, Ramirez-Schrempp D, et al. Effect of bedside ultrasound on management of pediatric soft-tissue infection. J Emerg Med 2010;39(5):637–43.

10. Marin JR, Dean AJ, Bilker WB, et al. Emergency ultrasound-assisted examination of skin and soft tissue infections in the pediatric emergency department. Acad Emerg Med 2013;20(6):545–53.

11. Pereda MA, Chavez MA, Hooper-Miele CC, et al. Lung ultrasound for the diagnosis of pneumonia in children: a meta-analysis. Pediatrics 2015;135(4):714–22.

12. Barata I, Spencer R, Suppiah A, et al. Emergency ultrasound in the detection of pediatric long-bone fractures. Pediatr Emerg Care 2012;28(11):1154–7.

13. Chaar-Alvarez FM, Warkentine F, Cross K, et al. Bedside ultrasound diagnosis of nonangulated distal forearm fractures in the pediatric emergency department. Pediatr Emerg Care 2011;27(11):1027–32.

14. Chen L, Kim Y, Moore CL. Diagnosis and guided reduction of forearm fractures in children using bedside ultrasound. Pediatr Emerg Care 2007;23(8):528–31.

15. Galletebeitia Laka I, Samson F, Gorostiza I, et al. The utility of clinical ultrasonography in identifying distal forearm fractures in the pediatric emergency department. Eur J Emerg Med 2017. [Epub ahead of print].

16. Joshi N, Lira A, Mehta N, et al. Diagnostic accuracy of history, physical examination, and bedside ultrasound for diagnosis of extremity fractures in the emergency department: a systematic review. Acad Emerg Med 2013;20(1):1–15.

17. Kozaci N, Ay MO, Akcimen M, et al. Evaluation of the effectiveness of bedside point-of-care ultrasound in the diagnosis and management of distal radius fractures. Am J Emerg Med 2015;33(1):67–71.

18. Patel DD, Blumberg SM, Crain EF. The utility of bedside ultrasonography in identifying fractures and guiding fracture reduction in children. Pediatr Emerg Care 2009;25(4):221–5.

19. Poonai N, Myslik F, Joubert G, et al. Point-of-care ultrasound for nonangulated distal forearm fractures in children: test performance characteristics and patient-centered outcomes. Acad Emerg Med 2017;24(5):607–16.

20. Rabiner JE, Friedman LM, Khine H, et al. Accuracy of point-of-care ultrasound for diagnosis of skull fractures in children. Pediatrics 2013;131(6):e1757–64.

21. Rowlands R, Rippey J, Tie S, et al. Bedside ultrasound vs X-ray for the diagnosis of forearm fractures in children. J Emerg Med 2017;52(2):208–15.

22. Weinberg ER, Tunik MG, Tsung JW. Accuracy of clinician-performed point-of-care ultrasound for the diagnosis of fractures in children and young adults. Injury 2010;41(8):862–8.

23. Lau CS, Chamberlain RS. Ultrasound-guided central venous catheter placement increases success rates in pediatric patients: a meta-analysis. Pediatr Res 2016;80(2):178–84.

24. Doniger SJ, Ishimine P, Fox JC, et al. Randomized controlled trial of ultrasound-guided peripheral intravenous catheter placement versus traditional techniques in difficult-access pediatric patients. Pediatr Emerg Care 2009;25(3):154–9.

25. Vinograd AM, Zorc JJ, Dean AJ, et al. First-attempt success, longevity, and complication rates of ultrasound-guided peripheral intravenous catheters in children. Pediatr Emerg Care 2018;34(6):376–80.

26. Gorn M, Kunkov S, Crain EF. Prospective investigation of a novel ultrasound-assisted lumbar puncture technique on infants in the pediatric emergency department. Acad Emerg Med 2017;24(1):6–12.

27. Neal JT, Kaplan SL, Woodford AL, et al. The effect of bedside ultrasonographic skin marking on infant lumbar puncture success: a randomized controlled trial. Ann Emerg Med 2017;69(5):610–9.e1.

28. Kwon H, Jung JY, Lee JH, et al. Sonographic aorta/IVC cross-sectional area index for evaluation of dehydration in children. Am J Emerg Med 2016;34(9):1840–4.

29. Levine AC, Shah SP, Umulisa I, et al. Ultrasound assessment of severe dehydration in children with diarrhea and vomiting. Acad Emerg Med 2010;17(10):1035–41.

30. Chen L, Hsiao A, Langhan M, et al. Use of bedside ultrasound to assess degree of dehydration in children with gastroenteritis. Acad Emerg Med 2010;17(10):1042–7.

31. Jauregui J, Nelson D, Choo E, et al. The BUDDY (bedside ultrasound to detect dehydration in youth) study. Crit Ultrasound J 2014;6(1):15.

32. Ng L, Khine H, Taragin BH, et al. Does bedside sonographic measurement of the inferior vena cava diameter correlate with central venous pressure in the assessment of intravascular volume in children? Pediatr Emerg Care 2013;29(3):337–41.

33. Pallin DJ, Dwyer RC, Walls RM, et al. Techniques and trends, success rates, and adverse events in emergency department pediatric intubations: a report from the national emergency airway registry. Ann Emerg Med 2016;67(5):610–5.e1.

34. Eisenberg MA, Green-Hopkins I, Werner H, et al. Comparison between direct and video-assisted laryngoscopy for intubations in a pediatric emergency department. Acad Emerg Med 2016;23(8):870–7.

35. Abdelgadir IS, Phillips RS, Singh D, et al. Videolaryngoscopy versus direct laryngoscopy for tracheal intubation in children (excluding neonates). Cochrane Database Syst Rev 2017;(5):CD011413.

36. Park R, Peyton JM, Fiadjoe JE, et al. The efficacy of GlideScope(R) videolaryngoscopy compared with direct laryngoscopy in children who are difficult to

intubate: an analysis from the paediatric difficult intubation registry. Br J Anaesth 2017;119(5):984–92.

37. Berg R, Hemphill R, Abella BS, et al. Part 5: adult basic life support: 2010 American Heart Association Guidelines for Cardiopulmonary Resuscitation and Emergency Cardiovascular Care. Circulation 2010;122(18 Suppl 3):S685–705.

38. Kleinman ME, Brennan EE, Goldberger ZD, et al. Part 5: adult basic life support and cardiopulmonary resuscitation quality: 2015 American Heart Association Guidelines Update for Cardiopulmonary Resuscitation and Emergency Cardiovascular Care. Circulation 2015;132(18 Suppl 2):S414–35.

39. Sutton RM, Niles D, French B, et al. First quantitative analysis of cardiopulmonary resuscitation quality during in-hospital cardiac arrests of young children. Resuscitation 2014;85(1):70–4.

40. Sutton RM, Niles D, Nysaether J, et al. Quantitative analysis of CPR quality during in-hospital resuscitation of older children and adolescents. Pediatrics 2009; 124(2):494–9.

41. Cave DM, Gazmuri RJ, Otto CW, et al. Part 7: CPR techniques and devices: 2010 American Heart Association Guidelines for Cardiopulmonary Resuscitation and Emergency Cardiovascular Care. Circulation 2010;122(18 Suppl 3):S720–8.

42. Putzer G, Fiala A, Braun P, et al. Manual versus mechanical chest compressions on surfaces of varying softness with or without backboards: a randomized, crossover manikin study. J Emerg Med 2016;50(4):594–600.e1.

43. Bonnes JL, Brouwer MA, Navarese EP, et al. Manual cardiopulmonary resuscitation versus CPR including a mechanical chest compression device in out-of-hospital cardiac arrest: a comprehensive meta-analysis from randomized and observational studies. Ann Emerg Med 2016;67(3):349–60.e3.

44. Buckler DG, Burke RV, Naim MY, et al. Association of mechanical cardiopulmonary resuscitation device use with cardiac arrest outcomes: a population-based study using the CARES Registry (Cardiac Arrest Registry to Enhance Survival). Circulation 2016;134(25):2131–3.

45. Sugarman L, Hedley D, Crowe S. Mechanical CPR in a child: can one size fit all? BMJ Case Rep 2017;2017 [pii:bcr-2017-219728].

46. Cheng A, Brown LL, Duff JP, et al, International Network for Simulation-Based Pediatric Innovation, Research, & Education (INSPIRE) CPR Investigators. Improving Cardiopulmonary Resuscitation with a CPR Feedback Device and Refresher Simulations (CPR CARES Study): a randomized clinical trial. JAMA Pediatr 2015;169(2):137–44.

47. Hostler D, Everson-Stewart S, Rea TD, et al. Effect of real-time feedback during cardiopulmonary resuscitation outside hospital: prospective, cluster-randomised trial. BMJ 2011;342:d512.

48. Yeung J, Meeks R, Edelson D, et al. The use of CPR feedback/prompt devices during training and CPR performance: a systematic review. Resuscitation 2009; 80(7):743–51.

49. Cheng A, Overly F, Kessler D, et al. Perception of CPR quality: influence of CPR feedback, Just-in-Time CPR training and provider role. Resuscitation 2014;87C: 44–50.

50. Claesson A, Fredman D, Svensson L, et al. Unmanned aerial vehicles (drones) in out-of-hospital-cardiac-arrest. Scand J Trauma Resusc Emerg Med 2016; 24(1):124.

51. Day LM, Wang SX, Huang CJ. Nonmydriatic fundoscopic imaging using the pan optic iExaminer system in the pediatric emergency department. Acad Emerg Med 2017;24(5):587–94.

52. Richards JR, Gaylor KA, Pilgrim AJ. Comparison of traditional otoscope to iPhone otoscope in the pediatric ED. Am J Emerg Med 2015;33(8):1089–92.

53. U.S. Congress. American Recovery and Reinvestment Act of 2009. Available at: http://www.healthit.gov/policy-researchers-implementers/hitech-act-0. Accessed October 30, 2017.

54. Nakamura MM, Harper MB, Castro AV, et al. Impact of the meaningful use incentive program on electronic health record adoption by US children's hospitals. J Am Med Inform Assoc 2015;22(2):390–8.

55. Kharbanda AB, Madhok M, Krause E, et al. Implementation of electronic clinical decision support for pediatric appendicitis. Pediatrics 2016;137(5) [pii: e20151745].

56. Tuuri RE, Gehrig MG, Busch CE, et al. "Beat the shock clock": an interprofessional team improves pediatric septic shock care. Clin Pediatr (Phila) 2016; 55(7):626–38.

57. Yadav K, Chamberlain JM, Lewis VR, et al. Designing real-time decision support for trauma resuscitations. Acad Emerg Med 2015;22(9):1076–84.

58. Deakyne SJ, Bajaj L, Hoffman J, et al. Development, evaluation and implementation of chief complaint groupings to activate data collection: a multi-center study of clinical decision support for children with head trauma. Appl Clin Inform 2015;6(3):521–35.

59. Goldberg HS, Paterno MD, Grundmeier RW, et al. Use of a remote clinical decision support service for a multicenter trial to implement prediction rules for children with minor blunt head trauma. Int J Med Inform 2016;87:101–10.

60. Dayan PS, Ballard DW, Tham E, et al. Use of traumatic brain injury prediction rules with clinical decision support. Pediatrics 2017;139(4) [pii:e20162709].

61. Dexheimer JW, Abramo TJ, Arnold DH, et al. Implementation and evaluation of an integrated computerized asthma management system in a pediatric emergency department: a randomized clinical trial. Int J Med Inform 2014;83(11): 805–13.

62. Bahm A, Freedman SB, Guan J, et al. Evaluating the impact of clinical decision tools in pediatric acute gastroenteritis: a population-based cohort study. Acad Emerg Med 2016;23(5):599–609.

63. Alvarez SM, Poelstra BA, Burd RS. Evaluation of a Bayesian decision network for diagnosing pyloric stenosis. J Pediatr Surg 2006;41(1):155–61 [discussion: 155–61].

64. Doan S, Maehara CK, Chaparro JD, et al. Building a natural language processing tool to identify patients with high clinical suspicion for Kawasaki disease from emergency department notes. Acad Emerg Med 2016;23(5):628–36.

65. Governale LS, Hoffman JM. Meaningful use: an electronic medical record tool for cerebrospinal fluid shunt history. J Neurosurg Pediatr 2017;19(4):391–8.

66. Ramnarayan P, Winrow A, Coren M, et al. Diagnostic omission errors in acute paediatric practice: impact of a reminder system on decision-making. BMC Med Inform Decis Mak 2006;6:37.

67. Committee on Pediatric Emergency Medicine, American Academy of Pediatrics, Krug SE, Frush K. Patient safety in the pediatric emergency care setting. Pediatrics 2007;120(6):1367–75.

68. Porter SC, Manzi SF, Volpe D, et al. Getting the data right: information accuracy in pediatric emergency medicine. Qual Saf Health Care 2006;15(4):296–301.

69. Sethuraman U, Kannikeswaran N, Murray KP, et al. Prescription errors before and after introduction of electronic medication alert system in a pediatric emergency department. Acad Emerg Med 2015;22(6):714–9.

70. Porter SC. Patients as experts: a collaborative performance support system. Proc AMIA Symp 2001;548–52.

71. Fine AM, Kalish LA, Forbes P, et al. Parent-driven technology for decision support in pediatric emergency care. Jt Comm J Qual Patient Saf 2009;35(6):307–15.

72. Spellman Kennebeck S, Timm N, Farrell MK, et al. Impact of electronic health record implementation on patient flow metrics in a pediatric emergency department. J Am Med Inform Assoc 2012;19(3):443–7.

73. Lo MD, Rutman LE, Migita RT, et al. Rapid electronic provider documentation design and implementation in an academic pediatric emergency department. Pediatr Emerg Care 2015;31(11):798–804.

74. Dexheimer JW, Kennebeck S. Modifications and integration of the electronic tracking board in a pediatric emergency department. Pediatr Emerg Care 2013;29(7):852–7.

75. Ai AC, Maloney FL, Hickman TT, et al. A picture is worth 1,000 words. The use of clinical images in electronic medical records. Appl Clin Inform 2017;8(3):710–8.

76. Landman A, Emani S, Carlile N, et al. A mobile app for securely capturing and transferring clinical images to the electronic health record: description and preliminary usability study. JMIR Mhealth Uhealth 2015;3(1):e1.

77. Mann T, Colven R. A picture is worth more than a thousand words: enhancement of a pre-exam telephone consultation in dermatology with digital images. Acad Med 2002;77(7):742–3.

78. Meyer BC, Raman R, Hemmen T, et al. Efficacy of site-independent telemedicine in the STRokE DOC trial: a randomised, blinded, prospective study. Lancet Neurol 2008;7(9):787–95.

79. Dayal P, Hojman NM, Kissee JL, et al. Impact of telemedicine on severity of illness and outcomes among children transferred from referring emergency departments to a children's hospital PICU. Pediatr Crit Care Med 2016;17(6):516–21.

80. Dharmar M, Kuppermann N, Romano PS, et al. Telemedicine consultations and medication errors in rural emergency departments. Pediatrics 2013;132(6):1090–7.

81. Dharmar M, Romano PS, Kuppermann N, et al. Impact of critical care telemedicine consultations on children in rural emergency departments. Crit Care Med 2013;41(10):2388–95.

82. Fugok K, Slamon NB. The effect of telemedicine on resource utilization and hospital disposition in critically ill pediatric transport patients. Telemed J E Health 2018;24(5):367–74.

83. Yang NH, Dharmar M, Kuppermann N, et al. Appropriateness of disposition following telemedicine consultations in rural emergency departments. Pediatr Crit Care Med 2015;16(3):e59–64.

84. Yang NH, Dharmar M, Yoo BK, et al. Economic evaluation of pediatric telemedicine consultations to rural emergency departments. Med Decis Making 2015;35(6):773–83.

85. McConnochie KM, Wood NE, Herendeen NE, et al. Acute illness care patterns change with use of telemedicine. Pediatrics 2009;123(6):e989–95.

86. Schoenfeld AJ, Davies JM, Marafino BJ, et al. Variation in quality of urgent health care provided during commercial virtual visits. JAMA Intern Med 2016;176(5):635–42.

87. Uscher-Pines L, Mulcahy A, Cowling D, et al. Access and quality of care in direct-to-consumer telemedicine. Telemed J E Health 2016;22(4):282–7.

88. Sharma R, Fleischut P, Barchi D. Telemedicine and its transformation of emergency care: a case study of one of the largest US integrated healthcare delivery systems. Int J Emerg Med 2017;10(1):21.

89. Conners GP, Kressly SJ, Perrin JM, et al. Nonemergency acute care: when it's not the medical home. Pediatrics 2017;139(5) [pii:e20170629].

90. Eckleberry-Hunt J, Tucciarone J. The challenges and opportunities of teaching "generation Y". J Grad Med Educ 2011;3(4):458–61.

91. Ilgen J, Sherbino J, Cook DA. Technology-enhanced simulation in emergency medicine: a systematic review and meta-analysis. Acad Emerg Med 2013;20: 117–27.

92. Norman G, Dore K, Grierson L. The minimal relationship between simulation fidelity and transfer of learning. Med Educ 2012;46(7):636–47.

93. Cheng A, Lang TR, Starr SR, et al. Technology-enhanced simulation and pediatric education: a meta-analysis. Pediatrics 2014;133(5):e1313–23.

94. Adler M, Trainor JL, Siddall VJ, et al. Development and evaluation of high-fidelity simulation case scenarios for pediatric resident education. Ambul Pediatr 2007; 7(2):182–6.

95. Mills DM, Wu CL, Williams DC, et al. High-fidelity simulation enhances pediatric residents' retention, knowledge, procedural proficiency, group resuscitation performance, and experience in pediatric resuscitation. Hosp Pediatr 2013;3(3): 266–75.

96. Cheng A, Hunt EA, Donoghue A, et al. Examining pediatric resuscitation education using simulation and scripted debriefing: a multicenter randomized trial. JAMA Pediatr 2013;167(6):528–36.

97. Eppich WJ, Hunt EA, Duval-Arnould JM, et al. Structuring feedback and debriefing to achieve mastery learning goals. Acad Med 2015;90(11):1501–8.

98. Kneebone R. Evaluating clinical simulations for learning procedural skills: a theory-based approach. Acad Med 2005;80(6):549–53.

99. Kessler D, Auerbach M, Pusic M, et al. A randomized trial of simulation-based deliberate practice for infant lumbar puncture skills. Simul Healthc 2011;6(4): 197–203.

100. Barsuk J, Cohen ER, Feinglass J, et al. Use of simulation-based education to reduce catheter-related bloodstream infections. Arch Intern Med 2009; 169(15):1420–3.

101. Barsuk J, McGaghie WC, Cohen ER, et al. Simulation-based mastery learning reduces complications during central venous catheter insertion in a medical intensive care unit. Crit Care Med 2009;37(10):2697–701.

102. Chang T, Pusic MV, Gerard JL. Screen-based simulation and virtual reality. In: Grant VJ, Cheng A, editors. Comprehensive healthcare simulation - pediatrics. 1st edition. Switzerland: Springer International Publishing; 2016. p. 686.

103. Chang TP, Weiner D. Screen-based simulation and virtual reality for pediatric emergency medicine. Clin Pediatr Emerg Med 2016;17(3):224–30.

104. Mohan D, Angus DC, Ricketts D, et al. Assessing the validity of using serious game technology to analyze physician decision making. PLoS One 2014;9(8): e105445.

105. Biese K, Moro-Sutherland D, Furberg RD, et al. Using screen-based simulation to improve performance during pediatric resuscitation. Acad Emerg Med 2009; 16:S71–5.

106. Bond WF, Lammers RL, Spillane LL, et al. The use of simulation in emergency medicine: a research agenda. Acad Emerg Med 2007;14(4):353–63.

107. Schwid H, Rooke GA, Michalowski P, et al. Screen-based anesthesia simulation with debriefing improves performance in a mannequin-based anesthesia simulator. Teach Learn Med 2001;13(2):92–6.

108. Schwaab J, Kman N, Nagel R, et al. Using second life virtual simulation environment for mock oral emergency medicine examination. Acad Emerg Med 2011; 18:559–62.

109. Joshi NK, Yarris LM, Doty CI, et al. Social media responses to the Annals of Emergency Medicine residents' perspective article on multiple mini-interviews. Ann Emerg Med 2014;64(3):320–5.

110. Cadogan M, Thoma B, Chan TM, et al. Free Open Access Meducation (FOAM): the rise of emergency medicine and critical care blogs and podcasts (2002-2013). Emerg Med J 2014;31(e1):e76–7.

111. Lumba-Brown A, Tat S, Auerbach MA, et al. PEMNetwork: barriers and enablers to collaboration and multimedia education in the digital age. Pediatr Emerg Care 2016;32(8):565–9.

112. Krishnan K, Thoma B, Trueger NS, et al. Gestalt assessment of online educational resources may not be sufficiently reliable and consistent. Perspect Med Educ 2017;6(2):91–8.

113. Lin M, Joshi N, Grock A, et al. Approved instructional resources series: a national initiative to identify quality emergency medicine blog and podcast content for resident education. J Grad Med Educ 2016;8(2):219–25.

The Impact of the Evolving Health Care System on Pediatric Emergency Care

Lalit Bajaj, MD, MPH

KEYWORDS

- Pediatric emergency medicine • Health care reform • Value-based care
- Affordable Care Act • High-deductible health plans • Accountable care organizations

KEY POINTS

- The changing payment landscape in the US will impact the Pediatric Emergency Department in a variety of ways.
- Expansion of Medicaid in some states may increase PED volume; while high deductible plans may decrease PED volume or cause delays in seeking care.
- Accountable care organizations are being developed in order to shift care out of costly PEDs and into the primary care medical home.

INTRODUCTION

Cases

A 7-year-old boy is brought to the emergency department (ED) for abdominal pain. He developed periumbilical abdominal pain a few hours after eating at a local restaurant. He then developed nonbilious vomiting and nonbloody diarrhea. The family is very concerned about appendicitis, and you feel reassured that the patient is very unlikely to have a surgical condition. The family is uncomfortable with leaving without further testing and imaging. You discuss the case with the primary care provider over the telephone, and he speaks to the family. They continue to insist, and he asks you to perform the laboratory tests and ultrasound. You tell him that the hospital is now tracking the use of imaging in patients with a low pediatric appendicitis score, and if his rate is too high, he will not be eligible for a bonus.

A 4-year-old girl is brought to the ED for difficulty breathing with the onset of an upper respiratory infection. She is treated according to the asthma care pathway at your institution and is improving. You notice she has had multiple ED visits and admissions over the past year, and that she is not using a controller medicine as prescribed by her primary care provider. You feel she could benefit from an inpatient admission for

Disclosure: The author has no commercial or financial conflicts of interests to disclose.
Clinical Effectiveness, University of Colorado School of Medicine, Children's Hospital Colorado, 13123 East 16th Avenue B400, Aurora, CO 80045, USA
E-mail address: Lalit.bajaj@childrenscolorado.org

Pediatr Clin N Am 65 (2018) 1247–1256
https://doi.org/10.1016/j.pcl.2018.07.007
pediatric.theclinics.com

asthma education. You discuss your concerns with the primary care provider, who asks you to discharge the patient and he will see the child in clinic tomorrow. He mentions that the insurance company is looking at his rate of admission for ambulatory-sensitive conditions and he does not want to get scrutinized over this case.

A 10-year-old boy is brought to the ED for fever and worsening leg pain over his right distal lower leg. You are concerned that he may have osteomyelitis and recommend that the patient get laboratory tests and an MRI. The father asks you how much all of this will cost, because he has a high deductible plan, and he will pay out of pocket until he reaches $6750.

BACKGROUND

Health care reform efforts have taken a more prominent role in US society over the past decade. Even before the Affordable Care Act (ACA), efforts were underway to decrease rising health care costs. Much of the early efforts focused on high-cost adult care, including reducing readmissions to the hospital for a variety of conditions, adherence to established quality metrics, and building accountable care organizations (ACOs) to integrate care across the care continuum. Efforts to implement similar structures and care measurement strategies have lagged behind in pediatrics but are beginning to become more important as payers, including Medicaid, are developing alternative payment models. Commercial payers, which have increasingly moved their products to high deductible plans and narrow network plans, have become more interested in partnering with providers and hospitals on programs that incent quality and lower cost. The term "value-based care" refers to high-quality care at the lowest cost to maintain excellent outcomes or demonstrate improved quality of care. The relevance to the pediatric emergency department (PED) becomes more evident as many of the incentives to providers and patients coalesce around decreasing the use of costly laboratory and radiology tests, decreasing hospital admissions, and revisits and readmissions to the hospital. These types of initiatives can be a difficult place for hospitals to focus when they are primarily reimbursed by a fee-for-service (FFS) payment mechanism that makes it financial rewarding to deliver high-cost care and admit patients to the hospital.

This article begins with a brief discussion on the comparison of health care cost and quality of care delivered in the United States as compared with other developed nations. This article looks at how several of these developments in the health care market are impacting the PED, including ACA Medicaid expansion, high deductible plans, and the creation of ACOs and new payment mechanisms. This article concludes with thoughts on how PEDs should align their efforts with the local efforts to create ACOs and integrated networks.

HEALTH CARE COSTS AND THE QUALITY OF CARE

Rising health care costs and how best to address these issues have become huge issues of debate at every level of government and in much of the private sector. The United States has consistently grown the percentage of the US Gross Domestic Product it spends on health care to almost 17%, double the average of comparison developed countries. Much of this increase has been blamed on the perpetuation of the FFS payment mechanism, and has equated to a spending of more than $9000 per person per year in the United States (**Fig. 1**). Recent reports estimate that the out-of-pocket percentage has also grown to almost 12% of the total individual health care spending.[1] The cost of children is approximately 8.4% of the total spending, which is about $800 per child in the United States. This amount is higher for commercially insured patients than for governmental insured patients and is concentrated in the

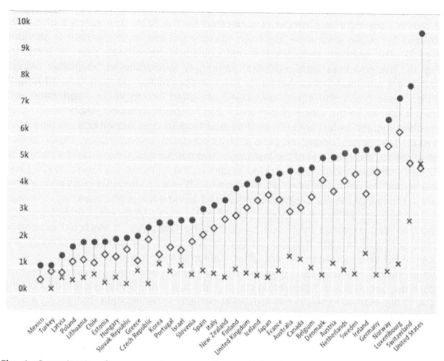

Fig. 1. Organization for economic cooperation and development cost comparisons. (*Data from* OECD (2018), Health spending (indicator). Available at: https://data.oecd.org/healthres/health-spending.htm. Accessed July 20, 2018. https://doi.org/10.1787/8643de7e-en.)

early years of life. It is estimated that the United States spends $70 billion in pediatric inpatient care and $23 billion on pediatric emergency care for children a year.[2] The percentage of children who have governmental insurance (primarily Medicaid) has also been steadily growing and then increased dramatically with the ACA. The costly care that is delivered in the United States is unfortunately not tied to better health outcomes. The United States ranks 26th among developed nations in life expectancy, and 29th in infant mortality.[3] In addition, higher physician spending per patient does not correlate with improved patient outcomes.[4]

THE IMPACT ON THE PEDIATRIC EMERGENCY DEPARTMENT

The ED has long been looked at as an expensive place to receive care, especially when this care is not deemed "emergent." The PED evolved as a subspecialty to address the unique needs of sick and injured children, and in many areas, especially urban areas, has become an expected resource. In areas with a high percentage of Medicaid-covered children, there is often a lack of accessible primary care for sick visits, so much of this volume comes to the local PED. It has been shown that children with public insurance have much higher rates of ED utilization that those with private insurance, especially for low acuity issues.[5]

THE AFFORDABLE CARE ACT AND THE IMPACT ON PEDIATRIC EMERGENCY DEPARTMENT VISITS

The ACA, passed in 2010, dramatically reduced the number of uninsured in the United States from 49 million to 29 million through Medicaid expansion and the development of health care insurance products supported by the ACA. The percent of people covered by public insurance has been steadily growing over the past 2 decades (**Fig. 2**). The greatest reductions in the uninsured have been seen in the poor (**Fig. 3**). The new insurance products, commonly referred to as "exchange plans," as they are purchased in exchange for subsided premiums, result in more affordable plans. These plans and others developed are often limited in coverage, especially when it comes to the range of providers and hospitals included. Many large PEDs are often located in tertiary care centers that tend to cost more because they have to fund many poorly funded missions such as education and advocacy. These centers are at risk for being left out of the less expensive narrow network plans. The impact on ED visits has been looked at, and the results of the analyses are mixed. Nikpay and colleagues[6] recently published an analysis of ED use in Medicaid expansion states versus those that did not expand Medicaid and found expansion states had increases of 2.5/1000 population over those that did not expand Medicaid. Barakat and colleagues[7] also explored this issue by comparing California, a Medicaid expansion state, to Florida, a state that did not expand Medicaid, and found that although the rates of ED visit increases did not differ, California saw a decrease in self-pay visits and an increase in Medicaid covered visits. Analyses performed on Maryland and Illinois data, both Medicaid expansion states, did show that ED visits increased after the ACA.[8,9] No studies have directly looked at pediatric-specific data, but young adults, aged 19 to 25, did have a reduction in ED visits after ACA in an analysis of data from the Health Cost and Utilization Project.[10] There have been studies demonstrating that well child visits have increased after ACA, but there are still significant ethnic disparities that have seen such improvements. Ortega and colleagues[11] published in

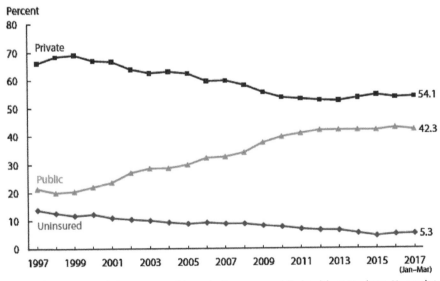

Fig. 2. The percent of those covered by private versus public health care plans. Note: data are based on household interviews of a sample of the civilian noninstitutionalized population. (*From* Cohen RA, Zammitti EP, Martinez ME, et al. Health coverage early release of estimates from the National Health Interview Survey, January – March 2017. CDC: National Health Interview Survey. Available at: https://www.cdc.gov/nchs/data/nhis/earlyrelease/insur201708.pdf. Accessed December 1, 2017; and NCHS, National Health Interview Survey, 1997-2017, Family Core component.)

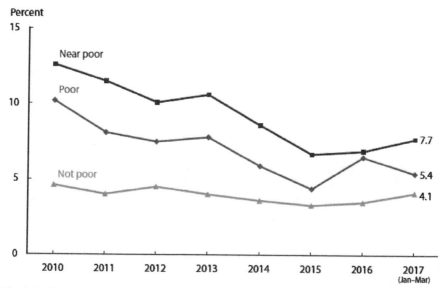

Fig. 3. Reductions in the percent uninsured by socioeconomic status. Note: data are based on household interviews of a sample of the civilian noninstitutionalized population. (*From* Cohen RA, Zammitti EP, Martinez ME, et al. Health coverage early release of estimates from the National Health Interview Survey, January – March 2017. CDC: National Health Interview Survey. Available at: https://www.cdc.gov/nchs/data/nhis/earlyrelease/insur201708.pdf. Accessed December 1, 2017; and NCHS, National Health Interview Survey, 2010–2017, Family Core component.)

2017 a study of data from the 2011 to 2015 National Health Interview Survey, that Latino youth had the largest absolute gain in insurance coverage, but they continued to have the largest proportion of uninsured children after ACA implementation. It appears that changes in pediatric ED volume with greater coverage are dependent on many factors, including location, race/ethnicity, and likely access to primary care in their communities. Ongoing research into how the impacts of insurance expansion will certainly shed more evidence on how pediatric EDs will be impacted.

HIGH DEDUCTIBLE HEALTH PLANS

The rising costs of health care have resulted in increasingly high health care premiums from employers, that are passed on to the patients and families. Health insurers that offer high deductible health plans (HDHPs) have become more popular and are often mandated by employers. These plans will offer less expensive premiums in exchange for a deductible. The Internal Revenue Service sets the minimum and maximum deductible amounts. For 2018, a family's minimum is $2700 and maximum is $13,300.[12] The purchaser of the plan is therefore responsible for the amount spent on health care up to the deductible amount before getting any payment from the insurer. Most recent data from Quarter 1 of 2017 show that 42.3% of those with private health insurance are enrolled in an HDHP, up from 25.3% in 2010.[13] (**Fig. 4**) Many of the HDHPs will offer preventative visits that are not included in the deductible, but they are not mandated to provide that coverage.

In 2007, the American Academy of Pediatrics published a comment from the Committee on Child Financing, that warned that these programs may incent families to

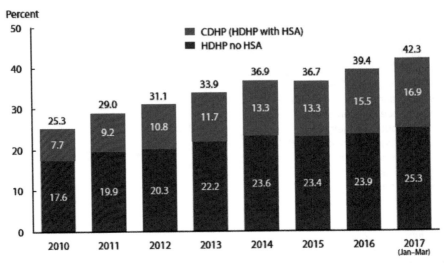

Fig. 4. Increase in percent of people covered by HDHPs. Notes: CDHP is consumer-directed health plan, which is an HDHP with a health savings account (HSA). HDHP no HSA is a high-deductible health plan without an HSA. The individual components of HDHPs may not add to total due to rounding. Data are based on household interviews of a sample of the civilian noninstitutionalized population. (*From* Cohen RA, Zammitti EP, Martinez ME, et al. Health coverage early release of estimates from the National Health Interview Survey, January – March 2017. CDC: National Health Interview Survey. Available at: https://www.cdc.gov/nchs/data/nhis/earlyrelease/insur201708.pdf. Accessed December 1, 2017; and NCHS, National Health Interview Survey, 2010–2017, Family Core component.)

delay or avoid seeking care, especially if the preventative services are not exempted from the deductible.[14] In 2011, Wharam and colleagues[15] published a large study looking at the impact of ED visits on patients mandated to use an HDHP, and they found sustained reductions in ED visits especially in nonemergent, and intermediate-severity visits, but no reductions in emergent visits was seen. Hospitalization rates decreased in the first follow-up year, but hospitalizations and cost reductions were not seen by the second follow-up year. The investigators caution that the effect of deferred utilization is still not well understood. Kozhimannil and colleagues[16] published in 2013 a study of members in the Harvard Pilgrim Health Care system that had moved to an HDHP and found that ED visits for adult men of any severity went down, including a decrease of 34% in high severity cases. Women selectively lowered ED visits for low severity cases, but not high severity visits. In men, hospitalizations decreased in the first year (24%) and were followed by a sharp increase (30%) in year 2. Women showed a similar, but not as drastic a pattern.

Consumer analysis has also demonstrated that patients are increasingly considering price in their decision to choose health care services, and that they are talking to providers about it; up to 30% report putting off services until they can afford it.[17] Concerns that patients of lower socioeconomic status will be adversely impacted by HDHPs come from 2 perspectives. Galbraith and colleagues[18] reported that patients in low-income neighborhoods were more likely to be switched to HDHPs than those in higher-income neighborhoods. In addition, Wharam and colleagues[19] published in 2013 that after switching to an HDHP, patients in low socioeconomic categories decreased all types of severity ED visits, but high economic status patients did not decrease high severity visits. In addition, the low socioeconomic patients with HDHPs demonstrated a sharp increase in hospitalizations in year 2. In aggregate, the evidence points toward a delay in care that is more detrimental in patients of low socioeconomic status from the incorporation of HDHPs.

Specific impacts of HDHP on pediatric care are not well studied. Galbraith and colleagues[20] published in 2010 that HDCP members did not have significant reductions in well child visits as compared with controls, although this HDHP did not include preventative care in the deductible and had similar co-pays to the control group. When the evidence is taken as a whole, it does appear that the risks that the AAP was concerned about in their 2007 statement have been substantiated in the research. Although there are initial decreases in high-cost care in low acuity ED visits, the resultant delays in seeking care do seem to result in more costly care in the long term. Although research on the impact of HDHPs on pediatric ED care still needs to be done, it is safe to say that the conversations around how the visit will impact the family's out-of-pocket expense will continue to grow.

PAYMENT REFORM AND ACCOUNTABLE CARE

Chamberlain and colleagues[21] described a series of issues that impact pediatric emergency care in the United States in 2013. They pointed out that most children are not seen in PEDs, that quality of care is quite variable, that incentives reward high-cost care, and that there are significant barriers to access to primary care in the underinsured. In addition, they mention that overcrowding of EDs and lack of performance metrics are significant issues that need to be addressed. The development of pediatric ACOs is an attempt to address many of these challenges and has lagged behind that of the creation of adult-based ACOs. In conjunction with the ACA, incentives were created for community care practices and hospitals to form partnerships and work together with both commercial and governmental (Medicaid) payers. In these partnerships, many alternative payment models have been created to incent lower cost, improved health, and improve patient experience. The goal of the ACO is to address the value of the care delivered and has prompted the creation and testing of alternate payment mechanisms that diverge from the traditional FFS models. After the failed trial of managed care in the late 1980s/early 1990s, most health care payments reverted to the FFS model, whereby payments were based on negotiated reimbursements based on charges developed by the provider entities. This activity-based reimbursement is often blamed for the sharp spike seen in health care spending, and for the poor outcomes associated with care for the "ill," as opposed to investing in care to keep patients well.

Primary care providers within, and not within, ACOs in pediatrics are increasing being asked to participate in alternate payment strategies such as "Pay for Performance" programs, which have become more popular, as have programs that provide upfront increases in per member per month payments to add provider resources to better manage complex patients, and keep patients out of costly EDs and avoid unnecessary hospitalizations. The programs often come with a potential of "shared savings," where any lowering of high-cost care from the program can be shared with the members of the ACO. Many suggest that these payment mechanisms signify the progression to increasingly placing the financial accountability onto the providers to keep costs low (**Fig. 5**). In addition, the ACOs need to create measurement systems and quality programs in order to demonstrate and incent best practice, as well as monitor their cost of care.

The evidence on whether these new payment models result in improvements in pediatric ED care, ED visits, and hospitalizations is sparse. One study of Blue

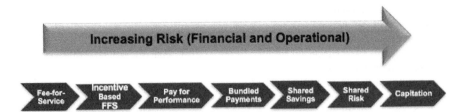

Fig. 5. Continuum of payment strategies.

Cross/Blue Shield in Massachusetts showed improvements in well child metrics tied to a P4P program. ED visits for asthma did decrease, but this metric was not tied to the program. In addition, the overall spending on the population did not decrease.[22] A recent study has looked at pediatric ACOs at different stages of development and characterized various themes. All sites identified the need for capital to support the clinical transformation of the practices, and most found the capital from hospitals. They all recognized that mental health costs need to be addressed in the development of these organizations, that costs of measurement and quality reporting are high, and that the relevant data are often difficult to find. Last, they all report that they are making large investments in care management to decrease ED utilization.[23] Scrutiny from payers and the ability to create meaningful contracts with them often means that the potential savings that the system can earn is judged on the "total cost of care." If there is no reduction in the overall "total cost of care," then the ACO is not eligible for any savings it may have achieved in reaching agreed upon quality measures.

These forces have placed the PED in a challenging position. If a system's PED is not part of an ACO or is excluded from the contract as part of a "narrow network," it can be adversely impacted. Many institutions rely on the ED to be a profit center for the system, because they are the point of entry of many admissions, perform reimbursable procedures, are trauma centers, and provide 24-hour access to all patients, including sick subspecialty patients. The efforts to reduce ED visits, reduce hospitalizations, and shift care to less expensive places such as urgent cares, and primary provider offices are forcing the EDs to look at operational efficiencies as well as clinical effectiveness improvements that increase the value of the care delivered.

QUALITY IMPROVEMENT INTERVENTIONS AND THE PEDIATRIC EMERGENCY DEPARTMENT

The PED has been on the forefront of quality improvement interventions for many years. In a review published in 2013, Macias[24] described the evolution of quality improvement in PEDs and the incorporation of these principles into improving efficiencies, decreasing variation in care, decreasing cost, and improving the outcomes for the patients.[24] The methods of LEAN and Six Sigma as well as the Model for Improvement from the Institute of Healthcare Improvement have been successfully applied in the pediatric ED to reduce utilization of high-cost care as well as to reduce admissions. It is beyond the scope of this article to go through all of the work that has been accomplished in this area. One issue that is important to mention is the power of the quality improvement collaborative programs to improve the quality of care delivered on a large scale through the use of shared improvement tools, and sharing of outcome data to identify best practices and promote rapid dissemination and implementation.[25,26] In order for these efforts to be sustainable, it will be important for these costly programs to be aligned with the financial incentives that are evolving. When the goals of the system promote the appropriate use of the ED, and the reimbursement strategies reward the efforts of the ED, then the incentive to partner with community health efforts to keep children healthy and out of the ED will flourish.

SUMMARY

The health care landscape is going through a transition from "ill" care to a value-based care system primarily in response to rising health care high costs and poor outcomes. Forces that are changing the pediatric ED include expansion of Medicaid and increasing insurance coverage, which may increase PED volumes. The increase in patient out-of-pocket financial responsibility will likely decrease some discretionary ED use, but may delay needed care and adversely impact outcomes, especially in low-income groups. The growing partnerships between community practices and hospitals will incent alignment of rewards, but may also restrict access to some high-cost centers in order to meet financial targets. It will be important that quality improvement initiatives in the PED be aligned with the overall goals of the system in order to be sustainable.

REFERENCES

1. Global Burden of Disease Health Financing Collaborator Network. Evolution and patterns of global health financing 1995-2014: development assistance for health, and government, prepaid private, and out-of-pocket health spending in 184 countries. Lancet 2017;389(10083):1981–2004.
2. Bui AL, Dieleman JL, Hamavid H, et al. Spending on children's personal health care in the United States, 1996-2013. JAMA Pediatr 2017;171(2):181–9.
3. Foundation UH. America's Health Rankings. 2016. Available at: https://www.americashealthrankings.org/learn/reports/2016-annual-report/comparison-with-other-nations. Accessed December 1, 2017.
4. Tsugawa Y, Jha AK, Newhouse JP, et al. Variation in physician spending and association with patient outcomes. JAMA Intern Med 2017;177(5):675–82.
5. Schlichting LE, Rogers ML, Gjelsvik A, et al. Pediatric emergency department utilization and reliance by insurance coverage in the United States. Acad Emerg Med 2017;24(12):1483–90.
6. Nikpay S, Freedman S, Levy H, et al. Effect of the affordable care act medicaid expansion on emergency department visits: evidence from state-level emergency department databases. Ann Emerg Med 2017;70(2):215–25.e6.
7. Barakat MT, Mithal A, Huang RJ, et al. Affordable care act and healthcare delivery: a comparison of California and Florida hospitals and emergency departments. PLoS One 2017;12(8):e0182346.
8. Feinglass J, Cooper AJ, Rydland K, et al. Emergency department use across 88 small areas after affordable care act implementation in Illinois. West J Emerg Med 2017;18(5):811–20.
9. Klein EY, Levin S, Toerper MF, et al. The effect of medicaid expansion on utilization in Maryland emergency departments. Ann Emerg Med 2017;70(5):607–14.e6.
10. Hernandez-Boussard T, Morrison D, Goldstein BA, et al. Relationship of affordable care act implementation to emergency department utilization among young adults. Ann Emerg Med 2016;67(6):714–20.e1.

11. Ortega AN, McKenna RM, Chen J, et al. Insurance coverage and well-child visits improved for youth under the affordable care act, but latino youth still lag behind. Acad Pediatr 2018;18(1):35–42.

12. Gisonny R, LB. IRS Announces 2018 limits for HSAs and HDHPs. 2017. Available at: https://www.towerswatson.com/en-US/Insights/Newsletters/Americas/insider/2017/05/irs-announces-2018-limits-for-hsas-and-hdhps. Accessed December 1, 2017.

13. Cohen RA, MM, Zammitti EP. Health insurance coverage: early release of estimates from the national health interview survey, January–March 2017. Available at: https://www.cdc.gov/nchs/data/nhis/earlyrelease/insur201708.pdf. Accessed December 1, 2017.

14. Johnson AD, Wegner SE. High-deductible health plans and the new risks of consumer-driven health insurance products. Pediatrics 2007;119(3):622–6.

15. Wharam JF, Landon BE, Zhang F, et al. High-deductible insurance: two-year emergency department and hospital use. Am J Manag Care 2011;17(10):e410–8.

16. Kozhimannil KB, Law MR, Blauer-Peterson C, et al. The impact of high-deductible health plans on men and women: an analysis of emergency department care. Med Care 2013;51(8):639–45.

17. Kullgren JT, Cliff EQ, Krenz C, et al. Consumer behaviors among individuals enrolled in high-deductible health plans in the United States. JAMA Intern Med 2017;178(3):424–6.

18. Galbraith AA, Ross-Degnan D, Soumerai SB, et al. High-deductible health plans: are vulnerable families enrolled? Pediatrics 2009;123(4):e589–94.

19. Wharam JF, Zhang F, Landon BE, et al. Low-socioeconomic-status enrollees in high-deductible plans reduced high-severity emergency care. Health Aff (Millwood) 2013;32(8):1398–406.

20. Galbraith AA, Ross-Degnan D, Soumerai SB, et al. Use of well-child visits in high-deductible health plans. Am J Manag Care 2010;16(11):833–40.

21. Chamberlain JM, Krug S, Shaw KN. Emergency care for children in the United States. Health Aff (Millwood) 2013;32(12):2109–15.

22. Chien AT, Song Z, Chernew ME, et al. Two-year impact of the alternative quality contract on pediatric health care quality and spending. Pediatrics 2014;133(1):96–104.

23. Perrin JM, Zimmerman E, Hertz A, et al. Pediatric accountable care organizations: insight from early adopters. Pediatrics 2017;139(2) [pii:e20161840].

24. Macias CG. Quality improvement in pediatric emergency medicine. Acad Pediatr 2013;13(6 Suppl):S61–8.

25. Lannon CM, Peterson LE. Pediatric collaborative networks for quality improvement and research. Acad Pediatr 2013;13(6 Suppl):S69–74.

26. Parikh K, Biondi E, Nazif J, et al. A multicenter collaborative to improve care of community acquired pneumonia in hospitalized children. Pediatrics 2017;139(3) [pii:e20161411].

Pediatric Urgent Care—New and Evolving Paradigms of Acute Care

Usha Sankrithi, MBBS, MPH, MD[a],*, Jeffrey Schor, MD, MPH, MBA[b]

KEYWORDS

- Pediatrics • Urgent care • Acute care • Emergency medicine • Clinics
- Medical home

KEY POINTS

- Parents of pediatric patients seek and value appropriate high-quality care that is timely, convenient, and cost effective.
- Pediatric urgent care offers new and evolving paradigms that serve the growing demand and complement services provided by the medical home and by pediatric emergency departments.
- The clinical spectrum is variable but mimics the more frequent presentations of acute pediatric injuries and illnesses that present to the pediatric emergency department.
- Categories of pediatric urgent care services in the nonprofit and for-profit sectors include hospital and satellite clinics, free-standing clinics, retail-based clinics, and telemedicine services.
- Research and the development of results-based training and standards are warranted.

INTRODUCTION

The delivery of acute care in the United States is evolving rapidly.[1–3] For the better part of the last half of the twentieth century, sick or injured patients had 2 choices—they could make an appointment with their primary care provider or they could visit an emergency department (ED) for immediate evaluation. The explosion of alternative delivery models over the past 2 decades has created other options. This article discusses these alternative models, focusing on the development of urgent care in the United States, especially pediatric-specific urgent care.

Disclosure Statement: U. Sankrithi—None; J. Schor—financial interest in PM Pediatrics, a private pediatric urgent care company.
[a] Urgent Care Services, Division of Emergency Medicine, Seattle Children's Hospital, MB.7.520, 4800 Sand Point Way, Northeast, Seattle, WA 98105, USA; [b] PM Pediatrics Management Group, One Hollow Lane, Suite 301, Lake Success, NY 11042, USA
* Corresponding author. 11914 Maplewood Avenue, Edmonds, WA 98026.
E-mail address: usha.sankrithi@gmail.com

THE EVOLUTION OF ACUTE CARE IN THE UNITED STATES

Emergency care, defined by distinct areas in a hospital staffed by designated providers, has evolved since its inception in the 1960s. EDs no longer just care for the critically ill or injured but also routinely evaluate those whose illnesses or injuries can be managed in a non-ED setting. Alternative delivery models began to develop in the 1980s, driven by needs for improved resource utilization as well as entrepreneurial innovation. Hospitals established lower-acuity areas within the ED, called fast tracks, which were designed to decompress the main ED. Simultaneously, freestanding urgent care centers (UCCs) began opening their doors, typically led by physicians seeking innovative practice opportunities.[4,5] The current model eventually emerged, offering services that vary widely but typically fall between a primary care office and an ED. Most general UCCs open and close early and most have weekend and holiday hours. Typically, UCCs have expanded capabilities, such as on-site laboratories and x-ray, wound management, and extended treatments. Staffing varies by size and scope, with most using physicians and advanced practitioners. Since 2000, there has been a steady increase in the number of UCCs, with an estimated 7000 to 10,000 locations today.[6–8] This number is difficult to quantify because there remains a lack of standardization in states' regulation of UCCs, and many states characterize UCCs as simply a physician office with extended hours.[9] Yearly volumes per location can be up to 50,000.[10]

The past 25 years have also seen continued evolution of other delivery models that focus on convenience and an improved experience. Retail-based clinics (RBCs) began providing care in 2001 and currently have approximately 2000 locations and more than 10,000,000 visits annually.[11] Like UCCs, RBCs offer walk-in care with extended evening and weekend hours. Generally located in pharmacies, big-box retail stores, or supermarkets, their emphasis is on treating a limited number of low-complexity acute conditions as well as providing select preventive health care services, such as vaccinations. Typically, the providers are advanced practitioners. There is some evidence that the growth of this type of care is slowing.[12–15] Similarly, the scope is changing to one involving partnership with larger health care institutions[12,16] and a more dedicated approach to wellness.[17]

Free-standing EDs (FSEDs) have also proliferated in many parts of the country. Initially a way to provide access to rural communities that could not sustain a full-service hospital, FSEDs now number more than 500 nationally and are often located in the same areas where RBCs and urgent care have proliferated.[18] At a minimum, FSEDs provide 24/7 access to emergency physicians and nurses, higher-level laboratories, advanced imaging (eg, ultrasound and CT), and care for most emergent illnesses. Although generally run well, there has been concern expressed about their high charges relative to the services provided.[19–23]

While these models proliferated, entities dedicated to providing acute care services for children have been a more recent phenomenon. Pediatric urgent care (PUC) offers a new and evolving paradigm of service that complements traditional models of acute care and are discussed.

WHY HAVE ALTERNATIVE MODELS PROLIFERATED?

Two important factors have converged to drive these changes in acute care delivery, especially urgent care[11,24–28]:

- Consumer demand for a more efficient and comprehensive system: this mirrors the growth of retail sectors, such as 24-hour grocery stores, fast-food restaurants,

fast package delivery for online orders, and immediate smartphone-leveraging communications, including information, social media, and entertainment.
- Generational expectations that health services will be as responsive and accessible as other service industries

In a recent poll conducted by National Public Radio, the Robert Wood Johnson Foundation, and the Harvard T.H. Chan School of Public Health,[10] most people reported going to urgent care because they believe it is more convenient and takes less time than going to see their regular doctor. This is also true in pediatrics.[29,30] Garbutt and colleagues[30] found that approximately 23% of approximately 1500 parents surveyed while in the waiting rooms of 19 primary care pediatrics practices had used an RBC in the past year for their child's care and approximately 50% of those had multiple visits. The primary reason was convenience (37%), even though their primary care practices were open for approximately half of the visits. Other reasons were lack of appointment availability (25%), not wanting to bother a pediatrician after hours (15%), or believing the problem was not serious enough to bother the pediatrician (13%).

Other factors stimulating growth of alternative models include the following:

- Personal health care costs have increased as patients are increasingly responsible for a larger portion of their health care expenses. For urgent but not life-threatening situations, UCCs and RBCs are far less expensive per visit than FSEDs and EDs.[31–33] A study by CVS Health in 2013[34] also showed lower annual cost of care for patients who used RBCs, primarily because people received treatment of issues before they became costlier chronic conditions.
- Hospitals are embracing the concept of alternative delivery models and choosing to develop them on their own and/or partner with (or purchase) existing providers.[35–40] Not only does this expand awareness and reach but also it will become increasingly important as value-based payments that levy financial penalties for costly and unnecessary ED visits or hospitalizations increase.[41]
- Many insurers see UCCs as attractive for a variety of reasons, in particular the potential to save on costs by directing patients to the right setting. Several plans have made significant investments or purchases of exiting UCCs (Optum/United, BlueCross BlueShield of South Carolina, BlueCross BlueShield of North Carolina, and others) have stated their intention to proceed on similar lines.[42]
- Billions of dollars in investment money have poured into the development of alternative delivery models, especially urgent care.

Use of alternative delivery models has become commonplace and most RBC users report being satisfied with their care.[43] This is true in the pediatric populations as well.[29,30] More recent evidence has speculated, however, that RBCs may not decrease health spending or decrease ED utilization.[30] Similarly, although the cost of care per episode may be lower, there remains concern (especially among insurers) that ease of use and convenience lead to higher overall costs by increasing utilization.

CARE OF PEDIATRIC PATIENTS IN GENERAL RETAIL-BASED CLINICS AND URGENT CARE CENTERS

Approximately 28% of urgent care patients are less than 21 years old.[44,45] Although RBCs often restrict patients to 2 years and above, general UCCs typically do not. Most general UCCs do not have providers who are specifically trained in pediatrics although many use emergency medicine–trained physicians. The American Academy of Pediatrics (AAP) has released several statements regarding the provision of care to pediatric patients in these settings. In 2006, the AAP published a policy statement opposing RBCs as an appropriate source of medical care for infants, children, and adolescents and strongly discouraged their use.[46,47] Policy development after 2010 recognized that use of these facilities had increased significantly, and a 2014 policy statement on retail-based clinics[48] presents a few key points:

- RBCs are an inappropriate source of primary care for pediatric patients.
- Pediatricians need to improve convenience for their patients.
- Pediatricians should work with RBCs to ensure appropriate care and follow-up.
- Insurers should not give patients incentives like lower copays to utilize RBCs instead of their own primary care providers.

Also in 2014, the AAP released a policy statement on freestanding urgent care facilities,[7] in which they recognized that many children were being treated there and recommended that

- Freestanding UCCs can enhance the provision of urgent care services to children, be integrated into the medical community, and provide a safe and effective adjunct to the medical home.
- Staff should be trained in pediatrics, have pediatric guidelines, and be equipped and prepared for pediatric emergencies.
- The UCC must complement and support the medical home.

The policy also noted that there are few data on PUC and recommended that research should be a focus in the future.

In 2017, the AAP revisited these statements in a policy entitled, "Nonemergency Acute Care: When It's Not the Medical Home,"[49–51] suggesting that alternative acute care services can meet the needs of parents and patients while also being synergistic and complementary to the medical home. The policy noted that treatment of children in these settings should adhere to the "core principles of care and communication, best practices within a defined scope of services, pediatric-trained staff, safe transitions of care, and continuous improvement." It also strongly recommended that communication is needed from acute care entities back to the medical home to ensure continuity of care. Finally, the policy explicitly recommended that acute care providers that lack pediatric expertise should not provide care to children younger than 2 years in view of "the variability of presentation, difficulties in assessment of symptoms and often unpredictable response to treatment."

EVOLUTION OF PEDIATRIC URGENT CARE MODELS

The concept of urgent care services provided by pediatric-trained providers to pediatric patients has been around since the 1980s but it has only recently started to proliferate. Like other general EDs, many children's hospitals adopted the use of fast-track areas adjacent to their EDs beginning in the 1980s. A few (eg, Denver, Colorado, and Cincinnati, Ohio) also began adding freestanding UCCs. Beginning in the late 1980s and extending into the 1990s, a few privately based PUC practices opened in Maryland (Nighttime Pediatrics), Utah (Night Light Pediatrics), and Florida (After Hours Pediatrics). Over the past 10 years, there has been a proliferation of PUCs, and today there are approximately 320 individual locations in 35 states that identify themselves as such (Schor JA, PM Pediatrics, unpublished data, 2018). Of these, only 150 are affiliated with a hospital or health system, the rest being private. As with the general urgent care market, however, the number of private hospital partnerships is increasing.

Although there is a dearth of published data, some key operational characteristics of most PUCs are well known. PUC facilities in many instances have child-appropriate equipment, on-site or off-site laboratory testing, and imaging suitable for pediatric patients. Providers and staff typically include physicians who are trained in pediatrics and/or pediatric emergency medicine as well as pediatric nurse providers, nurses with pediatric training and experience, and supporting staff.

To avoid competition with a patient's medical home, most PUCs open and close later than taking advantage of the hours when no option other than an ED is available. In a similar vein, most recognize the need for continuity and provide copies of charts and laboratory results with primary care providers and communicate on a regular basis. Also, although many UCCs provide extra services, such as occupational medicine, school physicals, and immunizations, PUCs tend to avoid these because they infringe on what is generally provided in primary care. **Figure 1**[52–54] summarizes key differences between PUCs and general UCCs.

Fig. 1[49] There is considerable variability in the size and scope of PUC locations throughout the country. There are 18 hospitals and 8 private groups that have at least 4 freestanding locations (Schor JA, PM Pediatrics, unpublished data, 2018). Personal correspondence with several hospital and private PUCs suggests that most established private PUCs see volumes between 5000 and 15,000 visits per year whereas volume ranges in established hospital-based PUCs are slightly higher on average. Volumes throughout the country seem to be increasing, suggesting increased public awareness of PUC as a unique model.

Hospitals have unique reasons for expanding PUC services and several have set up on-site and/or satellite PUCs. One of the obvious significant synergistic benefits of a PUC proximate to a pediatric ED is a reduction in low-acuity patients. There is also

How Is Pediatric Urgent Care Different?

	General Urgent Care	Pediatric Urgent Care
Typical providers	Family practice, internal medicine, some ED; PA, FNP common	Pediatricians, PEM; PNP/FNP, PA common
Hours	Open and close earlier (most are 9:00 AM–9:00 PM)	Some open early but most open at noon or later and close later
Relationship with PCP	Competitive; often offer services that overlap (eg, immunizations, physicals)	A few that are competitive but most with emphasis on continuity
Scope of care	Variable; occupational medicine, workers' comp and primary care common	Range from extension of practice to ED-like; some offer primary care

Fig. 1. Differences between PUC and general urgent care. FNP, family nurse practitioner; PA, physician assistant; PCP, primary care provider; PEN, pediatric emergency nurse; PNP, pediatric nurse practitioner.

evidence that private freestanding PUCs have an impact on low-acuity ED volume (Northwell Health System, personal communication).

CLINICAL SCOPE

There is significant variability in level of acuity that can be seen among different PUCs although most claim to provide services similar to many of those seen in the ED. Almost all PUCs offer radiographs and basic laboratory tests (eg, complete blood cell counts, chemistries, urinalysis, and point-of-care testing for common infections, such as strep throat, influenza, respiratory syncytial virus infection, and infectious mononucleosis). Many offer intravenous (IV) hydration and IV medication, if necessary, and most offer extended treatments (eg, respiratory treatments).

The overall capabilities are dependent on several factors, including

- Skill level and comfort of providers
- Equipment
- Ancillary staffing
- Availability of radiograph over reads
- Availability of subspecialty care (eg, plastic surgeons, orthopedic surgeons)

OPERATIONAL CONSIDERATIONS
Benchmarking

Given that the scope of clinical care in a PUC is not unlike that given in an ED, many of the quality-of-care metrics tracked are similar. Many PEDs are also now place an emphasis on patient experience and the delivery of quality clinical care, for reasons discussed previously. In a PUC location, these concerns are paramount. As a result, tracking indicators like throughput, customer service, inventory management, and impact of marketing are crucial. **Box 1** includes some commonly tracked clinical and operational metrics.

Transfers

Although it is extrmely rare, critical patients sometimes present or deteriorate after arrival at PUC facilities with varying levels of ability to address higher-acuity conditions. In cases that exceed a particular PUC's capabilities, 911 is activated. Transfer preferences vary based on the PUC (eg, some institution-affiliated PUCs have their own transport teams and some transport teams are willing to come to private PUCs) but a majority of children are transferred via personal vehicle. In all cases, the hospital should be notified and a receiving doctor should be aware. Other considerations include

- Transferring patients by personal vehicle with a peripheral IV in place
- Direct admissions for stable patients sent for that reason
- Expedited care for stable patients sent for advanced diagnostic capabilities

Transfer rates among different PUCs vary between 1% and 5%, according to the scope of care provided. In a recent study (Mathison DJ, Ledoux AZ, Schor J: Interfacility patient transfers to hospitals from pediatric-specialized urgent care centers. Submitted for publication.), there were 3076 (1.01%) patient transfers among the 303,750 patient visits in the study period. Among the different locations, the median transfer rate was 0.95% ±0.36% (range = 0.6% to 1.7%). Personal car transport was used for 2547 (84.5%) cases; 50% of patients were transferred for respiratory (eg, status asthmaticus) or abdominal/pelvic concerns (eg, appendicitis and ovarian torsion) and 791 (25.7%) of transfers resulted in hospital admission, including 95 (3.1%) and 123 (4.0%) requiring ICU or operative care, respectively.

Box 1
Commonly tracked clinical and operational metrics

Patient visits

Actual vs projected

Hourly

Injury vs illness

New vs existing

Geographic distribution

Throughput

Time to registration

Time to room

Time to provider

Total length of stay

Customer service

Net promoter score

Specific complaints

Financial

Payor mix

Reimbursement per visit

Clinical

Transfers
   Rates/visits
   Mode of transfer
   Receiving hospital
   Disposition
   Organ system

Interesting cases

Radiograph utilization
   Monthly
   Fracture rates
   Body site
   Discrepancy with over read

Laboratory utilization
   Rapid strep test usage/yields
   Usage per test
   Treatment of positive test (eg, flu)

Procedural care
   Lacerations
   Other

See Ward and Canares[55–58] for an excellent detailed discussion of pediatric transfers from UCCs.

ACADEMICS IN PEDIATRIC URGENT CARE
Education and Training

The levels of education and training necessary in a PUC depend on the scope of care provided; on whether the PUC has an academic affiliation or is willing to devote other resources; and on statewide regulatory issues that may affect the delivery of care (eg, who is able to take radiograph and who can give medications). Examples of education and training include

- Pediatric advanced life support, advanced pediatric life support, and other nationally recognized courses
- Regular lectures
- Procedure workshops (eg, splinting, wound management, abscess drainage, and IV placement)
- X-ray or laboratory techniques

Most hospital-affiliated and some private PUCs have external students or trainees training within their environments. These include students in various disciplines (eg, medical and nursing) and residents (typically pediatric). The logistics of supervising in this environment is similar to those in EDs.

Depending on the scope of care offered, many PUCs have recognized that the standard residency training offered by most pediatric programs is not sufficient for a PUC environment. Specifically, there is a lack of experience with many procedures and a lack of comfort with providing higher-acuity care. As such, both hospital-affiliated and private PUCs have begun offering 1-year, nonaccredited fellowships in PUC.

Research

There is a dearth of published research on PUC. Fortunately, there is a significant amount of information available and many individuals and organizations that have begun to mine these data. Examples of areas currently under investigation include

- Benchmark and other descriptive data
- Quality indicators
- Impact of PUC on ED utilization
- Opportunity to replicate many ED clinical studies in community setting (eg, trauma data)
- Outcome comparisons between PUC and other delivery models
- Efficacy and cost comparisons
- Evaluation of innovative training programs

WHAT IS AHEAD FOR PEDIATRIC URGENT CARE?

PUC is a relatively new area of practice that continues to evolve. Although there is currently significant variation between different PUCs, standards are being developed. The Society for Pediatric Urgent Care was formed in 2014 as a forum to share challenges and issues associated with PUC as well as to develop best practices for ensuring clinical excellence and overall quality of care. In 2015, the Subcommittee on Pediatric Urgent Care was established within the Section on Emergency Medicine of the AAP. The subcommittee has been focused on creating standards and measures for PUC, developing educational guidelines for training future PUC providers, and launching advocacy efforts to educate the pediatric community about PUC. The *Journal of Urgent Care Medicine* now has a section dedicated to PUC and a distinct journal focusing on PUC. A textbook on PUC is also in process. In addition, there have been multiple well-attended national conferences on PUC held since 2014. Ultimately, expectations are that PUC will become an accredited subspecialty similar to hospital medicine.

As health care continues to evolve, there is no doubt that acute care (and PUC) will continue to evolve as well. The same forces that have driven the developments already described are still present and nascent models continue to appear. One example is telemedicine, a delivery model that is expected to grow rapidly in acceptance and usage over the next few years. Acute care telemedicine could include developing interactive video and remote diagnostic tools or peripherals, such as stethoscopes and otoscopes, equipment to store and forward diagnostic and imaging tests, and advanced data analytics (see Raskas and colleagues[59] for an in-depth discussion of telemedicine in PUC). Finally, there are several entrepreneurial ventures whose goal is to bring back the ultimate convenience—bringing the provider back to a patient's home. It is not inconceivable that in a world where an app can be used to have a car pick up in 5 minutes, the same can be done in requesting in-home medical care.

REFERENCES

1. "The State of Pediatric Urgent Care," Srikant Iyer, Society for Pediatric Urgent Care 3rd Annual Conference, Seattle, Washington, October 4–8, 2017.
2. "PM Pediatrics and the Evolving Acute Care Market," Jeffrey Schor, Society for Pediatric Urgent Care 3rd Annual Conference, Seattle, Washington, October 4–8, 2017.
3. Convenient Care: Growth and Staffing Trends in Urgent Care and Retail Medicine. Available at: https://www.amnhealthcare.com/uploadedFiles/MainSite/Content/Healthcare_Industry_Insights/Industry_Research/AMN%2015%20W001_Convenient%20Care%20Whitepaper(1).pdf. Accessed November 12, 2016.
4. Trafford A. For doctor's too, it's a surplus. US News and World Report 1982;62.
5. Goldsmith JC. The health care market: can hospitals survive? Harvard Business Review 1980;100–12.
6. Gale R. Your child is sick and the doctor's office is closed. what do you do? Washington Post 2017.
7. Committee on Pediatric Emergency Medicine. Pediatric care recommendations for freestanding urgent care facilities. Pediatrics 2014;133:950–3.
8. Hampers LC, Faries SG, Poole SR. Regional after-hours urgent care provided by a tertiary children's hospital. Pediatrics 2002;110:1117–24.
9. Fellows J. How urgent care clinics are evolving. Available at: http://www.medpagetoday.com/practicemanagement/practicemanagement/54023. Accessed October 11, 2016.
10. NPR, RWJ Foundation, Harvard TH Chan School of Public Health. Patients' Perspectives on Health Care in the United States: A Look at Seven States and the nation. Available at: https://cdn1.sph.harvard.edu/wp-content/uploads/sites/21/2016/02/Patients-Perspectives-on-Health-Care-in-the-United-States-National-Report-with-topline-Feb2016.pdf. Accessed May 10, 2016.
11. Carroll AE. The undeniable convenience and reliability of retail health clinics. Available at: http://www.nytimes.com/2016/04/13/upshot/the-undeniable-convenience-and-reliability-of-retail-health-clinics.html. Accessed April 12, 2016.
12. Schorsch K, Sweeney B. Walgreens is outsourcing its metro Chicago clinics to advocate. Chicago (IL): Modern Healthcare; 2016.
13. Duane Reade Shutters New York City Drug Store Clinics. Available at: http://wwww.jucm.com/duane-reade-shutters-new-york-city-drugstore-clinics/. Accessed January 13, 2017.
14. Raja P, Mehrotra A. The nuts and bolts of convenient care partnerships. Available at: http://catalyst.nejm.org/the-nuts-and-bolts-of-convenient-care-partnerships/. Accessed April 21, 2016.

15. Martsolf G, Fingar K, Coffey R, et al. Association between the opening of retail clinics and low-acuity emergency department visits. Ann Emerg Med 2017;69: 397–403.
16. Terlep S. CVS moves deeper into doctors' turf. Available at: https://www.wsj.com/articles/cvs-moves-deeper-into-doctors-turf-1502222169. Accessed August 8, 2017.
17. Bachrach D, Frohlich, Garcimonde A, et al. Building a culture of health: the value proposition of retail clinics. New York: Manatt Health/Robert Wood Johnson Foundation; 2015.
18. Harish N, Wiler JL, Zane R. How the freestanding emergency department boom can help patients. Available at: Catalyst.nejm.org. Accessed February 18, 2016.
19. Castellucci M. Out-of-network ER pay and charges fuel ire from docs and patients alike. Chicago (IL): Modern Healthcare; 2016. p. 14.
20. More data show freestanding ERs cost more than urgent care. Available at: http://www.jucm.com/data-show-freestanding-ers-cost-urgent-care/. Accessed July 15, 2016.
21. Freestanding ERs Criticized For Billing And Cherry Picking Wealthy Patients. Available at: http://www.jucm.com/freestanding-ers-criticized-billing-cherry-picking-wealthy-patients/. Accessed September 18, 2016.
22. Ho V, Metcalfe L, Dark C, et al. Comparing utilization and costs of care in freestanding emergency departments, hospital emergency departments, and urgent care centers. Ann Emerg Med 2017;70(6):846–57.e3.
23. Hogencamp TC, Montalbano A. The new medical neighborhood- where does pediatric urgent care fit in? Clin Pediatr Emerg Med 2017;18:4–13.
24. Ochs R. Urgent care centers booming on long Island. 2014. Available at: http://www.newsday.com/news/health/urgent-care-centers-booming-on-li-1.9425769. Accessed December 9, 2014.
25. Solomon B. Drive-thru health care: how McDonald's inspired an urgent care gold rush. New York: Forbes; 2014.
26. Neighmond P. Can't get in to see your doctor? Many patients turn to urgent care. Available at: http://www.npr.org/sections/health-shots/2016/03/07/469196691/cant-get-in-to-see-your-doctor-many-patients-turn-to-urgent-care. Accessed March 7, 2016.
27. Cunningham C. You shouldn't be afraid to use an urgent care. Available at: http://www.washingtonian.com/2016/03/16/urgent-care-is-the-surprisingly-good-answer-to-the-emergency-room-crisis-washington-dc/. Accessed March 16, 2016.
28. McCluskey PD, Luna T. Walk-in clinics force medicine to rethink. Boston (MA): Boston Globe; 2015.
29. Rohrer JE, Garrison GM, Angstman KB. Early return visits by pediatric primary care patients with otitis media: a retail nurse practitioner clinic versus standard medical office care. Qual Manag Health Care 2012;21:44–7.
30. Garbutt JM, Mandrell KM, Allen M, et al. Parents' experiences with pediatric care at retail clinics. JAMA Pediatr 2013;167:845–50.
31. Chang JE, Brundage SC, Burke GC, et al. Convenient care options in New York state: proliferation and performance of retail clinics and urgent care centers. New York: United Hospital Fund; 2015.
32. Sussman A, Dunham L, Snower K, et al. Retail clinic utilization associated with lower cost of care. Manag Care 2013;19:e148–57.
33. Mehotra A, Liu H, Adams JL, et al. Comparing costs and quality of care at retail clinics with that of other medical settings for 3 common illnesses. Ann Intern Med 2009;151:321–8.

34. Ashwood JS, Gaynor M, Setodji C, et al. Retail clinic visits for low acuity conditions increase utilization and spending. Health Aff (Millwood) 2016;35:449–55.

35. Johnson SR. Hospitals go different ways on urgent care. Chicago (IL): Modern Healthcare; 2015. p. 13.

36. Landro L. Traditional Providers Get Into The Urgent Care Game. Available at: http://www.wsj.com/articles/traditional-providers-get-into-the-urgent-care-game-1458525877. Accessed March 20, 2016.

37. Evans M. Warding Off Decline, Hospitals Invest in Outpatient Clinics. Available at: http://www.wsj.com/articles/warding-off-decline-hospitals-invest-in-outpatient-clinics-1506331804. Accessed September 25, 2017.

38. Barkholz D. HCA charging ahead with urgent care centers and freestanding ER openings. Chicago (IL): Modern Healthcare; 2017. p. 15.

39. Sweeney B. Patients are flocking to urgent care clinics- now hospitals are too. Chicago (IL): Modern Healthcare; 2017.

40. Suter RE. Emergency medicine in the United States: a systematic review. World J Emerg Med 2012;3:5–10.

41. Chang J, Brundage SC, Chokshi DA. Convenient ambulatory care- promises, pitfalls, and policy. N Engl J Med 2015;373:382–8.

42. Stempniak M. Urgent care 2.0- new entrants help spur the evolution of an old model. Available at: http://www.hhnmag.com/articles/3496-urgent-care-2-0-new-entrants-help-spur-the-evolution-of-an-old-model. Accessed May 12, 2015.

43. Hunter LP, Weber CE, Morreale AP, et al. Patient satisfaction with retail health clinic care. J Am Acad Nurse Pract 2009;21:565–70.

44. 2014 Urgent care chart survey. JUCM 2015;9(7):48.

45. Kimball R. Urgent Care Association of America: 2015 benchmarking survey report. Available at: http://www.ucaoa.org/?UCBenchmarking. Accessed January 16, 2017.

46. Retail-Based Clinic Policy Work Group, AAP. AAP principles concerning retail-based clinics. Pediatrics 2006;118:2561–2.

47. Shaw KN, American Academy of Pediatrics Committee on Pediatric Emergency Medicine. Pediatric care recommendations for freestanding urgent care facilities. Pediatrics 2005;116:258–60.

48. Laughlin JJ, Simon GR, Baker C, et al. AAP principles concerning retail-based clinics. Pediatrics 2014;133:e794–7.

49. Conners GP, Kressly SJ, Perrin JM, et al. Nonemergency acute care: when it's not the medical home. Pediatrics 2017;139(5). Available at: http://pediatrics.aappublications.org/content/139/5/e20170629.

50. Weinick RM, Betancourt RM. No appointment needed: the resurgence of urgent care centers in the United States. Oakland (CA): California HealthCare Foundation; 2007.

51. Pasquarelli A. Med clinics see feverish growth rate. New York: Crain's New York Business; 2014.

52. Schor JA. Pediatric urgent care: a rapidly developing specialty. Pediatric Urgent Care Conference, Tampa, FL, March 21, 2015.

53. Schor JA. Disrupting The Disrupters: The Evolving Acute Care Market. Plenary lecture at the Pediatric Urgent Care Conference, New York, June 24, 2016.

54. Schor JA. The Evolving Acute Care Market. Pediatric Urgent Care Conference, New Orleans, LA, March 29, 2017.

55. Ward C, Canares TL. Urgent care as intermediary care: how inbound and outbound transport can enhance care of community-based pediatrics emergencies. Clin Pediatr Emerg Med 2017;18:14–23.

56. Shufeldt J. EMTALA and transferring patients to the emergency department. JUCM 2009;1:43.
57. EMTALA and urgent care: three things to know. Available at: https://www.mcguirewoods.com/client-resources/alerts/2012/11/EMTALA-Urgent-Care-3-Things-Know.aspx. Accessed November 26, 2012.
58. Federal District Court Finds Hospital-Owned Urgent Care Center Must Comply With EMTALA. Available at: htpps://www.mlmic.com/blog/hospitals/urgent-care-centers-must-comply-with-emtala/. Accessed January 20, 2017.
59. Raskas MD, Gali K, Aronson DA, et al. Telemedicine and pediatric urgent care: a vision into the future. Clin Pediatr Emerg Med 2017;18(1):24–31.

Quality Improvement and Safety in Pediatric Emergency Medicine

Brandon C. Ku, MD[a],*, James M. Chamberlain, MD[b],
Kathy N. Shaw, MD, MSCE[a]

KEYWORDS

- Quality improvement • Safety • Pediatric emergency medicine
- Performance measures • Benchmarking

KEY POINTS

- Pediatric emergency departments should adopt the principles of high-reliability organizations to optimize a culture of safety and quality.
- Quality improvement efforts in pediatric emergency medicine should continue to focus on the challenging domains of providing equitable and patient-centered care.
- In order to continue improvement in quality and safety, the goal should not be limited to learning locally from our mistakes, but to working collaboratively with other institutions with a commitment to improve through transparency and benchmarking of performance measures.

BACKGROUND

The primary goal as practitioners is to provide high-quality, safe care for each child who arrives in the emergency department (ED). The National Academies of Sciences, Engineering, and Medicine (NASEM), formerly the Institute of Medicine (IOM), report, *Crossing the Quality Chasm*, identified 6 domains of health care quality: effectiveness, safety, efficiency, timeliness, equitability, and patient centeredness.[1] Quality improvement (QI) work within pediatric emergency medicine has largely focused on efficiency and timeliness and less on the other domains. For example, the 2 National Quality

Disclosures: None.
[a] Department of Pediatrics, Perelman School of Medicine, University of Pennsylvania, Children's Hospital of Philadelphia, 3401 Civic Center Boulevard, Philadelphia, PA 19146, USA;
[b] Department of Pediatrics, Division of Emergency Medicine, Children's National Medical Center, George Washington University School of Medicine, 111 Michigan Avenue NW, Washington, DC 20010, USA
* Corresponding author. Division of Emergency Medicine, Children's Hospital of Philadelphia, 3401 Civic Center Boulevard, Philadelphia, PA 19104.
E-mail address: kub@email.chop.edu

Pediatr Clin N Am 65 (2018) 1269–1281
https://doi.org/10.1016/j.pcl.2018.07.010
0031-3955/18/© 2018 Elsevier Inc. All rights reserved.

pediatric.theclinics.com

Forum metrics devoted to ED practice involve reducing times in ED flow.[2] There has been some work focusing on addressing the national issue of ED overcrowding, which is associated with reduced compliance with evidence-based care,[3] medical errors, prolonged length of stay, and decreased patient satisfaction.[4] The EDs are using Lean methodology and other process QI methods to aid in optimizing resources in ED operations (see Russell Migita and colleagues' article, "Quality Improvement Methodologies: Principles and Applications in the Pediatric Emergency Department," in this issue). Ongoing quality work within pediatric emergency medicine should focus on providing the infrastructure for evidence-based safe and effective care, with attention also devoted to equity and patient centeredness.

The more recent NASEM report, *Pediatric Emergency Care: Growing Pains*, identified significant variability in the quality of pediatric emergency care across the United States. There continue to be significant differences in how care is provided between dedicated pediatric EDs and general EDs. All EDs caring for children should be pediatric-ready.[5,6] The American Academy of Pediatrics (AAP), the American College of Emergency Physicians (ACEP), and the Emergency Nursing Association have published joint guidelines for the care of children in EDs.[7] These guidelines focus on the structure and processes required in all EDs necessary to drive high-quality outcomes. In an assessment of the nation's ED's implementation of the guidelines, the presence of physician and nurse pediatric emergency care coordinators and QI committees were identified as essential to pediatric readiness, and these are associated with improved compliance with pediatric guidelines.[8]

With regard to patient safety, the principles of high-reliability organizations seem to be particularly relevant to the ED environment. High-reliability organizations acknowledge that human beings inevitably make mistakes, and systems should be designed proactively to help them avoid or mitigate errors.[9] A commitment to high reliability includes awareness and acceptance of human fallibility and development of a safety infrastructure that encourages reporting as well as actions on near-miss events to prevent future errors. Although large variation exists among EDs, the presence of an ED quality and safety committee is associated with an improved climate of safety.[10] EDs with a nonpunitive reporting system for front-line clinicians to identify actual or potential safety events, active QI committees with the ability to investigate near miss and actual events, and leadership that is present and modeling safety behaviors are critical to the development of a culture maximizing patient safety in the ED[11] (**Table 1**).

CURRENT EPIDEMIOLOGY AND RESEARCH ON PEDIATRIC EMERGENCY DEPARTMENT–BASED QUALITY AND SAFETY

The NASEM has disseminated 4 important publications regarding the quality of health care delivery in the United States. The first, *To Err is Human*, identified the vast scope of medical errors and pervasive threats to patient safety. *Crossing the Quality Chasm* defined 6 domains of quality: safety, effectiveness, efficiency, timeliness, adequate ability, and patient-centeredness, and identified strategies for improvement. *Unequal Treatment: Confronting Racial and Ethnic Disparities in Healthcare* focused on disparities in health care and concluded that racial and ethnic minorities are less likely to receive routine medical procedures and experience lower-quality health care. Finally, *Emergency Care for Children: Growing Pains* identified the high variability in the quality of pediatric emergency care and recommended strategies for improvement.

Seventeen years after *To Err is Human*, and 16 years after *Crossing the Quality Chasm*, practitioners are still far from achieving optimal patient safety and quality. In fact, medical errors are now the third leading cause of death in the United States.[12]

Table 1
Pediatric emergency department safety recommendations

Safety Recommendations	Examples
Raise awareness of safety as everyone's highest priority	Provide education on core patient safety concepts, provide performance metrics and incentives related to patient safety
Participate in, and model, important safety practices	Hand washing, time-outs before procedures, structured communication during hand-offs/transitions of care
Implement activities to identify risk and concerns	Safety Walk Rounds or Huddles
Encourage nonpunitive voluntary reporting of medical errors and near-misses	Develop system for voluntary, anonymous reporting and process for addressing and tracking trends
Provide training in teamwork and communication	SBAR (situation, background, assessment, recommendation) technique, I-PASS (illness severity, patient summary, action list, situational awareness and contingency planning, synthesis by receiver) handoffs
Recognize fatigue as an important safety risk and implement strategies for reducing fatigue	Consider the impact of length of shift on staff performance; recognize effects of shift sequence and rotation on provider fatigue
Develop, implement, evaluate, and update multidisciplinary evidence-based clinical practice guidelines for pediatric emergency care	Evidence-based ED pathways, CDS, and order sets readily available or linked to EHR
Encourage the use of clinical tools to aid medication dosing and administration	Educate ED staff on the correct use of length-based tape
Link efforts to improve safety within the ED to those in other units or departments caring for children	ED as part of a multidisciplinary hospital Patient Safety Committee
Build a partnership to improve the quality and safety of care provided by prehospital and intrahospital providers	Work with EMS professionals to develop evidence-based prehospital care protocols for the treatment, triage, and transport of children
Define pediatric emergency care competencies for all disciplines and provide initial and continuing education necessary to achieve and maintain those competencies	Require regular training for key cognitive and technical skills and updates on resuscitation guidelines
Integrate patient- and family-centered care into all aspects of pediatric care and in all settings	Provide timely access for emergency care providers to qualified language-translation support
Advocate for formal training in transparency and disclosure of medical errors	Engage parents and families in training to convey the patient/family perspective to staff
Support the IOM recommendation that federal agencies and private industry should fund research on pediatric-specific technologies, equipment, and medications used by emergency providers to improve patient safety	Implement computerized physician order entry and decision-support systems to aid in pediatric dosing

Adapted from Krug SE, Frush K, Committee on Pediatric Emergency Medicine, et al. Patient safety in the pediatric emergency care setting. Pediatrics 2007;120(6):1367–75.

Adverse events have decreased for some conditions but not for others.[13] Specifically related to pediatric emergency care, patients are still treated differently based on their location or their race/ethnicity.[14–18] The quality of pediatric resuscitation for critically ill children varies widely in simulation scenarios.[19] There is still poor adherence to evidence-based guidelines.[20] The long awaited implementation of the electronic health record (EHR) has improved some aspects of care, but may be costly in terms of provider efficiency and cognitive load.[21,22] Medication errors can be reduced,[23] for example, but communication with patients may suffer after implementation of the EHR.[24] Diagnostic accuracy in the ED setting may be improved because of the availability of more complete information.[25] Use of data derived from the EHR has facilitated QI efforts in pediatric emergency medicine.[26–28]

Health care institutions are complex sociotechnical systems that need to design and implement work-related tools and processes to enhance human capability for critical thinking and adaptability. Some hospitals have incorporated clinical decision support (CDS) within the EHR to provide additional cognitive support to support best practice.[29–31] The implementation of traumatic brain injury prediction rules in CDS within the EHR and the activation of electronic sepsis alerts to enhance early sepsis recognition are examples of the use of clinical practice guidelines and best practice alerts to serve as decision support tools to enhance clinical critical thinking and improve compliance with published guidelines.[26,28–34]

One of the principles of high-reliability organizations is a preoccupation with failure.[9] One of the most common failure modes in emergency medicine is in transitions of care, either to the next shift of ED staff or in transitioning the patient to the inpatient unit or back to the primary care provider.[35,36] Practitioners have learned from other high-risk industries, including aerospace, nuclear power, and aviation, to emphasize the importance of structured transitions of care or handoffs.[37,38] These structured handoffs result in concise, 2-way communication that enhances the use of checklists and memory triggers, limits experience and authoritative gradients and diagnostic momentum, and promotes family-centered care.[37] QI efforts designed to improve ED-to-inpatient handoffs can reduce care failures,[39] but, unfortunately, structured handoffs occur in less than 20% of handoffs from ED to inpatient care.[40] Attempts to extract data from the EHR to facilitate structured handoffs have met with variable success.[41–43]

Critical illness is uncommon in the pediatric ED,[44] and therefore, simulation has been used to improve and maintain technical and team communication skills.[45] Simulation has been used to improve specific safety behaviors[46] and to identify latent safety threats.[47,48] Simulation has helped to identify threats to safety in the use of epinephrine for anaphylaxis and the management of hypoglycemic seizures.[49,50] Structured simulation has also allowed investigators to identify the cause for pauses in pediatric cardiac arrest, and the use of deliberate practice through simulation has demonstrated improved compliance with American Heart Association guidelines for CPR that are associated with better outcomes.[51,52]

The nature of emergency medicine is such that many studies of quality have focused on timeliness of care.[53] For life-threatening emergent illnesses, improvements in timeliness may result in real improvements in morbidity and mortality, and timeliness is certainly important to patients.[54,55] In pediatric emergency care specifically, patient outcomes are often excellent despite less than optimal care, and mortality is rare, so studies are underpowered to detect effects on mortality or morbidity. Therefore, investigators often rely on process measures rather than outcome measures to measure quality.[56–58] Studying processes of care is acceptable when processes are tightly linked to outcomes.[59,60]

More recently, QI work in pediatric emergency medicine has focused on the other domains of quality, specifically providing equitable and patient-centered care. Recent research has continued to identify racial and ethnic differences in care provided in the pediatric ED with antibiotic use for viral acute respiratory tract infection, cranial computed tomography use among children with minor blunt head trauma, and analgesic use and length of stay for abdominal pain.[17,61,62] However, QI efforts targeted toward reducing racial and ethnic disparities are complex and challenging. QI projects aimed at improving quality overall may not improve disparities, and may even worsen them, depending on the intervention and population differences.[63] As a result, the medical literature has yet to reveal a demonstrable impact of QI interventions on reducing disparities, but restructured QI aimed at improved rigor of selecting and evaluating interventions, increased consideration of context and social determinants of health, and integrating community resources may be promising for the successful implementation of QI in reducing health disparities.[63,64] The role of implicit bias as a contributing and potentially modifiable factor in disparities in care remains to be fully elucidated.[65]

Both the AAP and ACEP have emphasized the importance of patient-centered care in the pediatric ED because knowledge of the patient's experience and perspective is essential to the practice of culturally effective care that promotes patient dignity, comfort, and autonomy.[66] Shared decision making is associated with lower costs and reduced ED use.[67] Patient experience surveys, such as National Research Corporation Picker and Press-Ganey Satisfaction Survey, have becoming increasingly prevalent in the pediatric ED. The relationship between patient satisfaction and objective measures of quality is complex and data are conflicting,[68] but patient satisfaction is correlated with reduced utilization and improved postdischarge adherence to prescribed medical plans.[69,70] ED quality committees should review data to guide areas for optimization, such as informing about delays, responding to pain, postdischarge communication with patients' primary providers.[71] Feedback from patients and families should continue to inform QI efforts, and by listening to patients and their families through focus groups, patient surveys, and patient-representatives, patient satisfaction and patient care can be optimized.[72]

PEDIATRIC PERFORMANCE MEASURE AND CURRENT BENCHMARKING

Local quality measurement and improvement efforts have been enhanced by leveraging data available from the EHR.[26–28] Advances in computer technology have also facilitated the measurement of quality from large databases, such as statewide[73] or national data,[16,18,74] or data shared among hospitals.[75] One serious limitation to the use of these large datasets is the lack of information with which to measure baseline severity of illness. In this regard, it is exciting to see the development of multi-institutional patient registries based on data from the EHR.[76] Data from the EHR can include vital signs, pain scores, asthma scores, coma scores, and other indicators of severity, and natural language processing can parse information from clinical documents to facilitate QI or research.[34,76,77] The use of provider report cards can help improve performance for some quality metrics.[27]

In order to improve the ability to provide continued high-quality safe care, the goal should not be limited to learning locally, but also to work collaboratively with other institutions with transparency to develop systems to improve quality and safety.[27] The Institute for Healthcare Improvement (IHI) offers courses and a roadmap for collaborative health care improvement.[78] The Accreditation Council for Graduate Medical Education has partnered with IHI to ensure that the next generation of trainees has received adequate education in quality and safety.[79] In response to the 2006 NASEM *Emergency Care for Children: Growing Pains* report and recommendation for the development of national standards for emergency are performance measurement, projects have been undertaken to define and organize pediatric emergency care performance measures.[6] The Pediatric Emergency Care Applied Research Network (PECARN) is a federally funded multicenter research network that has developed and implemented organizational evaluation tools to measure performance and to promote high-quality research.[80] Specifically, a project to define, classify, and prioritize pediatric emergency care performance measures was funded by a Targeted Issues Grant from the Emergency Medical Services for Children program.[51] Through a query of the medical literature, organizational Web sites, and communications with PECARN ED medical directors, a total of 405 measures from 643 sources were identified, and these measures were classified based on the Donabedian structure/process/outcome framework and the 6 NASEM domains of quality, with about half of those measures related to effectiveness and 17.3% related to safety.[51] Representatives from national organizations formed a working group to rate these measures based on NASEM domains of quality and the Donabedian framework, and 60 performance measures, subdivided based on 11 areas of interests, were identified as comprehensively reflecting pediatric emergency care.[81] Fifteen of these performance measures were prioritized for testing and improvement based on their importance to emergency medical services for children, scientific acceptability, usability, and feasibility by a diverse stakeholder group (**Table 2**).

This framework for the measurement of pediatric emergency care has facilitated the development of national benchmarking. Current research is being performed to identify benchmarks across institutions within the PECARN network and provide individual provider feedback.[76] Using the balanced performance report card, performance measures were selected to encompass the domains of quality in the NASEM report and include both medical and trauma-related diagnoses.[82] Select measures were chosen based on individual provider's control and ability for behavioral modification after receiving feedback,[82] and both providers and ED directors/managers are given monthly individual performance percentiles as well as network performance and achievable benchmarks of care based on best practice of top provider performance (see **Table 2**). The effectiveness of these report cards in improving care is being evaluated in a randomized trial using a step-wedge design among the 7 participating EDs.

POLICY IMPLICATIONS FOR REIMBURSEMENT

The NASEM's 6 domains of quality—safety, timeliness, effectiveness, efficiency, equitability, and patient centeredness—are not reflected in current incentives for emergency providers. By using relative value unit–based reimbursement, payers provide incentives that favor overtesting, which is inefficient, is potentially unsafe, and is not patient centered. Fear of malpractice claims provides similar incentives. Many hospitals, confusing customer service with patient centeredness, offer incentives for providers to perform unnecessary testing and to prescribe unnecessary therapies to avoid customer complaints. Physician income may also be tied to efficient staffing, which may come at the expense of safety because of lower staff-to-patient ratios. Policymakers should consider changing these financial incentives to promote quality and safety. Because private insurers generally follow rules enacted by government payers, implementation of these changes by the Centers for Medicare and Medicaid Services (CMS) could promote change on the national level.

Table 2
Top 15 measures in 9 areas of interest

Performance Measure	IOM Quality Domain	Donabedian Framework	Diagnosis Category
Initial care for every ED patient			
Measuring weight in kilograms for patients <18 y of age[a]	Effective, safe	Process	General
Presence of a method to identify age-based abnormal pediatric vital signs[a]	Effective, safe	Structure	General
ED infrastructure and personnel			
Pediatric equipment in the ED	Effective, safe	Structure	General
Presence of on-site pediatric coordinators	Effective, safe, patient-centered	Structure	General
Patient-centered ED care			
Parent/caregiver understanding of discharge instructions	Effective, safe, patient-centered	Process	General
ED flow			
Door to provider[a]	Timely, patient-centered	Outcome	General
Total length of stay[a]	Effective, timely, efficient, patient-centered	Outcome	General
Pain and sedation			
Reducing pain in children with acute fractures[a]	Effective, timely, patient-centered	Process	Cross-cutting (pain), fractures
Trauma			
Children with minor head trauma receiving a head computed tomographic scan	Safe, efficient	Process	Head trauma
Protocol for suspected child abuse in place	Effective, safe	Structure	Child abuse
Respiratory diseases			
Systemic corticosteroids in asthma patients with acute exacerbation[a]	Effective	Process	Asthma

(continued on next page)

Table 2
(continued)

Performance Measure	IOM Quality Domain	Donabedian Framework	Diagnosis Category
Evidence-based guideline for bronchiolitis	Effective, efficient	Structure	Bronchiolitis
Childhood infections			
Reducing antibiotic use in children with viral illnesses[a]	Effective, efficient	Process	Viral illness, upper respiratory infection
Quality and safe care of all patients			
Return visits within 48 h resulting in admission[a]	Effective, safe	Outcome	General
Medication error rates	Safe	Outcome	Cross-cutting (medications)

[a] Designates measures identified for benchmarking through PECARN.
Adapted from MCHB EMSC Innovation and Improvement Center (EIIC). Pediatric performance measures toolbox. Available at: https://emscimprovement.center/resources/toolboxes/emergency-department-pediatric-performance-measures-toolbox/. Accessed October 15, 2017.

In the future, many commercial payers will be exploring alternative payment methodologies based on performance or value-based reimbursement. Consumers of health care and employers providing health insurance are demanding a commitment to improving the value of care, and payers, including CMS, are beginning to link quality or value to reimbursement. As value and quality are being defined and measures are linked to reimbursements, it will be important to have providers and other stakeholders at the table rather than allowing payers to define these unilaterally. Pediatric emergency medicine providers should be proactive in improving the quality, value, and transparency of care before legislation demands it.

REFERENCES

1. Kohn L, Corrigan J, Donaldson M. Institute of medicine committee on quality of health care in America. Crossing the quality chasm. Washington, DC: National Academy Press; 2001.
2. National quality forum: measures, reports & tools. 2017. Available at: http://www.qualityforum.org/Measures_Reports_Tools.aspx. Accessed October 20, 2017.
3. Sills MR, Fairclough D, Ranade D, et al. Emergency department crowding is associated with decreased quality of care for children. Pediatr Emerg Care 2011;27(9):837–45.
4. Rutman L, Migita R, Spencer S, et al. Standardized asthma admission criteria reduce length of stay in a pediatric emergency department. Acad Emerg Med 2016;23(3):289–96.
5. Institute of Medicine, Committee of the Future of Emergency Care in the United States Health System. Hospital based emergency care: at the breaking point. Washington, DC: National Academy Press; 2006.
6. Institute of Medicine, Committee on the Future of Emergency Care in the United States Health System. Emergency care for children: growing pains. Washington, DC: National Academies Press; 2006.

7. American Academy of Pediatrics, Committee on Pediatric Emergency Medicine, American College of Emergency Physicians, et al. Joint policy statement–guidelines for care of children in the emergency department. J Emerg Nurs 2013;39(2): 116–31.

8. Gausche-Hill M, Ely M, Schmuhl P, et al. A national assessment of pediatric readiness of emergency departments. JAMA Pediatr 2015;169(6):527–34.

9. Weick KE, Sutcliffe KM. Managing the unexpected: sustained performance in a complex world. Hoboken (NJ): John Wiley & Sons; 2015.

10. Shaw KN, Ruddy RM, Olsen CS, et al. Pediatric patient safety in emergency departments: unit characteristics and staff perceptions. Pediatrics 2009;124(2): 485–93.

11. Committee on Pediatric Emergency Medicine, American Academy of Pediatrics, Krug SE, Frush K. Patient safety in the pediatric emergency care setting. Pediatrics 2007;120(6):1367–75.

12. Makary MA, Daniel M. Medical error-the third leading cause of death in the us. BMJ 2016;353:i2139.

13. Wang Y, Eldridge N, Metersky ML, et al. National trends in patient safety for four common conditions, 2005–2011. N Engl J Med 2014;370(4):341–51.

14. Walls TA, Chamberlain JM, Strohm-Farber J, et al. Improving pretransport care of pediatric emergency patients: an assessment of referring hospital care. Pediatr Emerg Care 2010;26(8):567–70.

15. Goyal MK, Hayes KL, Mollen CJ. Racial disparities in testing for sexually transmitted infections in the emergency department. Acad Emerg Med 2012;19(5): 604–7.

16. Chamberlain JM, Teach SJ, Hayes KL, et al. Practice pattern variation in the care of children with acute asthma. Acad Emerg Med 2016;23(2):166–70.

17. Goyal MK, Johnson TJ, Chamberlain JM, et al. Racial and ethnic differences in antibiotic use for viral illness in emergency departments. Pediatrics 2017; 140(4) [pii:e20170203].

18. Mannix R, Bourgeois FT, Schutzman SA, et al. Neuroimaging for pediatric head trauma: do patient and hospital characteristics influence who gets imaged? Acad Emerg Med 2010;17(7):694–700.

19. Auerbach M, Whitfill T, Gawel M, et al. Differences in the quality of pediatric resuscitative care across a spectrum of emergency departments. JAMA Pediatr 2016; 170(10):987–94.

20. Jain S, Cheng J, Alpern ER, et al. Management of febrile neonates in us pediatric emergency departments. Pediatrics 2014;133(2):187–95.

21. Ahmed A, Chandra S, Herasevich V, et al. The effect of two different electronic health record user interfaces on intensive care provider task load, errors of cognition, and performance. Crit Care Med 2011;39(7):1626–34.

22. Mathison D, Chamberlain J. Evaluating the impact of the electronic health record on patient flow in a pediatric emergency department. Appl Clin Inform 2011;2(1):39.

23. Sethuraman U, Kannikeswaran N, Murray KP, et al. Prescription errors before and after introduction of electronic medication alert system in a pediatric emergency department. Acad Emerg Med 2015;22(6):714–9.

24. Shachak A, Reis S. The impact of electronic medical records on patient–doctor communication during consultation: a narrative literature review. J Eval Clin Pract 2009;15(4):641–9.

25. Ben-Assuli O, Sagi D, Leshno M, et al. Improving diagnostic accuracy using ehr in emergency departments: a simulation-based study. J Biomed Inform 2015;55: 31–40.

26. Nigrovic LE, Stack AM, Mannix RC, et al. Quality improvement effort to reduce cranial cts for children with minor blunt head trauma. Pediatrics 2015;136(1): e227–33.

27. Jain S, Frank G, McCormick K, et al. Impact of physician scorecards on emergency department resource use, quality, and efficiency. Pediatrics 2015;136(3): e670–9.

28. Atabaki SM, Jacobs BR, Brown KM, et al. Quality improvement in pediatric head trauma with pecarn rules implementation as computerized decision support. Pediatr Qual Saf 2017;2(3):e019.

29. Dayan PS, Ballard DW, Tham E, et al. Use of traumatic brain injury prediction rules with clinical decision support. Pediatrics 2017;139(4):e20162709.

30. Sheehan B, Nigrovic LE, Dayan PS, et al. Informing the design of clinical decision support services for evaluation of children with minor blunt head trauma in the emergency department: a sociotechnical analysis. J Biomed Inform 2013;46(5): 905–13.

31. Balamuth F, Alpern ER, Abaddessa MK, et al. Improving recognition of pediatric severe sepsis in the emergency department: contributions of a vital sign–based electronic alert and bedside clinician identification. Ann Emerg Med 2017;70(6): 759–769.e2.

32. Demonchy E, Dufour J-C, Gaudart J, et al. Impact of a computerized decision support system on compliance with guidelines on antibiotics prescribed for urinary tract infections in emergency departments: a multicentre prospective before-and-after controlled interventional study. J Antimicrob Chemother 2014; 69(10):2857–63.

33. Gupta A, Ip IK, Raja AS, et al. Effect of clinical decision support on documented guideline adherence for head ct in emergency department patients with mild traumatic brain injury. J Am Med Inform Assoc 2014;21(e2):e347–51.

34. Yadav K, Chamberlain JM, Lewis VR, et al. Designing real-time decision support for trauma resuscitations. Acad Emerg Med 2015;22(9):1076–84.

35. Beach C, Croskerry P, Shapiro M. Profiles in patient safety: emergency care transitions. Acad Emerg Med 2003;10(4):364–7.

36. Horwitz LI, Moin T, Krumholz HM, et al. Consequences of inadequate sign-out for patient care. Arch Intern Med 2008;168(16):1755–60.

37. American Academy of Pediatrics Committee on Pediatric Emergency Medicine, American College of Emergency Physicians Pediatric Emergency Medicine Committee, Emergency Nurses Association Pediatric Committee. Handoffs: transitions of care for children in the emergency department. Pediatrics 2016;138(5): e20162680.

38. Gopwani PR, Brown KM, Quinn MJ, et al. Sound: a structured handoff tool improves patient handoffs in a pediatric emergency department. Pediatr Emerg Care 2015;31(2):83–7.

39. Bigham MT, Logsdon TR, Manicone PE, et al. Decreasing handoff-related care failures in children's hospitals. Pediatrics 2014;134(2):e572–9.

40. Kessler C, Scott NL, Siedsma M, et al. Interunit handoffs of patients and transfers of information: a survey of current practices. Ann Emerg Med 2014;64(4): 343–9.e5.

41. Flanagan ME, Patterson ES, Frankel RM, et al. Evaluation of a physician informatics tool to improve patient handoffs. J Am Med Inform Assoc 2009;16(4): 509–15.

42. Davis J, Riesenberg LA, Mardis M, et al. Evaluating outcomes of electronic tools supporting physician shift-to-shift handoffs: a systematic review. J Grad Med Educ 2015;7(2):174–80.

43. Wohlauer MV, Arora VM, Horwitz LI, et al. The patient handoff: a comprehensive curricular blueprint for resident education to improve continuity of care. Acad Med 2012;87(4):411.

44. Mittiga MR, Geis GL, Kerrey BT, et al. The spectrum and frequency of critical procedures performed in a pediatric emergency department: implications of a provider-level view. Ann Emerg Med 2013;61(3):263–70.

45. Schmidt E, Goldhaber-Fiebert SN, Ho LA, et al. Simulation exercises as a patient safety strategy: a systematic review. Ann Intern Med 2013;158(5_Part_2):426.

46. Pian-Smith MCM, Simon R, Minehart RD, et al. Teaching residents the two-challenge rule: a simulation-based approach to improve education and patient safety. Simul Healthc 2009;4(2):84–91.

47. Patterson MD, Geis GL, Falcone RA, et al. In situ simulation: detection of safety threats and teamwork training in a high risk emergency department. BMJ Qual Saf 2013;22(6):468–77.

48. Farnan JM, Gaffney S, Poston JT, et al. Patient safety room of horrors: a novel method to assess medical students and entering residents' ability to identify hazards of hospitalisation. BMJ Qual Saf 2016;25(3):153–8.

49. Walsh BM, Gangadharan S, Whitfill T, et al. Safety threats during the care of infants with hypoglycemic seizures in the emergency department: a multicenter, simulation-based prospective cohort study. J Emerg Med 2017;53(4):467–74.

50. Chime NO, Riese VG, Scherzer DJ, et al. Epinephrine auto-injector versus drawn up epinephrine for anaphylaxis management: a scoping review. Pediatr Crit Care Med 2017;18(8):764–9.

51. Kessler DO, Peterson DT, Bragg A, et al. Causes for pauses during simulated pediatric cardiac arrest. Pediatr Crit Care Med 2017;18(8):e311–7.

52. Cheng A, Brown LL, Duff JP, et al. Improving cardiopulmonary resuscitation with a cpr feedback device and refresher simulations (cpr cares study): a randomized clinical trial. JAMA Pediatr 2015;169(2):137–44.

53. Chang AM, Lin A, Fu R, et al. Associations of emergency department length of stay with publicly reported quality-of-care measures. Acad Emerg Med 2017; 24(2):246–50.

54. Al Owad A, Karim M, Ma L. Integrated lean six sigma approach for patient flow improvement in hospital emergency department. Advanced Materials Research 2014;834–836:1893–902.

55. Byczkowski TL, Fitzgerald M, Kennebeck S, et al. A comprehensive view of parental satisfaction with pediatric emergency department visits. Ann Emerg Med 2013;62(4):340–50.

56. Alessandrini E, Varadarajan K, Alpern ER, et al. Emergency department quality: an analysis of existing pediatric measures. Acad Emerg Med 2011;18(5):519–26.

57. Stang AS, Straus SE, Crotts J, et al. Quality indicators for high acuity pediatric conditions. Pediatrics 2013;132(4):752–62.

58. Stang AS, Hartling L, Fera C, et al. Quality indicators for the assessment and management of pain in the emergency department: a systematic review. Pain Res Manag 2014;19(6):e179–90.

59. Parshuram CS, Dryden-Palmer K, Farrell C, et al. Evaluating processes of care and outcomes of children in hospital (epoch): study protocol for a randomized controlled trial. Trials 2015;16(1):245.

60. Barata I, Brown KM, Fitzmaurice L, et al. Best practices for improving flow and care of pediatric patients in the emergency department. Pediatrics 2015; 135(1):e273–83.

61. Natale JE, Joseph JG, Rogers AJ, et al. Cranial computed tomography use among children with minor blunt head trauma: association with race/ethnicity. Arch Pediatr Adolesc Med 2012;166(8):732–7.

62. Johnson TJ, Weaver MD, Borrero S, et al. Association of race and ethnicity with management of abdominal pain in the emergency department. Pediatrics 2013;132(4):e851–8.

63. Lion KC, Raphael JL. Partnering health disparities research with quality improvement science in pediatrics. Pediatrics 2015;135(2):354–61.

64. McPheeters ML, Kripalani S, Peterson NB, et al. Closing the quality gap: revisiting the state of the science (vol. 3: quality improvement interventions to address health disparities). Evid Rep Technol Assess (Full Rep) 2012;(208.3):1–475.

65. Johnson TJ, Ellison AM, Dalembert G, et al. Implicit bias in pediatric academic medicine. J Natl Med Assoc 2017;109(3):156–63.

66. American Academy of Pediatrics Committee on Pediatric Emergency Medicine, American College of Emergency Physicians Pediatric Emergency Medicine Committee, O'Malley P, et al. Patient- and family-centered care and the role of the emergency physician providing care to a child in the emergency department. Pediatrics 2006;118(5):2242–4.

67. Fiks AG, Mayne S, Localio AR, et al. Shared decision-making and health care expenditures among children with special health care needs. Pediatrics 2012; 129(1):99–107.

68. Farley H, Enguidanos ER, Coletti CM, et al. Patient satisfaction surveys and quality of care: an information paper. Ann Emerg Med 2014;64(4):351–7.

69. Boudreaux ED, O'Hea EL. Patient satisfaction in the emergency department: a review of the literature and implications for practice. J Emerg Med 2004;26(1): 13–26.

70. Nelson TD, Steele RG. Beyond efficacy and effectiveness: a multifaceted approach to treatment evaluation. Prof Psychol Res Pr 2006;37(4):389.

71. Locke R, Stefano M, Koster A, et al. Optimizing patient/caregiver satisfaction through quality of communication in the pediatric emergency department. Pediatr Emerg Care 2011;27(11):1016–21.

72. Augustine EM, Kreling BA, Chamberlain JM. Caretakers' perspectives on return pediatric emergency department visits: a qualitative analysis of focus groups. Pediatr Emerg Care 2016;32(9):594–8.

73. Berry EA, Kelton CM, Guo JJ, et al. Adaptation and application of the agency for healthcare research and quality's asthma admission rate pediatric quality indicator to ohio medicaid claims data. Res Social Adm Pharm 2013;9(3):240–50.

74. Goyal MK, Kuppermann N, Cleary SD, et al. Racial disparities in pain management of children with appendicitis in emergency departments. JAMA Pediatr 2015;169(11):996–1002.

75. Mannix R, Meehan WP, Monuteaux MC, et al. Computed tomography for minor head injury: variation and trends in major united states pediatric emergency departments. J Pediatr 2012;160(1):136–9.e1.

76. Grundmeier RW, Masino AJ, Casper TC, et al. Identification of long bone fractures in radiology reports using natural language processing to support healthcare quality improvement. Appl Clin Inform 2016;7(4):1051–68.

77. Yadav K, Sarioglu E, Choi H, et al. Automated outcome classification of computed tomography imaging reports for pediatric traumatic brain injury. Acad Emerg Med 2016;23(2):171–8.
78. The breakthrough series: Ihi's collaborative model for achieving breakthrough improvement. Boston: Institute for Healthcare Improvement; 2003. Available at: http://www.ihi.org/resources/Pages/IHIWhitePapers/TheBreakthroughSeriesIHIs CollaborativeModelforAchievingBreakthroughImprovement.aspx.
79. Wagner R, Weiss KB, Passiment ML, et al. Pursuing excellence in clinical learning environments. J Grad Med Educ 2016;8(1):124–7.
80. Stanley R, Lillis KA, Zuspan SJ, et al. Development and implementation of a performance measure tool in an academic pediatric research network. Contemp Clin Trials 2010;31(5):429–37.
81. Emergency medical services for children innovation and improvement. Available at: https://emscimprovement.center/resources/toolboxes/emergency-department-pe diatric-performance-measures-toolbox/. Accessed October 20, 2017.
82. Alpern ER, AE, Casper TC, et al. Benchmarks in pediatric emergency medicine performance measures derived from an multicenter electronic health record registry. Paper presented at: E-PAS2015. April 25–28, San Diego, CA.

Quality Improvement Methodologies

Principles and Applications in the Pediatric Emergency Department

Russell Migita, MD[a,b,]*, Hiromi Yoshida, MD, MBA[a],
Lori Rutman, MD, MPH[a], George A. Woodward, MD, MBA[a]

KEYWORDS

- Quality improvement • Lean • Pediatrics • Emergency medicine

KEY POINTS

- Improvement science has a long history in health care and methods, such as Six Sigma, Lean, and the Model for Improvement, have been successfully applied to improve health care processes over time.
- Patients and families are the focus for all improvement efforts; they are the "customer." When a process is examined from the point of view of the patient and family, interdepartmental and interdisciplinary silos are more difficult to defend.
- Standardization is essential for improvement, but it is only the first step in improvement. To achieve provider acceptance of standardization, one must use the standardization as a basis for ongoing improvement.

INTRODUCTION

As the debate over health care finance rages on, arguments about the quality of health care have become a political trope. Although the US health care system is a leader in scientific innovation and providing highly specialized care, it rates poorly in most other dimensions of health care despite per capita spending that is nearly double that of most other developed nations.[1] The United States falls behind in ratings of access, administrative efficiency, equity, and health care outcomes.[2] In 1999, the Institute of Medicine (now known as the National Academies of Sciences Engineering and Medicine) catalyzed in its report entitled "To Err is Human" the need for improvement of US

[a] Department of Pediatrics, Division of Emergency Medicine and Emergency Department, Seattle Children's Hospital, University of Washington School of Medicine, MB.7.520, PO Box 5371, Seattle, WA 98145-5005, USA; [b] UW Medicine Center for Scholarship in Patient Care Quality and Safety, UWMC Health Sciences, BB1240, Campus Box #356526, 1959 NE Pacific Street, Seattle, WA 98195, USA
* Corresponding author. Emergency Department, Seattle Children's Hospital, MB.7.520, PO Box 5371, Seattle, WA 98145-5005.
E-mail address: Russ.migita@seattlechildrens.org

Pediatr Clin N Am 65 (2018) 1283–1296
https://doi.org/10.1016/j.pcl.2018.07.011
0031-3955/18/© 2018 Elsevier Inc. All rights reserved.

pediatric.theclinics.com

health care systems and delivery by estimating that nearly 100,000 patients died of medical errors every year.[3] Although some improvements, notably in reduction of hospital-acquired infections, have been made in the past two decades, the pace has been slower than desired.[4] Health care systems are complex, often convoluted, and wasteful. Improvement efforts are often poorly implemented and sustained. Finally, many clinicians do not have the requisite skills or tools to work effectively and efficiently without compromising quality and patient safety. Emergency medicine is well suited as a testing and proving ground for quality improvement (QI) methodologies because of its high patient volume and rapid turnover.

HISTORY OF IMPROVEMENT SCIENCE IN HEALTH CARE

Medicine has a long history of innovation to improve outcomes. Joseph Lister combined germ theory with carefully codified standard practice to introduce the principles of antisepsis to surgery.[5] Florence Nightingale used data to drive organizational improvement to reduce mortality during the Crimean War and created the first performance measures of hospitals in 1859.[6] However, the origins of QI in health care in the twentieth century are traced back to industry.

Walter A. Shewhart was a physicist who worked at Bell telephone laboratories in the 1920s. He was the first to distinguish "attributable," or special cause variation, an infrequent or nonrandom event that can be eliminated from processes to improve reliability, from common cause variation, which is statistical noise or natural variation in a process.[7] Shewhart influenced Joseph Juran, who worked at the Western Electric Hawthorne plant. Juran built on work by the nineteenth century Italian economist, Vilfredo Pareto. In working to understand the causes of variation, he developed Pareto charts, which help identify the most frequent cause of defects, and clarified the applicability of the 80:20 rule in health care, that 80% of results come from 20% of causes.[8] W. Edwards Deming was another protégé of Shewhart. Deming's system of profound knowledge forms the theoretic basis for current improvement science. He popularized the Plan-Do-Check-Act (PDCA) or Plan-Do-Study-Act (PDSA) cycle, which is the concept of iteratively implementing a change, followed by assessing the impact of that change to continuously improve.[9] This idea is fundamental to all modern QI approaches.

OVERVIEW OF IMPROVEMENT METHODOLOGIES
Six Sigma

Although there is considerable overlap between improvement methodologies, Six Sigma is focused on reducing defects. This approach uses principles derived from Shewhart (to reduce variation) and learnings from Juran (to understand the causes of variation) to reduce error rates to Six Sigma levels (a maximum of 3.4 errors per million opportunities). In contrast, health care error rates are estimated to be between 2700 and 45,500 errors per million opportunities (between 2 and 3 sigma).[10] Six Sigma was first introduced in industry by Bill Smith and Mikel J. Harry at Motorola in the 1980s and subsequently by Jack Welch at General Electric in the 1990s before being adopted by health care systems. The Six Sigma equivalent of PDCA cycles is represented by the acronym DMAIC (**Box 1**).

Institute for Healthcare Improvement Model for Improvement

The Institute for Healthcare Improvement (IHI) approach to QI is strongly based on the principles of Shewhart, Juran, and Deming, most particularly Deming's theory of profound knowledge. It is a conceptual, holistic framework to understanding systems, people, and experimentation that has been developed over the past 25 years in

---

Box 1
Definition of the DMAIC improvement cycle

Define
- Clearly define the project and its scope
- Determine the requirements of the customer
- Establish the value proposition of the proposed project

Measure
- Clearly establish baseline performance using run or statistical process control charts that display mean or median
- Understand baseline performance with regards to error rate

Analyze
- Use tools, such as Ishikawa (fishbone) diagrams, to understand cause and effect
- Use multivariate analysis to understand variability and failure modes and effect analysis to identify failures in a process

Improve
- Create, test, and implement solutions

Control
- Monitor and sustain improvement using statistical process control charts or run charts

---

collaboration with Tom Nolan, Ron Moen, and Lloyd Provost at Associates in Process Improvement and IHI.[11] At its heart is the Model for Improvement. Model for Improvement is an easily understandable framework for improvement that starts with three simple questions that are linked to a continuous PDSA cycle (**Box 2**). In IHI-QI, improvement is not a static process. Instead, it is a continuous process of small tests of change that are tracked over time.[12]

Queuing Theory

Queuing theory was developed by Agner Krarup Erlang, a Danish mathematician, in 1909 when he was studying waiting times for telephone calls for the Copenhagen Telephone Company. He wanted to determine the optimal number of circuits needed to handle a variable number of calls coming into the company.[13] The queuing theory can be applied to any system that involves wait times. Through a variety of formulas and simulations, queuing theory attempts to minimize waiting times while maximizing the use of resources.[14] As batch sizes increase (surge) and variability increases (lack of standardization), the effects of crowding increase exponentially. The effects of these principles on the emergency department (ED) are clear. The ED has an obvious queuing system: the patient arrives, then waits, is seen by a provider, then may wait several more times before getting laboratory work or imaging, and then eventually leaves the ED, whether it be going home or getting admitted. Queuing theory can be applied to each of these steps to minimize wait times for the patient; to ensure that the physicians and nurses are being used appropriately; and to figure out if there are enough resources, such as radiology equipment and inpatient bed available, to care for the patient.[15]

Lean

The origins of Lean are traced to the "flow production" system of the Ford Model-T assembly line in Michigan in the early twentieth century. Soon after, Lean principles, such as "*jidoka*," a system in which automated processes stop when problems arise, were incorporated into processes at the Toyoda Automatic Loom Works in Japan. In the 1940s, Taiichi Ohno began laying the foundations of the Toyota Production System

---

Box 2
IHI Model for Improvement framework. Each question is linked to a continuous PDSA cycle

What are we trying to accomplish?

- For significant work, start with a charter
- Establish boundaries
- Ensure that the right people are involved
- Ensure leadership support
- Craft a SMART AIM statement that clearly defines what you are trying to do
  - Specific
  - Measurable
  - Achievable
  - Relevant
  - Time-based
- Example: "We will improve average time to antibiotics for febrile neutropenic patients from its current baseline of 75 minutes to a target of 45 minutes by June 2018."

How will we know that change is an improvement?

- Define measures
  - Outcome measures: relate directly to the experience of the customer
  - Process measures: measures the functioning of your system
  - Balancing measures: tracks unintended effects of the change
- Display data in longitudinal form whenever possible. This is important to assess the effect of serial changes over time. Confounders cannot be eliminated in a system that is committed to continuous improvement.
  - Run charts
  - Statistical process control charts

What change can we make that will result in an improvement?

- Draw from the many QI or safety tools that exist
  - Process maps
  - Use standards to reduce the effect of queues
  - Six Sigma tools to reduce variation
  - Lean tools to remove waste
  - Remove bottlenecks

---

including standardized work, single-piece flow, and just-in-time. These principles were further influenced by W. Edwards Deming's visits in the 1950s to what would later become the Japanese Union of Scientists and Engineers. The principles of the Toyota Production System largely existed as implicit knowledge within the Toyota Corporation. They were almost unknown in the West until the seminal work, *The Machine that Changed the World*, by Womack and Jones introduced the term "Lean" to the world in 1990.[16,17] By the time *Lean Thinking*[18] was published in 1996, these principles were in widespread use in industry and health care institutions, such as Virginia Mason,[19] Theda Care,[20] and Seattle Children's Hospital,[21–23] began using Lean extensively to improve their daily operations. A deeper exploration of Lean principles is discussed next.

Lean Principles

Lean is not just about waste reduction. When successfully applied in health care, it is a system that fosters continuous improvement while involving "respecting" staff and the patients they care for. There are several key principles that we describe in greater detail:

- Define value from the point of view of the customer
- Respect the people who are doing the work
- Create standard work
- Iteratively identify and remove waste
- Create a system that naturally flows and reveals further opportunities for improvement

Define value from the point of view of the customer

In the pediatric ED, it is easy to fall into the trap of customer confusion. Is our customer the patient and family? Or is it our trainees, other hospital staff, referring providers, or our payers? In Lean thinking, the answer is simple. Our customer is the patient and their family. This does not mean that everything else is unimportant. However, clearly defining the customer and looking at the experience from their point of view simplifies the approach and analysis. When conflict arises between departmental silos, reminding oneself of who the customer is makes it more difficult to retreat back to silos.

Respect the people who are doing the work: going to Gemba

An essential principle of Lean is to involve (respect) the people who do the work and know that work best. Going to *Gemba* means going to the actual workplace, to watch the actual work, with the people who do that work. Simulation can be used when a process is rare or difficult to observe, but it should not be the starting point. From these observations, a process map is developed (**Fig. 1**).

Create standard work

The Lean term for improvement is *kaizen*. Taiichi Ohno said "without standards, there can be no *kaizen*." A process in which every provider does things in a unique way or in a different order is difficult to improve and to resource. When nurses know what to expect next, they are better able to carry out their tasks and keep families informed. A related concept is *jidoka*, which is generally translated as "automation with a human touch." An example from the early days of Toyota manufacturing is a spinning machine that spins multiple cotton threads at the same time. The machine was designed to function automatically most of the time. When a thread breaks, it becomes obvious that a specific spindle has stopped. This signals the operator to fix the problem. In the ED, clinical standard pathways or protocols allow patients to continuously move forward in their care and makes it easier to identify patients who are not responding as expected. When this system works well, interruptions are less frequent, and when they happen, they are more relevant. It also decreases cognitive clutter.

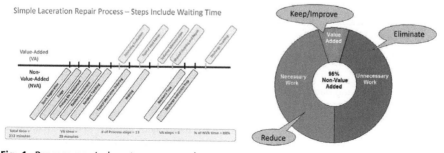

Fig. 1. Process map/value stream example.

Standard work also allows better matching of resource to demand. *Takt* time is a measure of customer demand. If 10 patients arrive in 1 hour, the *takt* time is 6 minutes. If we are not able to discharge one patient every 6 minutes, the waiting room will start to fill. Having predictable cycle times and lead times and understanding your historical arrival patterns allows an ED administrator to staff the ED to maximize productivity and efficiency (**Fig. 2**).

Iteratively identify and remove waste

Process mapping The process map defines the steps in the process. Each step should be observed and measured. The time it takes to perform each step, including waiting time, is the cycle time for that step. The sum of all of the cycle times is the lead time, which corresponds to the patient's experience with our care. There is likely to be some variability with cycle times. It is difficult to remove all of the variability because each patient's needs are different. However, one should work to remove variability that is caused by provider variation to allow for a more predictable process.

Value Each step is then classified as value-added or non-value-added from the point of view of the customer. A value-added step is one in which a patient moves closer toward complete care. This could include examination, education, or delivery of a medication. Another way of defining a value-added step is simple: would the family be willing to pay for that step on an itemized bill? **Fig. 1** shows a typical ED experience

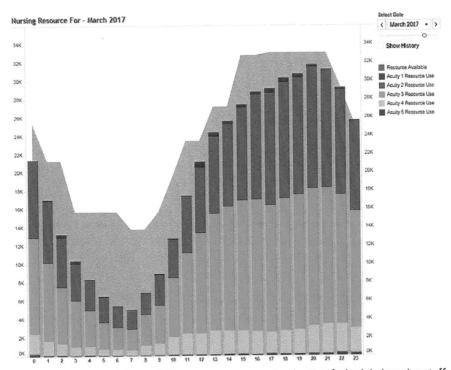

Fig. 2. RN resource and demand. The gray area represents minutes of scheduled nursing staffing per hour of day over the course of a month. Each *bar* represents the average amount of nursing work required per hour based on observed patient arrivals. This was generated through direct observation of nursing work time for a variety of patients in each Emergency Severity Index triage level. Some buffer is required to allow staff to be able to respond to unpredictable surges in demand. Poorly staffed late-night hours require additional buffer.

including lead times, value-added, and non-value-added steps. In a typical health care process, 90% to 95% of time is estimated to be non-value-added.[22] This does not mean that one can eliminate every non-value-added step (see **Fig. 1**). Some steps are non-value-added, but necessary. This includes such steps as registration or check steps to ensure safety. The unnecessary non-value-added steps may be easy opportunities for improvement. Eliminating these steps allows one to spend more time with patients or on important non-value-added steps, such as instructing trainees.

Waste There are many types of waste in health care and the pediatric ED (**Table 1**).

Create a system that naturally flows and reveals further opportunities for improvement

Pull and flow Ultimately, the goal of Lean is to create a system that flows naturally. Many people's introduction to Lean is an exercise in which a team of people folds paper into paper airplanes.[24] Each person is responsible for making a fold. At first each person works as quickly as they can. Airplanes stack up at the constrained steps. Quality suffers. Next, the team is asked to only produce when the next person in line is ready. This is "one-piece" or "single-piece" flow. It is also a classic example of a "pull" system in which an item is not produced until a *kanban* or signal is given that the next station is ready. The counterintuitive finding of this exercise is that the lead time decreases significantly and more planes are completed despite the fact that everyone feels that their work is easier.

Too often, however, the exercise stops there. An important concept is that "pull" is not the ultimate goal. Rather, it is an intermediate step on the way to flow. When pull is interpreted as "do not send a patient to the inpatient unit until they are completely ready," patients stack up in the ED. The true goal of a pull system is to identify why the inpatient team cannot pull and problem solve the issues so that patients can continue to receive efficient and progressive care. Perhaps they do not have enough environmental services staff to clean rooms, or the pharmacy is not staffed to handle the demand of discharge prescriptions. These are issues that can be acknowledged and addressed to help improve flow. In the Toyota manufacturing system, the line does not stop moving unless a problem cannot be fixed. There is a great deal of emphasis on identification and mitigation of issues. For Lean to reach its highest potential in health care, there is a need to support a system that identifies and addresses issues. Each time waste is removed, it

Table 1	
Types of waste and examples in the pediatric ED	
Type of Waste	**Example**
Processing	Duplicated documentation
Correction	Recovery efforts when an error is made
Inventory	Difficulty finding a specific supply because there is too much stock
Wait time	Unintended waiting associated with results being available to act on, but providers are unaware Patients waiting to be admitted when ED care complete
Search time	Looking for staff members to all be available for a procedure
Transportation	Unnecessary patient movement
Space	Too many may rooms hides flow issues
Complexity	Complicated admission process
Underused people	Employees not being used to their full capacity

reveals the next opportunity for improvement. Lean is not a "one and done" process, but a commitment to continuously improve over time.

Other Tools

5S

5S is translated in several different ways. One translation is "sort, straighten, scrub, standardize, sustain." 5S is a tool that is used to organize a workplace with a goal of having a place for everything and for everything to be in its place. 5S is much more than placing tape on the floor to indicate where a piece of equipment should be. It is also about removing unnecessary items and maintaining the desired state. When 5S is done well, search time decreases.

Kaizen or rapid process improvement workshop

These events are typically week-long workshops where the goal is to bring a team together and implement a change by the end of the workshop week. The first part of the week involves going to *Gemba* with the people who do the work to observe and better understand the current state. Then an ideal future state is envisioned and the team systematically goes about creating standards and removing waste.

A3

This methodology refers to A3 paper size, roughly 11 × 17 inches (**Fig. 3**). An A3 is a miniature *kaizen* activity that is owned by a single person or a small group. A target condition is established along with an understanding of the current state. The team documents their "5 whys," an exercise designed to get to root cause of challenges in the current state by asking "why." The team then designs and trials countermeasures to get the process closer to its ideal state.

Value stream map

This is an expanded process map that outlines the entire patient experience along their continuum of care. It also documents flows of people and information and current state data (**Fig. 4**). It is used for planning project work and for engaging staff by making it clear that the patient's experience goes beyond the walls of their silo.

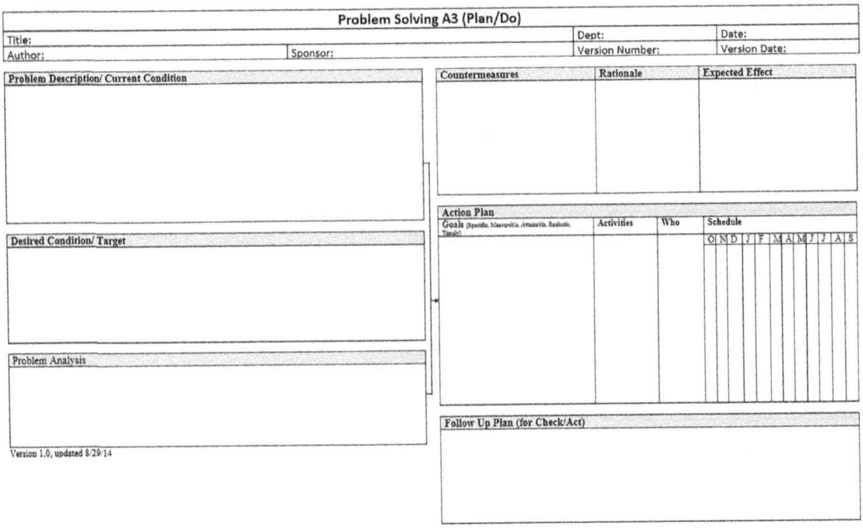

Fig. 3. A3 template.

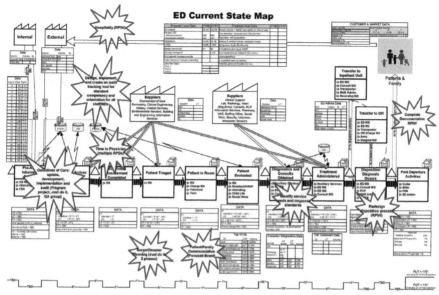

Fig. 4. Value stream map.

TYING IT ALL TOGETHER: APPLICATIONS IN THE PEDIATRIC EMERGENCY DEPARTMENT

There are numerous examples of how QI methodologies have been implemented to improve patient care. Every ED has unique answers to similar problems because every system is unique in the challenges that it faces. However, by approaching an issue with Lean or other QI methodologies, improvements are achieved. In a pediatric ED in Sweden, they were able to improve wait times and time to physicians by creating physician-nurse teams to improve evaluation and communication, defining roles, getting senior physicians involved sooner, and having overlapping physician schedules. They were able to maintain their improvements by ensuring that front line staff met every 2 weeks and the ED team met with management monthly.[25] EDs have also been able to decrease length of stay, time to physician, and left without being seen (LWBS) by using Lean principles to identify low-acuity patients who can be evaluated and discharged by a physician in the triage area.[26,27] Other common improvements include revamping the triage and registration process and having flexible room assignments to get patients into rooms faster and creating procedure carts and ensuring rooms are stocked with appropriate supplies to decrease search time.[27–29] Our institution has applied Lean methodologies to numerous improvement projects, impacting clinical and operational practice. We describe three examples from our experience at Seattle Children's Hospital in greater detail next.

Seattle Children's Hospital Emergency Department Front-End Model Redesign

A 26-member multidisciplinary team met over 5 days to redesign our front-end ED care team structure and workflow using Lean methodologies (rapid process improvement workshop).[30] The goal of the redesign process was to create a new model that reduced time to be seen by a licensed ordering provider to 30 minutes or less for 80% of patients. Lean design principles included careful observation of current state processes and analysis of each step in the process to determine if they are completely unnecessary, unnecessary but unavoidable, or necessary (ie, Value Stream Mapping). Based on a review of ED front-end literature, mapping of the current system through direct observation, and methodical elimination of non-value-added steps, a new model was designed.

In our "current state" we used a traditional front-end model found in many academic EDs. "Current state" patient flow was mapped out as follows. On arrival, patients were greeted by security and administrative staff in the waiting room. Next, they saw the triage nurse who obtained vital signs and assigned a triage level. If a room was not immediately available, patients were sent to the waiting room after triage. Once roomed, patients were seen by registration staff; medication intake coordinators (trained pharmacy technicians who verify and enter all home medications, dose and frequency into the computer); nurses; and multiple physicians or trainees including medical students, residents, fellows, and attendings in a series of often redundant encounters.

Non-value-added steps identified in this model included: delay from patient arrival to provider, patient wait times to nursing assessment, travel times, redundant questioning about medications and historical information, and providers not always available to see patients when they arrive to a patient room. To minimize or eliminate these non-value-added steps, a new front-end model was adopted.

Patient flow through the new front-end model is as follows. On arrival, patients are first seen by a lobby nurse who does a rapid visual assessment that includes assessing the patient's level of consciousness, work of breathing, and perfusion. The lobby nurse then performs a quick registration that involves entering name, date of birth, and whether an interpreter is needed into the electronic medical record. Nurses are geographically zoned in the ED and have an electronic mechanism for visually indicating on the tracking system when they are ready for a new patient ("Pull" system). Medication intake coordinators then transport patients (minimizing underused staff and transport time) to an open room, where they are greeted by a nurse who obtains vital signs, thereby eliminating traditional triage for most patients. Medication intake is completed by the medication intake coordinators simultaneously with vital signs. In our ideal state, the medical provider care team is also present to assess the patient once they are placed in a room. The care team listens to the presenting complaint, performs a focused physical examination, and verbalizes an initial plan to the nurse and family. If a physician care team is not available, a separate "Early Initiation" team (physician or nurse practitioner plus a registered nurse) is often available to meet and assess patients, place orders, and start treatments.

The new model was tested over two pilot periods and compared with a similar period of control days. ED census and patient acuity were similar during both pilot periods. Eighteen patients were included in pilot one and 80 patients were included in the expanded second pilot. Patients seen within 30 minutes improved from a baseline of 33% to 93% in pilot two. Time to a visual assessment by a nurse, to a room, and to a licensed independent provider all decreased. The largest decrease was in median time to provider, from 43 minutes in the current state to 7 minutes during pilot two.

Emergency Department Asthma Clinical Standard Work

Asthma is the most common chronic illness in children and accounts for greater than 600,000 ED visits in the United States each year.[31] At our institution, asthma is the leading ED diagnosis resulting in hospital admission. We recognized that reducing ED length of stay for patients with moderate to severe asthma would improve ED throughput (flow) and patient care for this high-risk population. Our institution has used the Respiratory Clinical Score since 2002 to guide treatment on our standardized clinical pathway for asthma.[32] Documentation of respiratory scores before and after treatments allowed a review of patients with asthma presenting to our pediatric ED over a 7-month period in 2010 to 2011. We reviewed respiratory score on arrival to the ED, score after the first and second hours of treatment, disposition (admit/discharge), and ED length of stay for all patients with a diagnosis of asthma who presented to the ED from October 2010 through April 2011. This analysis revealed that 90% of patients with high scores (9–12) after 1 hour of treatment were ultimately admitted to the hospital; however, these patients had variable and often prolonged lengths of stay in the ED before admission (non-value-added step). To expedite care and improve ED efficiency, standardized respiratory score–based admission criteria were added to our asthma clinical pathway in September 2011. Mean ED length of stay and time to bed request for admitted patients with asthma both decreased by 30 minutes after implementing the modified asthma pathway with standardized admission criteria. Thus, by standardizing care for patients with asthma to include objective admission criteria early in the ED course, we optimized patient care and improved ED flow.

Lean-Focused Simulation and Emergency Department Resuscitation Room Redesign (5S)

Seattle Children's Hospital has also integrated Lean methodology with simulation methodology.[30] In situ simulation is used as an adjunct to going to *Gemba* for rare or complex processes, to help identify waste and constraints, design standard work, and perform an initial PDSA cycle, even before rolling-out a new process. We have created a simulation process that incorporates Lean tools and a Lean-focused debrief. The goal of Lean-focused simulation is to efficiently identify and address systems and quality issues.

A 13-member multidisciplinary team that included physicians, nurses, and facilities personnel met over 2 days to redesign an existing resuscitation room through the use of in situ simulation and Lean methodologies. The goal of the redesign process was to reduce search and set-up time for materials and to remove waste in the process of administering resuscitative care. The first step in the process was video review of multiple different resuscitations to understand the current state and identify opportunities for improvements. Then, two in situ simulations, an infant in cardiogenic shock and a toddler with multiple traumatic injuries, were conducted to supplement the team's understanding of current state. At the start of these simulations, participants were oriented to the systems-focus of the simulation and provided with the medical case scenario and specific targets for the team (eg, defibrillation of the infant when in pulseless ventricular tachycardia). This type of participant orientation is unique in Lean or systems simulation and takes the focus off the medical care itself to allow emphasis on the system and process of delivering care. Lean-focused debriefing was used to systematically identify waste and to identify opportunities to streamline care. To encourage participant focus on waste, a poster with the types of waste and examples of each were available for reference.

In addition to the identification of waste in the delivery of resuscitative care, the event team conducted a 5S exercise of the entire room and its contents. A total of 42 types of waste were identified in areas of inventory, transportation, and motion. Examples of waste included: unnecessary duplication of medications in the code cart and in-room supply dispensing station, the need for the nurse to leave the room to obtain critical resuscitative medications only located in the central ED medication room, the lack of standard intravenous setup to allow efficient access to needed intravenous and laboratory supplies, and the lack of team role clarity resulting in role confusion and care delays. The 5S exercise resulted in several additional improvements including: decreased par level of respiratory supplies in the room (sort), identification of a stepstool on the patient's right side for compressions (straighten), removal of an asthma algorithm from 1998 (scrub), clarified code team role locations around the patient (standardize), and created room readiness checklist (sustain). Simulations conducted at the end of the event identified overall improvement in the delivery of resuscitative care.

REFLECTIONS AND LESSONS LEARNED

The science of QI has been developing over the last 100 years. Application to delivery of medical care has also grown exponentially over the last 15 to 20 years. From unknown/seldom used formal methodologies in medicine, QI techniques have changed the way many see their job, deliver care, and assess successes. No longer should individual experiences be the driver for quality. This has been challenging for some, because personal experiences impact greatly when one encounters what may be a similar situation. QI and standardization enable one to take individual experiences and overlay them on a framework of evidence-based standardization. Only then can one replicate, standardize, measure, and learn. It may be that anecdotal experiences are not represented well in the literature and perhaps could/should be published, to provide critical peer review. Developing standard work is vital and needs to include all evidence or best accepted practices when evidence is sparse or conflicting. Measuring, however, and communicating this information may be the most vital part of the process. There are multiple was to assess, identify, and remove waste and work toward adding value to the primary customer. Robust QI assessment, however, allows one to critically review whether they have made a difference and if that difference is specifically attributable to a change, the result of random variation, or perhaps a fleeting improvement secondary to observational bias (ie, the Hawthorne effect). For years, clinicians have reported case studies and local interventions without robust measurable outcomes. Being able to continue to try and report novel approaches for care and operations is vital, but having the appropriate methodology to assess and critique is vital. Part of academic and clinical training needs to include the science of QI and the ability to critically assess change and new ideas. Without that rigor and understanding, clinicians risk venturing back into anecdotal care and delivery of medicine.

The application of QI methodologies and process improvement require an iterative and longitudinal approach. It also requires acceptance and support from all involved, especially leaders who can obtain and direct resources for the providers and processes to enable important change to occur and be sustained. The providers and staff need to believe in the process and be willing to work hard to identify opportunities for improvement, develop alternative strategies to trial, and develop measures that can be assessed prechange and post-change to identify successes and failures. Failures in these efforts are just as valuable as successes, and sometimes even more so. Failures provide an opportunity for the team to investigate new and perhaps novel approaches, which can engage the staff and help with thoughtful reassessment regarding why a process did not make the expected improvement. Often, those relooks at why something did not work provide further insights into opportunities. This is expected as part of the planning process in the "5 Why's" efforts, but one can provide enhanced engagement and enthusiasm when other "why's" are uncovered after a failed improvement effort.

It is also clear, that in this era of cost conscious medicine, large investments of time and money for the practice of process improvement may be limited. Clinicians need to learn about processes and find ways to discover, engage, and challenge staff and other vital stakeholders (eg, families, administrators) without a huge investment of time and resource. Rapid "just in time" events and change efforts can often serve as trials to identify opportunities to invest more time and effort. Although the "Plan" stage for change is vital, and "Do" portion of the PDSA (PDCA) process is often exciting and fun, the "Study" and "Act" components are what offer the opportunity for sustainable improvement. ED providers are especially good at exploring and trialing new ideas, but that excitement sometimes wanes when it comes to critical assessment and monitoring of a successful change. Without monitoring and the willingness to identify risks or difficulties with sustainability, improvements are potentially temporary and at the end of the day may not have a lasting impact. As clinicians proceed on their QI journeys, they should always have an eye on the future and identify how they are addressing the important IHI triple aim goals of best care and experience for the patient (and family), least cost, and population health improvement.

REFERENCES

1. Schneider EC, Squires D. From last to first: could the U.S. health care system become the best in the world? N Engl J Med 2017;377(10):901–4.
2. Schneider EC, Sarnak DO, Squires D, et al. Mirror, mirror 2017: international comparison reflects flaws and opportunities for better U.S. health care. New York: The Commonwealth Fund; 2017.
3. Kohn LT, Corrigan JM, Donaldson MS, editors. To err is human: building a safer health system. Washington, DC: National Academy Press; 2000.
4. Berwick DM, Shojania KG, Atchinson BK, et al. Free from harm: accelerating patient safety improvement fifteen years after to err is human. Boston (MA): National Patient Safety Foundation; 2015.
5. Worboys M. Joseph Lister and the performance of antiseptic surgery. Notes Rec R Soc Lond 2013;67(3):199–209.
6. Mitchell P. Defining patient safety and quality care. In: Hughes R, editor. Patient safety and quality: an evidence-based handbook for nurses. Rockville (MD): Agency for Healthcare Research and Quality; 2008.
7. Berwick DM. Controlling variation in health care: a consultation from Walter Shewhart. Med Care 1991;29(12):1212–25.
8. Best M, Neuhauser D. Joseph Juran: overcoming resistance to organisational change. Qual Saf Health Care 2006;15(5):380–2.
9. Perla RJ, Provost LP, Parry GJ. Seven propositions of the science of improvement: exploring foundations. Qual Manag Health Care 2013;22(3):170–86.
10. Chassin MR. Is health care ready for six sigma quality? Milbank Q 1998;76(4):565–91.
11. Scoville R, Little K. Comparing lean and quality improvement. Boston (MA): Institute for Healthcare Improvement; 2014.
12. Langley GJ, Moen RD, Nolan KM, et al. The improvement guide: a practical approach to enhancing organizational performance. 2nd edition. Hoboken (NJ): Jossey-Bass; 2009. p. 512.
13. Sundarapandian V. Probability, statistics and queueing theory. Delhi (India): PHI Learning; 2009. p. 820.
14. Murray M, Berwick DM. Advanced access: reducing waiting and delays in primary care. JAMA 2003;289(8):1035–40.

15. Fomundam S, Herrmann J. A survey of queueing theory applications in healthcare. College Park (MD): The Institute for Systems Research; 2007.

16. Womack JP, Daniel TJ, Roos D. The machine that changed the world. New York: Free Press; 1990. p. 352.

17. Holweg M. The genealogy of lean production. Journal of Operations Management 2007;25(2):420–37.

18. Womack JP, Jones DT. Lean thinking: banish waste and create wealth in your corporation. New York: Simon & Schuster; 1996.

19. Kenney C. Transforming health care: Virginia mason medical center's pursuit of the perfect patient experience. New York: Productivity Press; 2010. p. 248.

20. Toussaint JS. On the mend: revolutionizing healthcare to save lives and transform the industry. Cambridge (England): Lean Enterprise Institute, Inc.; 2010. p. 181.

21. Stapleton FB, Hendricks J, Hagan P, et al. Modifying the Toyota Production System for continuous performance improvement in an academic children's hospital. Pediatr Clin North Am 2009;56(4):799–813.

22. Hagan P. Waste not, want not: leading the lean health-care journey at Seattle Children's Hospital. Global Business and Organizational Excellence 2011;30(3):25–31.

23. Toussaint JS, Berry LL. The promise of Lean in health care. Mayo Clin Proc 2013; 88(1):74–82.

24. Elbadawi I, McWilliams DL, Tetteh EG. Enhancing Lean manufacturing learning experience through hands-on simulation. Simul Gaming 2010;41(4):537–52.

25. Mazzocato P, Holden RJ, Brommels M, et al. How does Lean work in emergency care? A case study of a Lean-inspired intervention at the Astrid Lindgren Children's hospital, Stockholm, Sweden. BMC Health Serv Res 2012;12:28.

26. Murrell KL, Offerman SR, Kauffman MB. Applying Lean: implementation of a rapid triage and treatment system. West J Emerg Med 2011;12(2):184–91.

27. Emerman CL, Laskey S, Warner C, et al. Lower ED walkout rates follow rapid improvement process changes. Sci Commun 2010;17(4):163–6.

28. White BA, Chang Y, Grabowski BG, et al. Using Lean-based systems engineering to increase capacity in the emergency department. West J Emerg Med 2014; 15(7):770–6.

29. Dickson EW, Singh S, Cheung DS, et al. Application of Lean manufacturing techniques in the emergency department. J Emerg Med 2009;37(2):177–82.

30. Rutman L, Stone K, Reid J, et al. Improving patient flow using Lean methodology: an emergency medicine experience. Curr Treat Options Pediatr 2015;(4):359–71.

31. Rutman L, Migita R, Spencer S, et al. Standardized asthma admission criteria reduce length of stay in a pediatric emergency department. Acad Emerg Med 2016;23(3):289–96.

32. Liu LL, Gallaher MM, Davis RL, et al. Use of a respiratory clinical score among different providers. Pediatr Pulmonol 2004;37(3):243–8.

Moving?

Make sure your subscription moves with you!

To notify us of your new address, find your **Clinics Account Number** (located on your mailing label above your name), and contact customer service at:

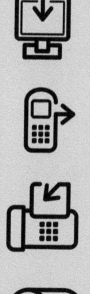

Email: journalscustomerservice-usa@elsevier.com

800-654-2452 (subscribers in the U.S. & Canada)
314-447-8871 (subscribers outside of the U.S. & Canada)

Fax number: 314-447-8029

Elsevier Health Sciences Division
Subscription Customer Service
3251 Riverport Lane
Maryland Heights, MO 63043

*To ensure uninterrupted delivery of your subscription, please notify us at least 4 weeks in advance of move.

Printed and bound by CPI Group (UK) Ltd, Croydon, CR0 4YY

22/10/2024

01777661-0002